SOCIAL WORK AND INTEGRATED HEALTH CARE

SOCIAL WORK AND INTEGRATED HEALTH CARE

FROM POLICY TO PRACTICE AND BACK

Edited by *Victoria Stanhope*

AND

Shulamith Lala Ashenberg Straussner

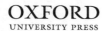

OXFORD

UNIVERSITY PRESS

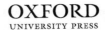

Oxford University Press is a department of the University of Oxford. It furthers
the University's objective of excellence in research, scholarship, and education
by publishing worldwide. Oxford is a registered trade mark of Oxford University
Press in the UK and certain other countries.

Published in the United States of America by Oxford University Press
198 Madison Avenue, New York, NY 10016, United States of America.

Library of Congress Cataloging-in-Publication Data
Names: Stanhope, Victoria, editor. | Straussner, Shulamith Lala Ashenberg, editor.
Title: Social work and integrated health care : from policy to practice and back /
edited by Victoria Stanhope and Shulamith Lala Ashenberg Straussner.
Description: New York : Oxford University Press, [2018] | Includes bibliographical references and index.
Identifiers: LCCN 2017012753 (print) | LCCN 2017022171 (ebook) | ISBN 9780190607302 (updf) |
ISBN 9780190607319 (epub) | ISBN 9780190607296 (alk. paper)
Subjects: LCSH: Integrated delivery of health care—United States. | Health services administration—United States.
Classification: LCC RA981.A2 (ebook) | LCC RA981.A2 S64 2018 (print) | DDC 362.10973—dc23
LC record available at https://lccn.loc.gov/2017012753

CONTENTS

PREFACE

Victoria Stanhope and Shulamith Lala Ashenberg Straussner

Since 2001, when the Institute of Medicine's report, *Crossing the Quality Chasm*, documented the ways in which the U.S. health care system is failing the American people, health care reform initiatives have been offered at federal, state, and local levels. The high costs of health care, coupled with strikingly poor outcomes in comparison with other high-income countries, have driven a serious reappraisal of how we distribute and structure care—particularly for people with complex health needs. There is widespread consensus about the need to shift the emphasis from acute care to prevention, which addresses the ongoing physical and behavioral health needs of the population. Reform efforts have resulted in the redesign of systems to integrate health care—with the ultimate goal of providing seamless primary care, mental health, and substance abuse services. Although services have traditionally addressed the mind and body separately, there is increasing recognition that they are inseparable with regard to the ways in which people experience health and wellness and how health problems affect their lives.

Recognizing the critical role that the social work profession plays in the health and behavioral health care sectors, we designed this book to help social workers understand the policies and practices that shape integrated health care. The Patient Protection and Affordable Care Act of 2010 promotes reforms to encourage public and private systems to integrate primary care and behavioral health care. Although the future of this legislation is uncertain due to continuing political opposition, the Act was built on reform initiatives that were already taking place throughout the country. The potential for integrated health care to simultaneously improve health outcomes at individual and population levels and significantly reduce costs means that the movement toward an integrated health care system will continue despite the constantly changing health policy landscape. As these changes occur, there is a great need in the social work field for resources that can provide the context for these changes and translate policies into daily social work practice. From policy to practice and back, this book presents the new social work environment emerging from these important shifts in health care. The focus is on health care for vulnerable populations, with a special emphasis on adults with severe mental illnesses and substance use disorders.

The book is divided into three parts. Part I establishes the need for integrated health care by describing the shortcomings of the current health care system. This section defines integrated health care and elucidates the models of care that have emerged in physical and mental health care to inform the integrated health care approach. Part II focuses on the policies that have shaped health care reform, including background information on public funding for health care, the development of behavioral health services in the community, and the passage of mental health parity legislation. Two chapters describe how the Affordable Care Act and new health care financing models have expanded access and promoted delivery system redesign. Part III presents an overview of integrated health care settings and describes evidence-based practices that are central to integrated health care, such as screening, person-centered care planning, motivational interviewing, and wellness self-management. Various aspects of working in integrated health care settings are detailed, including roles and tasks for social workers, interprofessional practice, and evaluation.

The terminology used to describe integrated health care is evolving as quickly as the health care environment itself. A glossary at the conclusion of this book provides what we understand by these terms at this moment in time. To describe someone who receives services, we have used the terms *individual* and *person* whenever possible. When this usage was ambiguous, we used the term *service user* to avoid the business connotations of *client* or *consumer*, which are terms commonly used in behavioral health. The word *patient* is used only to refer to medical settings or as part of a specific term such as *patient-centered medical home*.

ACKNOWLEDGMENTS

We would like to thank all of our authors who took time out of their busy schedules to make their valuable contributions to this book. We also thank Taylor Kravitz for editing the book with such care and attention. Finally, we thank Elizabeth Matthews, Lauren Jessell, Mimi Choy-Brown, Meredith Doherty, and Emily Hamovitch for their contributions to this book.

CONTRIBUTORS

Stacey L. Barrenger, PhD, AM, Assistant Professor, Silver School of Social Work, New York University, New York, NY.

Anna M. Blackburn, MSW, LCSW, ACM, Licensed Clinical Social Worker, Feinberg School of Medicine, Northwestern University, Chicago, IL.

Neil S. Calman, MD, FAAFP, President and CEO, Institute for Family Health, New York, NY; Professor and System Chair, Alfred and Gail Engelberg Department of Family Medicine and Community Health, Icahn School of Medicine at Mount Sinai, New York, NY.

Peter C. Campanelli, PsyD, Clinical and Consulting Psychologist, Principal, Strategic Organizational Development, New York, NY.

Jeff Capobianco, PhD, Senior Consultant, National Council for Behavioral Health, Washington, DC; Adjunct Lecturer, School of Social Work, University of Michigan, Ann Arbor, MI.

Julie A. Cederbaum, PhD, MSW, MPH, Associate Professor, Department of Children, Youth, and Families, Suzanne Dworack-Peck School of Social Work, University of Southern California, Los Angeles, CA.

Aminda Heckman Chomanczuk, PhD, LCSW, Assistant Professor and Faculty Fellow, Silver School of Social Work, New York University, New York, NY.

Mimi Choy-Brown, LMSW, Research Scientist and Doctoral Candidate, Silver School of Social Work, New York University, New York, NY.

Andrew F. Cleek, PsyD, Executive Officer, McSilver Institute for Poverty Policy and Research, Silver School of Social Work, New York University, New York, NY; Research Assistant Professor, School of Medicine, New York University, New York, NY.

Benjamin Clemens, LCSW, Director of Technology Implementation, Psychosocial Services Department, The Institute for Family Health, New York, NY.

Darla Spence Coffey, PhD, MSW, President and Chief Executive Officer, Council on Social Work Education, Alexandria, VA.

Meredith Doherty, LCSW, Silberman Doctoral Fellow, Silberman Aging: A Hartford Center of Excellence in Diverse Aging, School of Social Work, Hunter College, City University of New York, New York, NY.

Larry Fricks, BA, Director, Appalachian Consulting Group, Cleveland, GA.

Todd P. Gilmer, PhD, Professor and Chief, Division of Health Policy, Vice Chair for Faculty Affairs, Department of Family Medicine and Public Health, University of California—San Diego, San Diego, CA.

Benjamin F. Henwood, PhD, LCSW, Assistant Professor, Suzanne Dworak-Peck School of Social Work, University of Southern California, Los Angeles, CA.

Janna C. Heyman, PhD, LMSW, Chair and Professor, Henry C. Ravazzin Center on Aging & Intergenerational Studies, Graduate School of Social Service, Fordham University, New York, NY.

Heather Klusaritz, PhD, MSW, Associate Director, Center for Community and Population Health, Department of Family Medicine and Community Health, Perelman School of Medicine, University of Pennsylvania, Philadelphia, PA; Director of Community Engagement, Center for Public Health Initiatives, Perelman School of Medicine, University of Pennsylvania, Philadelphia, PA.

Max D. Krauss, MSW, Site Manager, Wediko Children's Services, Windsor, NH.

Virna Little, PsyD, LCSW-R, CCM, SAP, Senior Vice President, Institute for Family Health, New York, NY.

Virgen T. Luce, MSW, LCSW-R, Clinical Associate Professor, Silver School of Social Work, New York University, New York, NY.

Jennifer I. Manuel, PhD, LMSW, Assistant Professor, Silver School of Social Work, New York University, New York, NY.

Elizabeth B. Matthews, MSW, Research Scientist and Doctoral Candidate, School of Social Work, Rutgers University, New Brunswick, NJ.

Mary M. McKay, PhD, Dean, Brown School, Washington University in St. Louis, St. Louis, MO; Research Scientist, McSilver Institute for Poverty Policy and Research, Silver School of Social Work, New York University, New York, NY.

Diane M. Mirabito, DSW, LCSW, Clinical Associate Professor, Silver School of Social Work, New York University, New York, NY.

Peggy Morton, DSW, LCSW, Clinical Associate Professor and Assistant Dean, Field Learning & Community Partnerships, Silver School of Social Work, New York University, New York, NY.

Brenda Ohta, PhD, MS, MSW, Visiting Scholar, Silver School of Social Work, New York University, New York, NY; Private Consultant, Health Services Innovation, Care Integration, & Clinical Bioethics, New York, NY.

Jordana Rutigliano, LMSW, CHC, Assistant Vice President for Psychosocial Services, The Institute for Family Health, New York, NY.

Anthony Salerno, PhD, Practice and Policy Scholar, McSilver Institute for Poverty Policy and Research, Silver School of Social Work, New York University, New York, NY; Senior Integrated Health Consultant, National Council for Community Behavioral Healthcare, Washington, DC; Assistant Research Professor, Child and Adolescent Psychiatry, Langone Medical Center, New York University, New York, NY.

Evan Senreich, PhD, MSW, LCSW, CASAC, Associate Professor of Social Work, Lehman College, City University of New York, New York, NY.

Elizabeth Siantz, PhD, MSW, Postdoctoral Fellow, Department of Family Medicine and Public Health, University of California—San Diego, San Diego, CA.

Judith P. Siegel, PhD, LCSW, Professor, Silver School of Social Work, New York University, New York, NY.

Victoria Stanhope, PhD, MSW, Associate Professor, Silver School of Social Work, New York University, New York, NY.

Shulamith Lala Ashenberg Straussner, PhD, LCSW, Professor and Director, Post-Master's Certificate Program in the Clinical Approaches to Addictions, Silver School of Social Work, New York University, New York, NY; Founding Editor, *Journal of Social Work Practice in the Addictions*, New York, NY.

W. Patrick Sullivan, PhD, Professor and Director, Center for Social Health and Wellbeing, School of Social Work, Indiana University, Bloomington, IN.

Helle Thorning, PhD, MS, LCSW, Clinical Professor, Columbia University, New York, NY.

Lynn Videka, PhD, AM, Collegiate Professor and Dean, School of Social Work, University of Michigan, Ann Arbor, MI.

Shelly A. Wiechelt, MSW, PhD, Associate Professor, University of Maryland, Baltimore County, Baltimore, MD.

INTRODUCTION

Darla Spence Coffey

Passage of the Patient Protection and Affordable Care Act (ACA) in 2010 was a watershed moment in the United States and was arguably the most significant piece of legislation passed since the Social Security Act in providing care to U.S. citizens. As vitally important as this law is, it is essential to place it in the context of how our understanding of health and the ways in which health care is delivered in this country have been changing for some time. Changes have been prompted by a number of factors, including advances in science and technology, a more contextualized understanding of the determinants of health, and the rise of the consumerism movement. One of the most important reforms to emerge is the effort to integrate primary care and behavioral health care to promote a holistic perspective of what constitutes health and wellness.

Advances in the understanding of and approaches to health care have also created new and revitalized roles for the social work profession. Although the profession has been engaged in the health sector since its inception, the number of social workers employed and the roles that they have assumed in these settings have varied considerably. Today, social work has an opportunity to lead—and who better to lead in this new era of health care reform than the professionals and scholars who understand that quality care requires responsiveness to social determinants, attention to the risks inherent in transitioning from one form of care to another, and approaches that are culturally appropriate and community based? For social workers to be fully prepared to step into current and emerging roles in health, deliver integrated health care, and provide leadership for national health efforts, we need to focus our attention on the following specific areas.

INTERPROFESSIONAL EDUCATION

The National Center for Interprofessional Practice and Education, or Nexus (https://nexusipe.org/), asserts that improving the experience, outcomes, and costs of health care depends on high-functioning interprofessional teams. The Nexus has also explicitly incorporated the experience of the learner into their work, observing that "interprofessional, collaborative practice occurs when multiple health workers and students from different professional backgrounds provide comprehensive health services by working with patients, their families, carers (caregivers), and communities to deliver the highest quality of care across settings" (Brandt, 2016). Social work programs need to ensure that students are learning in interprofessional settings and are prepared to work in interprofessional teams. There is good evidence that this is already happening; however, we need to ensure that this becomes the rule rather than the exception for modern social work students (Council on Social Work Education [CSWE], 2014).

In 2015, CSWE became an institutional member of the Interprofessional Education Collaborative (IPEC). Its board of directors endorsed the Core Competencies for Interprofessional Collaborative Practice (IPEC, 2016), which include communication, roles and responsibilities, values and ethics, and teamwork, and they are closely aligned with the Educational Policy and Accreditation Standards to which all accredited social work education programs adhere (Commission on Accreditation & Commission on Educational Policy, 2015). Social work programs are encouraged to incorporate the IPEC competencies into their curricula to more thoroughly prepare students to work in interprofessional settings and teams.

SOCIAL WORK RESEARCH

Social work research has contributed to understanding the causes and appropriate interventions for some of the most complex social problems in the country's history (Sherraden, 2013). However, the value of social work research is often eclipsed because of the long-standing preference for pure science. It has become increasingly apparent that for scientific advances to reap their full benefits, we need a greater understanding of how efficacious interventions can be implemented in real-world settings to meet the needs of individuals and communities with full appreciation of their differences. To participate, social work researchers need to be bolder in their research questions and in the application of their findings. Aligning with the trend toward interprofessional delivery of care, social work education programs need to ensure that the next generation of students and scholars is prepared to engage in transdisciplinary research that will best attend to the complex social factors that influence health and health outcomes (Gehlert, Walters, Uehara, & Lawlor, 2015).

POLICY AND ADVOCACY

For social work to assume a leadership role in health, health care, and health care reform, educational programs need to ensure that students are equipped to effectively advocate for and influence policy at federal, state, local, and organizational levels. More than 16 million Americans gained health care coverage due to the ACA, but the legislation is vulnerable to repeal given the current, highly divided political context. Although parts of the legislation could be improved, we cannot stand idle and allow the country to revert to a time when health care was a privilege for the few rather than a right for all. Beyond the provisions to extend health care coverage to all Americans, the law moves us toward an integrated health care system that is a vast improvement over the costly, siloed, and fragmented system that has existed for decades.

The U.S. Bureau of Labor Statistics (2015) predicts that social work jobs will grow at a faster rate than all other occupations over the next 2 decades. Health care, mental health, and substance abuse social workers will have the largest rate of growth, almost 20%. It is our duty to ensure that social workers are equipped to meet the health challenges of the populace and the evolving practices and policies of the modern health care system.

REFERENCES

Brandt, B. F. (2016). *Memo to social work: It's about the collaboration and the redesign* [Powerpoint slides]. Retrieved from https://nexusipe-resource-exchange.s3.amazonaws.com/CSWE%2011.3.16%20 Brandt%20Memo%20to%20Social%20Work.pdf

Council on Social Work Education. (2014). *2013 statistics on social work education in the United States.* Retrieved from http://www.cswe.org/file.aspx?id=74478

Commission on Accreditation & Commission on Educational Policy, Council on Social Work Education. (2015). *Educational policy and accreditation standards for baccalaureate and master's social work programs.* Retrieved from http://cswe.org/File.aspx?id=81660

Gehlert, S., Walters, K., Uehara, E., & Lawlor, E. (2015). The case for a national health social work practice-based research network in addressing health equity. *Health & Social Work, 40,* 253–255. doi: 10.1093/hsw/hlv060

Interprofessional Education Collaborative (IPEC). (2016). Core competencies for interprofessional collaborative practice: 2016 update. Washington, DC: Interprofessional Education Collaborative. Retrieved from https://ipecollaborative.org/uploads/IPEC-2016-Updated-Core-Competencies-Report__ final_release_.PDF

Sherraden, M. (2013). *Grand accomplishments in social work* (Grand Challenges for Social Work Initiative, Working Paper No. 2). Baltimore, MD: American Academy of Social Work & Social Welfare. Retrieved from http://aaswsw.org/wp-content/uploads/2013/12/FINAL-Grand-Accomplishments-sb-12-9-13-Final.pdf

U.S. Bureau of Labor Statistics. (2015, December 17). *Occupational outlook handbook (2016-2017 ed.), social workers, U.S. Department of Labor.* Retrieved from http://www.bls.gov/ooh/community-and-social-service/social-workers.htm#tab-6

SOCIAL WORK AND INTEGRATED HEALTH CARE

PART I

INTRODUCTION TO INTEGRATED HEALTH CARE

CHAPTER 1

THE NEED FOR INTEGRATED HEALTH CARE IN THE UNITED STATES

Victoria Stanhope

There is a great divide between what people living in the United States expect from their health care and what is being delivered to them. People wish for health care that is timely, appropriate, effective, and safe. Instead, according to the Institute of Medicine (IOM, 2001), they receive health care that is "overly complex and poorly coordinated" (p. 1), resulting in between $17 billion and $29 billion in costs due to unnecessary care, lost productivity, and disability (IOM, 1999). The growing recognition that the U.S. health care system is in crisis has led to renewed reform efforts from the bottom up in terms of delivery system innovations and from the top down with system changes through legislation.

One of the best ways to understand the extent to which the U.S. health care system has underperformed is to compare it with the health care systems of other high-income democracies, such as Japan, Denmark, and Australia. The United States spends twice as much as most peer countries on health care, with an average spending per capita of $7538 per year (Squires, 2011). However, people who live in the United States have poorer outcomes on key health indicators, including life expectancy, rates of HIV infection and AIDS, drug-related deaths, and disability (IOM, 2013). Compared with 29 other member countries from the Organization for Economic Co-operation and Development (OECD), the United States ranks 22nd in maternal mortality, 23rd in life expectancy for women, and 25th in infant mortality (Schroeder, 2007). This discrepancy between spending and outcomes most clearly demonstrates the inefficiency of the U.S. health care system. The Commonwealth Fund, a private U.S. foundation, rated the U.S. system the lowest of 11 similar industrialized countries, finding that the poorest outcomes were related to access, efficiency, and equity (Davis, Stremikis, Squires, & Schoen, 2014). Weakness in equity signifies that the poor performance of the U.S. system is not uniform but instead rests on profound disparities in access and quality of care. These disparities lead to significant differences in health outcomes among racial groups. For instance, Asian Americans live 13 years longer than African Americans, and Native Americans live 4 years less than the national average (Lewis & Burd-Sharps, 2014).

What is driving this poor return on investment in health care for Americans? One theory is that the U.S. population has higher health care needs compared with the populations of other countries, but in fact the United States has a relatively young population and an average amount of chronic illness burden (Squires, 2011). More likely, the reasons stem from the way that we organize and deliver care, which differs from that of most peer countries. A key difference is that the United States does not provide universal access to health care through nationalized health care or government-sponsored insurance; as a result, 18.5% of the population was uninsured in 2010 (Holahan & McGrath, 2014). This lack of access occurs partly because most funding for U.S. health care is derived from private sources. In 2008, $3119 of the $7538 per capita health care spending was from private insurance, and the remainder was composed of Medicare, Medicaid, and out-of-pocket spending (Squires, 2011).

Even with this high level of private spending, the United States still spends more public funding on health care than do other similar countries. The diversity of funding streams leads to a highly complex and fragmented system that has to meet the demands of multiple payors. Many siloed systems of care have evolved that treat one aspect of a person's health without coordinating and communicating across systems. Moreover, funding streams determining how care is reimbursed often have more influence on which services people receive than do their actual health care needs. Payors have traditionally incentivized volume over quality, meaning that health care systems have tended to prescribe more care to generate additional funds without considering whether more is actually better (Song & Lee, 2013). Payors are more likely to reimburse acute care (which is often inpatient care) over preventive care, an approach that has driven up costs while not necessarily improving outcomes.

The IOM presented the blueprint for health care reform by setting six aims for high-quality health care (see Figure 1.1). These aims are the fundamental principles that can guide our efforts and the standards by which health care reforms will be judged to have been successful.

To meet these aims, the existing health care system needs major reforms, including insurance reform and expansion to improve access to health care, payment reform to incentivize care that improves outcomes, and system redesign to improve the coordination of health care (Rosenberg, 2013). Social workers are important to all aspects of reform, but our skills and knowledge can play particularly key roles in the coordination of care. This book demonstrates how social workers can solve some of the health care system's most pressing problems. The purpose of this chapter is to explore why the U.S. health care system is failing, to elucidate the particular problems related to integrated health care, and to discuss how these problems relate to social work.

SOCIAL DETERMINANTS OF HEALTH

Although most of us look to health care services to keep us well, health is largely determined by other factors that have traditionally been considered to be outside of the realm

Safe	• Care that is intended to be helpful should not injure service users in any way.
Effective	• Services should be based on scientific knowledge and provided to all who could benefit.
Patient-Centered	• Care should be respectful and attentive to individual service users' preferences and needs and should be guided by service users' values.
Timely	• Wait times and delays should be minimized.
Efficient	• Waste (of equipment, supplies, ideas, and energy) should be avoided.
Equitable	• Quality of care should not vary because of individual characteristics such as gender, ethnicity, location, or socioeconomic status.

FIGURE 1.1: Six characteristics of quality health care. Data from *Crossing the Quality Chasm: A New Health System for the 21st Century*, p. 2, by Institute of Medicine, 2001, Washington, DC: National Academies Press. Copyright 2000 by the National Academy of Sciences.

of health care. In a groundbreaking series of studies conducted in the United Kingdom, Marmot, Rose, Shipley, and Hamilton (1978) examined the health outcomes of 10,308 government workers over a period of 10 years. These cohort studies found that workers in janitorial jobs had three times the mortality rate of those in top administrative positions. This laid the initial foundation for the concept of the *social gradient*, the principle that there is a direct positive correlation between professional rank and mortality rate. Although the findings from comparing those in the highest and lowest employment levels might have been predictable, less predictable was that the relationship held through each level of employment. With each increase in seniority, people experienced improvements in health outcomes and life expectancy.

These studies paved the way for what have become known globally as the *social determinants of health* (SDH). This term refers to any nonmedical factors that impact health. A focus on SDH at the global level and in the United States led to a plethora of studies adding to our knowledge about the ways in which social factors influence health (Kawachi & Kennedy, 2002). Early studies focused mainly on how poverty and deprivation can lead to inequalities in health, whereas many later and more focused studies have investigated how race, gender, education, employment, housing, and citizenship influence health outcomes.

SDH has been conceptualized as including personal behavior, living and working conditions in homes and communities, and economic and social opportunities and resources (Braveman, Egerter, & Williams, 2011). Personal behavior encompasses health-related knowledge, beliefs, attitudes, and conduct, each of which influences a person's health choices and interactions with the health care system. These are *micro* or *downstream* SDH that social workers operating within the health care system and in communities can address through building relationships, helping people navigate health care systems, and educating and supporting people in their pursuit of healthier behaviors. However, healthier behaviors do not occur in isolation; people are influenced by their social contexts, which include the neighborhoods in which they live, community and social supports, education, and working conditions. These contexts also are shaped by larger *macro* or *upstream* SDH, which are the policies and organizational structures that provide or deny opportunities for people to thrive socially and economically. With this framework, health becomes inextricably connected to more macro policies that reach beyond the scope of health, including issues such as taxation, housing, the environment, and transportation. Understanding health within this person-in-environment perspective, which lies at the heart of SDH, is deeply congruent with the ecological approach of the social work profession (Stanhope, Videka, Thorning, & McKay, 2015).

In comparing SDH with health care itself, it becomes clear why health care reform must move beyond the traditional reach of the health care system. In determining life expectancy, health care plays only a small role (10%), whereas genetic disposition plays a much larger role (30%), and behavioral patterns are the biggest predictor (40%). Therefore, improved health care can make only a small dent in early mortality rates (Schroeder, 2007). The real opportunity to save lives lies in our ability to alter behaviors such as smoking, unhealthy diet, and lack of physical activity. Health care providers can no longer afford to regard people as the passive recipients of treatment (i.e., patients) but must instead recognize the importance of actively involving individuals in their own care and encouraging them to pursue wellness in their homes and communities. However, intervening only at the individual level is insufficient because the causal pathways to health are extremely complicated and influenced by myriad, multilevel factors.

The World Health Organization identified 10 key areas that need to be addressed to promote a healthy population: the social gradient, stress, early life, social exclusion, work, unemployment, social support, addiction, food, and transportation (Wilkinson & Marmot, 2003). All of these domains interact with each other. For instance, early life experiences affect educational life attainment, which can alter employment, earnings, and stress levels. Moreover, the impact of social factors extends far beyond a single person's life. Social disadvantage can span generations by not only affecting people's material circumstances but also altering their biology through epigenetic changes that diminish people's health and capacities (Conley & Rauscher, 2013). Given this broader understanding of SDH, there is great potential for social work interventions. Social workers in all sectors of the profession, including advocacy, community organizing, child welfare, education, health, and behavioral health, can play key roles in contributing to this expanded view of health promotion.

HEALTH CARE DISPARITIES

RACE AND ETHNICITY

One of the greatest challenges for health care reform is to achieve equity in the distribution and quality of care. Health care disparities arise when there are differences between groups in access and quality of care despite no differences between them in terms of preferences or needs (IOM, 2002). Although Americans experience poorer outcomes overall than people from other similar countries, there are significant variations in outcome across race and ethnicity that persist even after controlling for socioeconomic status, suggesting that the differences are driven by discrimination. This situation evokes grave concern about the adequacy of the health care system to meet the demands of an increasingly diverse society: 13 million residents of the United States were born in another country; one in three identifies as Hispanic or Latino, African American, or Asian; and by 2050, whites are estimated to comprise only 47% of the population (Moore, 2013).

People from minority backgrounds experience differences in how they perceive their health and in health outcomes. Among whites, 59.3% rate their health status as very good, compared with 55.8% of Asians, 44.4% of African Americans, 43.7% of Native Americans, and 33.6% of Hispanics or Latinos (Centers for Disease Control and Prevention, 2008). Perceptions of health reflect actual health outcomes. For example, in 2010, the infant mortality rate was 5.1 deaths per 1000 births among white mothers and 11.6 deaths per 1000 births among African-American mothers (Annie E. Casey Foundation, 2013). Overall, African Americans experience higher rates of heart disease, cancer, homicide, diabetes, and perinatal conditions compared with whites (Kochanek, Arias, & Anderson, 2013).

Despite having a longer life expectancy than other minorities, Asians are still at greater risk for cancer, heart disease, stroke, and diabetes compared with whites, and there are significant differences in health outcomes among Asian subgroups. Ten percent of all Asians and Pacific Islanders have diabetes, compared with 5.9% of the general population, and rates are especially high among American Samoans and Native Hawaiians (Ida, SooHoo, & Chapa, 2012). There are also significant disparities in physical health conditions among Latinos compared with non-Hispanic whites. Latinos are more likely to have liver disease, more likely to be diabetic, more than twice as likely to be diagnosed with HIV infection, and six times more likely to have tuberculosis ("Latino health disparities," 2014).

Mental health outcomes also vary according to race and ethnic group. Overall, the prevalence of lifetime mental disorders among minorities is lower than it is among whites, with the exception of Puerto Ricans, but there are still pronounced differences in terms of specific disorders (McGuire & Miranda, 2008). For example, American Indians and Alaska Natives experience higher rates of posttraumatic stress disorder and alcohol misuse, and are 6.1 times more likely to die of alcohol-related causes compared with the general population (Moore, 2013). African Americans have a higher incidence of schizophrenia than whites; some of this disparity may be attributable to overdiagnosis, but this is unlikely to account for the entire difference. Although Latinos and African Americans may have lower prevalences of mental health disorders than whites, they tend to have more severe and persistent symptoms. One of the most disconcerting findings among the Asian population is that elderly Chinese women are 10 times more likely to commit suicide than elderly white women (American Psychiatric Association, 2014). For adolescent immigrants, the risk of substance misuse increases as they acculturate, with the highest prevalence found among Spanish-speaking immigrants (Gfroerer & Tan, 2003). The picture of disparities in behavioral health is complex and may reflect how culture influences the ways in which symptoms are understood and reported. Nevertheless, there are specific racial and cultural vulnerabilities that persist even after other SDH are taken into account.

An important factor leading to disparities in health outcomes is treatment barriers. One barrier to receiving equal treatment for many minorities is lack of health care insurance. Even when minorities do have insurance, their plans often place more restrictions on the types of services they cover, and even if they have the same plans as whites, they still are not offered the same services by health care providers. Overall, Hispanics, American Indians, Alaska Natives, and African Americans score worse than whites on a variety of measures related to access and quality of care (Agency for Healthcare Research and Quality, 2011).

Examples of receiving lower quality of care include not receiving the best available treatments, lack of access to preventive care and screening, waiting long periods in clinics and hospitals, less chronic illness care, and poor coordination between primary and behavioral health care systems. One study found that office-based psychiatric visits for African Americans were 4.4 minutes shorter across all visits and 10.5 minutes shorter during first visits compared with whites (Olfson, Cherry, & Lewis-Fernández, 2009). In substance abuse treatment, whites are more likely to be recommended for residential treatment or methadone maintenance compared with Latinos and African Americans (Lundgren & Krull, 2014). Not surprisingly given the higher chances of receiving suboptimal care, the disengagement rates from treatment are higher among minorities than they are among whites (Dixon et al., 2011).

One of the most apparent failures of the health care system is its lack of adequate accommodation for people with limited English proficiency. In one study, 16% of Asian Americans who were not born in the United States said they were not able to understand the information given to them at their primary care clinic, and 46% said they found the doctor's advice hard to follow (Ida et al., 2012). People are often reluctant to ask questions when they do not understand something because of language barriers. Moreover, when there is uncertainty about a course of treatment, language problems and differences in the ways in which a person and a doctor understand the illness can result in a treatment plan that is not centered on the person's needs or preferences (IOM, 2002).

The role of culture runs much deeper than language differences; it extends to the ways in which people seek help, their values and beliefs about wellness, views about self-determination, approaches to decision-making, and personal experiences of illness. For instance, among the Hispanic community, *personalismo* (i.e., being warm and personable) is more important than formality and institutional conventions, and it can determine whether people choose to engage in treatment (Cabassa et al., 2014). On a more structural level, the constant pressure to keep costs down can lead to failure of physicians to offer all available treatments to those whom they perceive as less educated or less likely to request more services, and this disproportionately hurts minorities.

Disparities are driven by overt prejudice and bias, which results in providers' making decisions based on stereotypes rather than treating the individual. The pressure of time can exacerbate these tendencies, with providers not taking the time to understand the complexities of a person's specific experience. An example is the overdiagnosis of African Americans with psychotic disorders rather than mood disorders, which leads to higher rates of medication, hospitalization, and long-term involvement in the mental health system (Neighbors, Trierweiler, Ford, & Muroff, 2003).

Health care disparities are not limited to racial and ethnic minorities; women are also negatively impacted. Overall, U.S. adults die younger than adults in other high-income countries, but this difference is more accentuated for women, indicating underlying disparities (IOM, 2013). Women are vulnerable to a host of gender-specific risk factors that negatively impact their overall health, including higher rates of poverty, exposure to sexual and intimate partner violence, disproportionate burden of caregiving, and general experience of discrimination. Lack of financial resources often results in less access to care and leads women to delay care or not fill prescriptions (Salganicoff, Ranji, Beamesderfer, & Kurani, 2014). These stressors also affect mental health, with women experiencing much higher rates of depression and anxiety than men (Kessler, 2003), and can lead to higher rates of comorbidity. One study found a higher prevalence of mental health disorders among women, notably depression among women with chronic illnesses compared with men with chronic illnesses (Verhaak, Heijmans, Peters, & Rijken, 2005).

Health care disparities also affect lesbian, gay, bisexual, and transgender people, who face many similar challenges, report lower levels of health than cisgender heterosexuals, and are less likely to have insurance coverage or seek health care (Krehely, 2009). Despite differences in sexual orientation and gender, overall medical care has not accounted for these differences in its approach to diagnosis, treatment, or illness management. For instance, although the use of illicit drugs is higher among men than among women, women often encounter poorer treatment than men because interventions have been developed to treat men and do not take into account differences such as specific gender-based traumas, needs related to pregnancy, and child care needs (Substance Abuse and Mental Health Services Administration [SAMHSA], 2011).

The increasing recognition of disparities and the mechanisms that lie behind them has made clear the need for the health care system to pay attention to health care at the population level. Each individual should receive personalized care, but to fully understand and prevent illness, the health care system must also address the causes of disorders that function at the group level, which means tracking and analyzing health outcomes of specific groups. Health care reform is tasked with making the health care system more culturally responsive to achieve greater equity in access and quality of care, which will improve health outcomes for all Americans.

COMORBIDITY OF PHYSICAL, MENTAL, AND SUBSTANCE USE DISORDERS

The pressing need for health care reform has focused attention on one particular group of people whose plight illustrates the failure of the U.S. health care system:

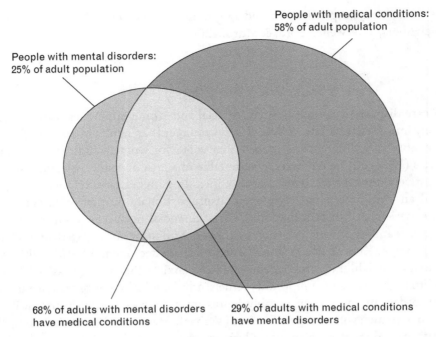

People with mental disorders:
25% of adult population

People with medical conditions:
58% of adult population

68% of adults with mental disorders
have medical conditions

29% of adults with medical conditions
have mental disorders

FIGURE 1.2: Percentages of people with mental disorders and/or medical conditions (2001–2003). Reprinted with permission from *Mental Disorders and Medical Comorbidity* (Research Synthesis Report No. 21), by B. G. Druss and E. Walker, 2011, Princeton, NJ: Robert Wood Johnson Foundation. Copyright 2011 by the Robert Wood Johnson Foundation.

those who suffer from comorbid mental, substance use, and medical health disorders. This group comprises an estimated 17% of the adult population (Druss & Walker, 2011). The 2001–2003 National Comorbidity Survey Replication epidemiological study, the most recent study to have examined the prevalence of behavioral health disorders in the general population, found high rates of physical illness among those with mental disorders. Among people with medical conditions, 29% also had mental disorders; more strikingly, 68% of those with mental disorders also had medical conditions (see Figure 1.2) (Alegria, Jackson, Kessler, & Takeuchi, 2007).

The disproportionate amount of care that this group receives has significant implications for federal and state budgets because most people with comorbid and chronic illnesses receive Medicaid and Medicare. Overall, people with disabilities (many of whom have comorbid illnesses) comprise only 15% of the Medicaid population, but they account for 44% of the Medicaid budget (Kaiser Commission on Medicaid and the Uninsured, 2013). The average cost of treating a chronic illness in a person who also has a mental health disorder is $560 more than the cost to treat the chronic illness alone (Druss & Walker, 2011). Increased understanding of the prevalence and service use patterns of people with comorbid and chronic illnesses has led health care reform initiatives to focus particularly on this population.

The interconnectedness of mind and body is borne out by the strong association between certain medical and mental health conditions. For example, having depression intensifies the risk of having worse physical illness outcomes. One study found that among individuals who were hospitalized for a heart attack, those with major depression were three times more likely to die of a future heart attack (Druss & Walker, 2011). Those with disabling psychiatric conditions are particularly vulnerable to chronic illnesses such as diabetes, chronic obstructive pulmonary disease, and cardiovascular disease. The risk among people with schizophrenia for congestive heart disease is 34% higher for males and 50% higher for females, compared with the general population (Goff et al., 2005). Overall, people with mental illnesses are more susceptible to obesity, cardiovascular diseases, diabetes, HIV infection, and pulmonary and gastrointestinal diseases.

A significant part of this comorbidity is driven by health risk behaviors, particularly tobacco use, substance misuse, lack of physical activity, and poor nutrition. Although these behaviors are prevalent among all populations, they are particularly common among people with mental health disorders. People with a mental health disorder are two to three times more likely to smoke than those without one, and they are more likely to be heavy smokers (Compton, Daumit, & Druss, 2006). Another important factor is that many psychiatric medications result in weight gain, increasing the rate of obesity among those with mental illnesses.

The relationship between mental illness and problems with substance use is complex, with some attributing substance misuse to self-medication for mental health symptoms and others viewing mental health symptoms as stemming from substance use disorders (SUDs). Whatever the cause, individuals with co-occurring disorders often have more significant impairment than those with a single psychiatric disorder, experiencing higher rates of unemployment, homelessness, and incarceration and diminished social support (Druss & Walker, 2011). Individuals with mental illness and substance use problems are at high risk for heart disease, asthma, gastrointestinal disorders, skin infections, and acute respiratory disorders (Hert et al., 2011). Overall, the health care system has struggled to serve people with comorbid mental health and substance use problems, leading to high disengagement rates and poor outcomes. Many attribute this failure to the bifurcated nature of mental health and substance abuse services, which prevents people from receiving comprehensive treatment.

People with severe mental illnesses (SMIs) have a particular vulnerability to chronic medical conditions, and as a result, they have shorter life expectancies. The landmark study by Colton and Mandersheid (2006) found that people with SMIs die on average 25 years before individuals in the general population, largely due to medical causes rather than accidents or suicide. A follow-up study examined excess mortality among people with SMIs using a national representative sample rather than only individuals receiving services and found that people with SMIs died 8.2 years earlier than the general population over a 17-year period (Druss, Zhao, Von Esenwein, Morrato, & Marcus, 2011).

Among the 9.8 million people in the United States with SMIs, approximately 2.3 million also have an SUD (Center for Behavioral Health Statistics and Quality, 2015). People with an SMI and an SUD also have particularly high rates of hospitalization, which is one of the main determinants of health care costs. Overall, people with an SMI and an SUD make an estimated 12 million visits annually to emergency departments (Gerrity, Zoller, Pinson, Pettinari, & King, 2014). Most of these visits and subsequent hospitalizations are for medical care, not psychiatric care; most importantly, they often could have been prevented with good primary care. These studies provide a wake-up call about the pressing need to coordinate behavioral health care and physical health care within delivery systems.

FRAGMENTATION OF HEALTH CARE

The intertwined nature of physical and behavioral health disorders is poorly served by a fragmented health care system, which reinforces the false dichotomy between mind and body. From federal agencies down, the United States has created a bifurcated system of behavioral and physical health, with further divisions between mental health and substance use. The evolution of these separate systems began with Descartes, the 17th century philosopher who stated that the mind and body were separate entities (Descartes, 1991). The medical profession has used these conceptual divisions to create distinct specialties, with illnesses considered to be disorders of the mind being treated by psychiatrists and behavioral health specialists, including psychologists and social workers. These divisions are reflected in the health care system: Most state and local health care systems have separate departments for behavioral health, and many have further divisions between mental health and substance use. At the federal level, behavioral health is overseen by SAMHSA, which exists as a separate department within the U.S. Department of Health and Human Services.

The fragmentation in the U.S. health care system is driven by siloing of care according to the disorder and by the way in which health care is funded, which together create a complicated web of services. As people seek treatment, they run the risk of accessing care in the wrong setting and having each aspect treated in isolation rather than receiving care from one provider who views their health holistically. This disjointed approach leads to poor quality of care and sometimes can be fatal. Seidenberg (2008) described the plight of his son, Noah, who was diagnosed with an SUD and bipolar disorder; Noah overdosed after being hospitalized 19 times and accruing 326 outpatient visits. Seidenberg ascribed the tragic failure of all this treatment to the inadequacy of acute care response, discontinuity of care, and lack of communication between substance abuse and mental health care providers.

ACUTE CARE VERSUS CHRONIC CARE

The U.S. health care system is largely designed to meet acute care needs rather than chronic care needs, and this orientation drives high health care costs and inhibits us from focusing on prevention and health maintenance. In his seminal article in *The New Yorker*, "The Hot Spotters," Gawande (2011) painted a compelling picture of how the U.S. health care system is fundamentally misaligned with the needs of its most vulnerable individuals with chronic illnesses. He described the work of Dr. Jeffrey Brenner from Camden, New Jersey, who studied patterns of hospitalizations. He discovered that people who experienced frequent hospitalizations were often concentrated in one geographic area and that only a few people accounted for most hospitalizations. Overall, Brenner found that 1% of service users in Camden accounted for 30% of all costs, with one person having been admitted 324 times in 5 years and another generating more than $3.5 million in health care costs. As he dug deeper into the histories of the high-cost service users of Camden, he found that instead of intractable acute conditions driving up their hospitalization rates, the cause was lack of quality care that could have been improved by relatively inexpensive low-tech solutions.

His response was to hire social workers to help people get insurance, connect to a consistent set of primary care providers, access housing and benefits, eat well and exercise, reduce their substance misuse, and improve their support in the community. Brenner's approach focused on building relationships and working with high-cost service users in the community; this basic social work approach was successful in reducing health care costs by more than 56% (Gawande, 2011).

Our care delivery system has been organized around illness, with each condition treated separately and care concentrated only when the illness is acute. Specialization within the medical profession has reflected and reinforced this approach, with various illnesses and diseases treated as separate entities by separate experts. Prestige and financial rewards often come with specialization, leading to a shortage of generalist doctors who practice in primary care settings (U.S. Department of Health and Human Services, 2013). This episodic and fragmented treatment approach, which is prevalent in the medical model, can be effective for individuals who encounter an illness that is discrete, is of short duration, and has limited consequences for work and family; however, it is rarely effective for people with chronic conditions.

For people with chronic illnesses, lack of care coordination places them at a much higher risk of emergency department visits and hospitalization. Reducing this high rate of often preventable hospitalizations is one of the primary goals of health care reform. One study of emergency visits in New York City found that 41.3% of visits were non-emergent, meaning that care was not needed within 12 hours; 33.5% were emergent but could have been treated in primary care; 7.3% were emergent but could have been avoided; and 17.3% were emergent and could not have been avoided (Billings, Parikh, & Mijanovich, 2000).

The U.S. health care system also has a high rate of rehospitalization, particularly among those with chronic illnesses. Forty percent of people with congestive heart failure who are discharged from a hospital are readmitted within 90 days, and many of these readmissions could have been avoided by coordinated discharge planning and follow-up care (Berwick, Nolan, & Whittington, 2008). Overall, readmissions account for 17% to 24% of the Medicare budget, with an estimate of 75% of those admissions being preventable (Barber, Coulourides Kogan, Riffenburgh, & Enguidanos, 2015).

IMPROVING HEALTH CARE WITH
THE TRIPLE AIM

The 2001 IOM report, *Crossing the Quality Chasm,* put the health care crisis in the United States firmly on the map, and since then, some progress has been made in the areas identified as key to quality health care: safety, effectiveness, person-centeredness, timeliness, efficiency, and equity (see Figure 1.1). However, real reform has been stalled by the fact that these efforts have occurred within isolated systems and settings, a symptom of the fragmented health care system. For example, a hospital setting can focus on improving care at its site without any improvements in care occurring in the other settings in which it interacts. This narrow approach to service delivery is caused by fragmentation and by fee-for-service payment mechanisms, which provide incentives for providers to expand services and increase costs rather than improve quality (Berwick et al., 2008). Although some have argued that universal access to health care is not affordable, it could be possible if the per capita costs of health care were reduced. This suggests that the problems of the U.S. health care system are intertwined and that the solution lies in setting goals beyond site-specific care.

In response, health care reform has focused on the Triple Aim, which states that initiatives must pursue the tripartite goal of improving the individual experience of care, improving the health of populations, and reducing the per capita cost of care (see Figure 1.3). These aims are interdependent, and all three must be addressed. This stipulation seeks to allay fears that health care reform will lead to wide-scale cost cutting and reductions in services. Instead, any demonstration of cost reduction must be accompanied by demonstration of improved quality of services at both individual and population levels. On the surface, the assertion that costs can be cut and quality improved seems counterintuitive, but because of fragmentation and supply-driven services, it is clear that more is not necessarily better in the present system. The linked nature of

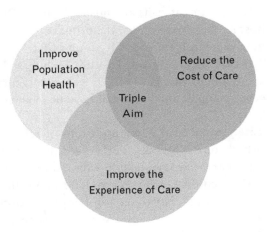

FIGURE 1.3: The Triple Aim. Data from "IHI Triple Aim Initiative," by Institute for Healthcare Improvement (IHI), n.d., (http://www.ihi.org/engage/initiatives/tripleaim/pages/default.aspx).

the Triple Aim goals ensures that one person or setting does not improve care at the expense of others.

The U.S. health care system can provide excellent high-end care but only to those few who have the necessary insurance or money to pay out-of-pocket. Such intense investment in resources for a select few individuals comes at the cost of adequate population-level care. Population, in this context, can mean a group of people who live in the same area, but it can also mean any defined group of people including those who share a common health care concern, or a group based on race, ethnicity, or financial status. The goal of improving the health of populations therefore forces health care systems to address health care needs collectively, which includes increasing outreach and prevention efforts.

Population-based care has been defined as an approach that "encompasses the ability to assess the health needs of a specific population, implement and evaluate interventions to improve the health of that population, and provide care for individual patients in the context of the culture, health status, and health needs of the populations of which that patient is a member" (Halpern & Boulter, 2000, p. 1). With its roots in public health, population-based health care requires a significant reorientation for the U.S. health care system that has traditionally treated people on an individual-by-individual basis and has failed to think about how certain groups of people share risk and protective factors that can be addressed more effectively and efficiently at the population level. Social workers, whose roots have been in individual care, must integrate this public health perspective into their approach and consider how social work practice can contribute to promoting health care at the population level.

To make progress toward the Triple Aim goals, we need to fundamentally change the design of the health care system and the way in which we pay for care by adopting a more systems approach that orients toward chronic illness and takes a holistic view of health and wellness (Dubusk & Snapp, 2015). Health care reform initiatives and the Affordable Care Act have embodied the implementation of global caps on spending for designated populations; the use of standardized measures of quality of care and health care costs and accountability to these measures; payment reform, which ensures that savings are shared across providers and invested in care improvement; and changes in professional education and training to ensure that providers, including social workers, are prepared for health care reform (Berwick et al., 2008). Social workers are gradually being affected by all of these developments, which are transforming the practice in health and behavioral health settings.

CONCLUSION

There is much to fix in the current U.S. health care system, which delivers poor-quality care at a higher cost than systems in other similar countries. Its fundamental problems can be summarized as lack of insurance for millions of people, overuse of unnecessary services that drive up costs, underuse of less costly preventive services, and medical errors due to poor coordination of care (Rosenberg, 2013). The result is a costly but ineffective system that delivers care of uneven quality and leads to significant health disparities. Moreover, growing evidence regarding SDH demonstrates that health care interventions play a relatively minor role in achieving good health. A host of other factors contribute to health status, including employment, income, education, housing, and residence. Some argue that the excess mortality seen among certain populations is, in fact, a problem of excess inequality, with the increasing divide between the wealthy and the rest of the population underlying stark health disparities (Porter, 2015). In addition to resources, behavior plays a major role in health, with smoking, substance misuse, poor nutrition, and lack of exercise significantly contributing to negative health outcomes.

At the system level, the way that health care is structured and paid for leads to high costs and an uneven distribution of services. Many of the problems with the health care system are demonstrated by how poorly people with comorbid and chronic illnesses are served. The excessive fragmentation that bifurcates physical and behavioral health and emphasizes acute care needs leads to episodic and poorly coordinated care. Health care services are shaped by the ways in which they are financed, with health care settings offering services that are reimbursed even if they are not needed. Changing the financial incentives to prioritize quality over quantity and rewarding providers for keeping people healthy and out of the hospital are important strategies for health care reform. To address these structural problems, health care reform encompasses policies that expand insurance, redesign systems, and refine payment mechanisms.

The Triple Aim has set the larger framework for health care reform by demonstrating how progress depends on holding and balancing three goals simultaneously: improving the experience of care at the individual level, improving outcomes at the population level, and reducing costs. To prepare for these changes, social workers must understand their practice within the context of the Triple Aim.

Andrews and colleagues (2013) identified four professional qualities of social workers that align with health care reform: understanding of the person-in-environment perspective, which supplies us with expertise in working with families and communities; training in navigation of complex social service systems to provide resources to our service users; a social justice framework, which helps us understand how health outcomes are shaped by SDH and how we can advocate for marginalized groups; and the social work evidence base that anchors our work in the rigorous study of practice in real-world settings. These qualities support the imperative role of social workers in health care policy, research, and practice, and they will ensure that the profession is part of the solution for the significant problems undermining the nation's health.

RESOURCES

Community Health Status Indicators 2015, Centers for Disease Control and Prevention (CDC) http://wwwn.cdc.gov/communityhealth

"Doctor Hotspot," PBS Frontline http://www.pbs.org/wgbh/pages/frontline/doctor-hotspot/

The Health and Medicine Division (HMD), National Academies of Science, Engineering, and Medicine https://www.nationalacademies.org/hmd/

"Health Disparities," Substance Abuse and Mental Health Services Administration (SAMHSA) http://www.samhsa.gov/health-disparities

Institute for Healthcare Improvement (IHI) Triple Aim Initiative http://www.ihi.org/Engage/Initiatives/TripleAim/pages/default.aspx

Social Determinants of Health (SDH) Program, World Health Organization (WHO) http://www.who.int/social_determinants/en/

REFERENCES

Agency for Healthcare Research and Quality. (2011). *National healthcare disparities report* (AHRQ Pub. No. 12-0006). Rockville, MD: Agency for Healthcare Research and Quality.

Alegria, M., Jackson, J. S., Kessler, R. C., & Takeuchi, D. (2007). National Comorbidity Survey Replication (NCS-R), 2001–2003. In M. Alegria, J. S. Jackson, R. C. Kessler, & D. Takeuchi. *Collaborative Psychiatric Epidemiology Surveys (CPES), 2001–2003 (United States)* [Computer file]. ICPSR20240-v5. Ann Arbor, MI: Institute for Social Research, Survey Research Center.

American Psychiatric Association. (2014). *Mental health disparities: Asian Americans*. Washington, DC: American Psychiatric Association.

Andrews, C. M., Darnell, J. S., McBride, T. D., & Gehlert, S. (2013). Social work and implementation of the Affordable Care Act. *Health & Social Work, 38*, 67–71. doi: 10.1093/hsw/hlt002

Annie E. Casey Foundation. (2013). *2013 KIDS COUNT data book: State trends in child well-being*. Baltimore, MD: The Annie E. Casey Foundation.

Barber, R. D., Coulourides Kogan, A., Riffenburgh, A., & Enguidanos, S. (2015). A role for social workers in improving care setting transitions: A case study. *Social Work in Health Care, 54*, 177–192. doi: 10.1080/00981389.2015.1005273

Berwick, D. M., Nolan, T. W., & Whittington, J. (2008). The Triple Aim: Care, health, and cost. *Health Affairs, 27*, 759–769. doi: 10.1377/hlthaff.27.3.759

Billings, J., Parikh, N., & Mijanovich, T. (2000). *Emergency department use in New York City: A substitute for primary care?* (Pub. No. 434). New York, NY: The Commonwealth Fund.

Braveman, P., Egerter, S., & Williams, D. R. (2011). The social determinants of health: Coming of age. *Annual Review of Public Health, 32*, 381–398. doi:10.1146/annurev-publhealth-031210-101218

Cabassa, L., Gomes, A. P., Meyreles, Q., Capitelli, L., Younge, R., Dragatsi, D., . . . Lewis-Fernández, R. (2014). Primary health care experiences of Hispanics with serious mental illness: A mixed-methods study. *Administration and Policy in Mental Health and Mental Health Services Research, 41*, 724–736. doi: 10.1007/s10488-013-0524-2

Center for Behavioral Health Statistics and Quality. (2015). *Behavioral health trends in the United States: Results from the 2014 National Survey on Drug Use and Health* (HHS Pub. No. SMA 15-4927, NSDUH Series H-50). Retrieved from http://www.samhsa.gov/data

Centers for Disease Control and Prevention. (2008). Racial/ethnic disparities in self-rated health status among adults with and without disabilities—United States, 2004–2006. *Morbidity and Mortality Weekly Report, 57*, 1069–1073. Retrieved from https://www.cdc.gov/mmwr/index.html

Colton, C. W., & Manderscheid, R. W. (2006). Congruencies in increased mortality rates, years of potential life lost, and causes of death among public mental health clients in eight states. *Preventing Chronic Disease, 3*, A42. Retrieved from https://www.cdc.gov/pcd/

Compton, M. T., Daumit, G. L., & Druss, B. G. (2006). Cigarette smoking and overweight/obesity among individuals with serious mental illnesses: A preventive perspective. *Harvard Review of Psychiatry, 14,* 212–222. doi: 10.1080/10673220600889256

Conley, D., & Rauscher, E. (2013). Genetic interactions with prenatal social environment: Effects on academic and behavioral outcomes. *Journal of Health and Social Behavior, 54,* 109–127. doi: 10.1177/0022146512473758

Davis, K., Stremikis, K., Squires, D., & Schoen, C. (2014). *Mirror, mirror, on the wall: How the performance of the U.S. health care system compares internationally.* (Pub. No. 1755). New York, NY: The Commonwealth Fund.

Descartes, R. (1991). *Principles of philosophy.* Norwell, MA: Kluwer Academic Publishing.

Dixon, L., Lewis-Fernández, R., Goldman, H., Interian, A., Michaels, A., & Kiley, M. C. (2011). Adherence disparities in mental health: Opportunities and challenges. *The Journal of Nervous and Mental Disease, 199,* 815–820. doi: 10.1097/NMD.0b013e31822fed17

Druss, B. G., & Walker, E. (2011). *Mental disorders and medical comorbidity* (Research Synthesis Report No. 21). Princeton, NJ: Robert Wood Johnson Foundation.

Druss, B. G., Zhao, L., Von Esenwein, S., Morrato, E.H., & Marcus, S. C. (2011). Understanding excess mortality in persons with mental illness: 17-Year follow up of a nationally representative U.S. survey. *Medical Care, 49,* 599–604. doi: 10.1097/MLR.0b013e31820bf86e

Dubusk, R., & Snapp, C. (2015). A systems medicine approach to behavioral health in the era of chronic disease (pp. 287–312). In M.A. Burg and O. Oyama (Eds.), *The behavioral health specialist in primary care: Skills for integrated practice* (pp. 1–20). Springer Publishing Company.

Gawande, A. (2011, January 24). The hot spotters: Can we lower medical costs by giving the neediest patients better care? *The New Yorker.* Retrieved from http://www.newyorker.com/magazine/2011/01/24/the-hot-spotters

Gerrity, M., Zoller, E., Pinson, N., Pettinari, C., & King, V. (2014). *Integrating primary care into behavioral health settings: What works for individuals with serious mental illness.* New York, NY: Milbank Memorial Fund.

Gfroerer, J. C., & Tan, L. L. (2003). Substance use among foreign-born youths in the United States: Does the length of residence matter? *American Journal of Public Health, 93,* 1892–1895. Retrieved from http://ajph.aphapublications.org/

Goff, D. C., Sullivan, L. M., McEvoy, J. P., Meyer, J. M., Nasrallah, H. A., Daumit, G. L., . . . Lieberman, J. A. (2005). A comparison of ten-year cardiac risk estimates in schizophrenia patients from the CATIE study and matched controls. *Schizophrenia Research, 80,* 45–53. doi: 10.1016/j.schres.2005.08.010

Halpern, R., & Boulter, P. (2000). *Population based health care: Definitions and applications.* Boston, MA: Tufts Managed Care Institute.

Hert, M., Correll, C. U., Bobes, J., Cetkovich-bakmas, M., Cohen, D. A. N., Asai, I., . . . Newcomer, J. W. (2011). Physical illness in patients with severe mental disorders. I: Prevalence, impact of medications and disparities in health care. *World Psychiatry, 10,* 52–77. doi: 10.1002/j.2051-5545.2011.tb00014.x

Holahan, J., & McGrath, M. (2014). *As the economy improves, the number of uninsured is falling but not because of a rebound in employer sponsored insurance* [Issue Brief]. Menlo Park, CA: Kaiser Family Foundation.

Ida, D. J., SooHoo, J., & Chapa, T. (2012). *Integrated care for Asian American, Native Hawaiian and Pacific Islander communities: A blueprint for action—Consensus statements and recommendations.* Rockville, MD: U.S. Department of Health and Human Services, Office of Minority Health.

Institute of Medicine. (1999). *To err is human: Building a safer health system.* Washington, DC: National Academy Press. doi: 10.17226/9728

Institute of Medicine. (2001). *Crossing the quality chasm: A new health system for the 21st century.* Washington, DC: National Academy Press. doi: 10.17226/10027

Institute of Medicine. (2002). *Unequal treatment: Confronting racial and ethnic disparities in healthcare.* Washington, DC: National Academy Press. doi: 10.17226/10260

Institute of Medicine. (2013). *U.S. Health in international perspective: Shorter lives, poorer health.* Washington, DC: National Academy Press. doi: 10.17226/13497

Kaiser Commission on Medicaid and the Uninsured. (2013). *Medicaid and its role in state/federal budgets & health reform* [Issue Brief]. Menlo Park, CA: Kaiser Family Foundation.

Kawachi, I., & Kennedy, B. P. (2002). *The health of nations: Why inequality is harmful to your health.* New York, NY: The New Press.

Kessler, R. C. (2003). Epidemiology of women and depression. *Journal of Affective Disorders, 74,* 5–13. doi: 10.1016/S0165-0327(02)00426-3

Kochanek, K., Arias, E., & Anderson, R. N. (2013). *How did cause of death contribute to racial differences in life expectancy in the United States in 2010?* (NCHS Data Brief No. 125). Hyattsville, MD: National Center for Health Statistics.

Krehely, J. (2009, December 21). How to close the LGBT health disparities gap. *Center for American Progress.* Retrieved from https://cdn.americanprogress.org/wp-content/uploads/issues/2009/12/pdf/lgbt_health_disparities.pdf

Latino health disparities compared to non-Hispanic whites. (2014, July). *Families USA.* Retrieved from http://familiesusa.org/product/latino-health-disparities-compared-non-hispanic-whites

Lewis, K., & Burd-Sharps, S. (2014). *The measure of America 2013–2014: American human development report.* Brooklyn, NY: Social Science Research Council.

Lundgren, L., & Krull, I. (2014). The Affordable Care Act: New opportunities for social work to take leadership in behavioral health and addiction treatment. *Journal of the Society for Social Work and Research, 5,* 415–438. doi: 10.1086/679302

Marmot, M. G., Rose, G., Shipley, M., & Hamilton, P. J. (1978). Employment grade and coronary heart disease in British civil servants. *Journal of Epidemiology and Community Health, 32,* 244–249. doi: 10.1136/jech.32.4.244

McGuire, T. G., & Miranda, J. (2008). New evidence regarding racial and ethnic disparities in mental health: Policy implications. *Health Affairs, 27,* 393–403. doi: 10.1377/hlthaff.27.2.393

Moore, R. H. (2013, September). *Addressing behavioral health disparities: Opportunities for a changing America.* Paper presented at the CSWE White House Briefing: Addressing the Social Determinants of Health in a New Era: The Role of Social Work Education, Washington, DC.

Neighbors, H. W., Trierweiler, S. J., Ford, B. C., & Muroff, J. R. (2003). Racial differences in DSM diagnosis using a semi-structured instrument: The importance of clinical judgment in the diagnosis of African Americans. *Journal of Health and Social Behavior, 44,* 237–256. Retrieved from http://www.jstor.org/stable/1519777

Olfson, M., Cherry, D. K., & Lewis-Fernández, R. (2009). Racial differences in visit duration of outpatient psychiatric visits. *Archives of General Psychiatry, 66,* 214–221.

Porter, E. (2015, April 28). Income inequality is costing the U.S. on social issues. *The New York Times.* Retrieved from http://www.nytimes.com/2015/04/29/business/economy/income-inequality-is-costing-the-us-on-social-issues.html?_r=0

Rosenberg, L. (2013, January). *Health care reform and behavioral health organizations.* Paper presented at the The Coalition for Behavioral Health Agencies Policy Conference, New York, NY.

Salganicoff, A., Ranji, U., Beamesderfer, A., & Kurani, N. (2014). *Women and health care in the early years of the Affordable Care Act: Key findings from the 2013 Kaiser Women's Health Survey.* Menlo Park, CA: Kaiser Family Foundation.

Schroeder, S. A. (2007). We can do better: Improving the health of the American people. *The New England Journal of Medicine, 357*, 1221–1228. doi: 10.1056/NEJMsa073350

Seidenberg, G. R. (2008). Personal accounts: Could Noah's life have been saved? Confronting dual diagnosis and a fragmented mental health system. *Psychiatric Services, 59*, 1254–1255. doi: 10.1176/appi.ps.59.11.1254

Song, Z., & Lee, T. H. (2013). The era of delivery system reform begins. *The Journal of the American Medical Association, 309*, 35–36. doi: 10.1001/jama.2012.96870

Squires, D. A. (2011). *The U.S. health system in perspective: A comparison of twelve industrialized nations.* New York, NY: The Commonwealth Fund.

Stanhope, V., Videka, L., Thorning, H., & McKay, M. (2015). Moving toward integrated health: An opportunity for social work. *Social Work in Health Care, 54*, 383–407. doi: 10.1080/00981389.2015.1025122

Substance Abuse and Mental Health Services Administration. (2011). *Addressing the needs of women and girls: Developing core competencies for mental health and substance abuse service professionals* (HHS Pub. No. SMA 11-4657). Rockville, MD: Substance Abuse and Mental Health Services Administration.

U.S. Department of Health and Human Services, Health Resources and Services Administration, and National Center for Health Workforce Analysis. (2013). *Projecting the supply and demand for primary care practitioners through 2020.* Rockville, MD: U.S. Department of Health and Human Services.

Verhaak, P. F., Heijmans, M. J., Peters, L., & Rijken, M. (2005). Chronic disease and mental disorder. *Social Science & Medicine, 60*, 789–797. doi: 10.1016/j.socscimed.2004.06.012

Wilkinson, R., & Marmot, M. G. (2003). *Social determinants of health: The solid facts* (2nd ed.). Copenhagen, Denmark: World Health Organization.

CHAPTER 2

INTEGRATED HEALTH CARE MODELS AND FRAMEWORKS

W. Patrick Sullivan

Few issues generate more debate and scrutiny in American society than health care. This topic has ignited a multifaceted discussion that ranges from the general health status of U.S. citizens to thorny matters of public and fiscal policy. The ends of this discourse are inextricably tied together: Health care policies impact quality of care, which in turn determines health and wellbeing, and ultimately the life and death, of the populace. As the population continues to grow and age, we can anticipate a greater demand for services, and by extension, increasing health care expenditures for both individuals and society at large (Milani & Lavie, 2015). However, French (2009) argued that we experience a value gap because increased spending on health care does not appear to improve the country's net overall health. Possible sources of this gap are an overriding preoccupation with treatment rather than prevention and the prevailing separation between physical and behavioral health care. In the absence of an integrated system, Kodner and Spreeuwenberg (2002) commented, "patients get lost, needed services fail to be delivered or are delayed, quality and patient satisfaction decline, and the potential for cost-effectiveness diminishes" (p. 2). They defined *integration* as

> a coherent set of methods and models on the funding, administrative, organizational, service delivery, and clinical levels designed to create connectivity, alignment, and collaboration within the cure and care sectors. The goal of these methods and models is to enhance quality of care and quality of life, consumer satisfaction, and system efficiency for patients with complex, long-term problems cutting across multiple services, providers, and settings. (p. 3)

Conceptual models and frameworks guide how health and illness are understood and responded to at both individual and policy levels. Consider an issue like substance misuse. Approaching substance misuse as an illness leads to certain policy and practice decisions that drastically differ from those that result from viewing it as the consequence of poor individual choices and willful behavior. Over time, these models can become embedded in practice and policy so deeply that their basic tenets are no longer questioned or debated, only ritualistically upheld. Thomas Kuhn (1970) wrote in *The Structure of Scientific Revolutions*:

> Paradigms gain their status because they are more successful than their competitors in solving a few problems that the group of practitioners has come to recognize as acute. To be more successful is not, however, to be either completely successful with a single problem or notably successful with any large number. (p. 23)

It appears that we have come to a key point in our health care history where what has been assumed is now being questioned and new approaches are being considered. Although the movement for integrated health care is motivated by many intuitions, it reflects a general acknowledgment that our current system is in urgent need of a major overhaul; however, balancing the many claims of diverse stakeholders is not an easy task.

The primary focus of this chapter is the underlying conceptual models and frameworks of our care system and how they may serve as platforms for new service delivery mechanisms on the horizon. Specifically, the chronic care and medical models are discussed, followed by a review of prevention and wellness frameworks and the recovery model. Additionally, exemplars are presented for programs and practices that fit under specific frameworks, and we will discuss the scope of care, the role of the service user, and the implications for policy.

THE MEDICAL MODEL

In June 1910, Abraham Flexner's report on the unfortunate state of medical education in the United States and Canada turned the field on its head. According to Flexner, comprehensive university training programs were needed, with heavy grounding in subjects such as chemistry, biology, and physics. The Flexner report resulted in increased rigor in these previously lenient programs and stricter requirements for admission (Chapman, 1974). With these reforms, medicine became a true profession and thrived thereafter.

Medicine (and by extension, the *medical model*) has since become synonymous with science and bestowed with prestige. The model is viewed as a scientific process that draws on observations and procedures that determine the causes of illness and lead to treatments that cure or ameliorate the effects of illness (see Clare, 1980). Shah and Mountain (2007) defined the medical model as "a process whereby, informed by the best evidence, doctors advise on, coordinate or deliver interventions for health improvement" (p. 375). A key aspect of the model in practice is *differential diagnosis*, which is based on symptoms and self-reports and further buttressed by tests and procedures. Although information is gathered from the service user's perspective, the treatment process is primarily decided by the professional who has accumulated expert knowledge. This is done in an effort to ensure that the selection of treatment or therapy is predicated on clinical experience and evidence and to strive for objectivity. However, an unfortunate result of this approach is that service users are excluded from decisions about their own care. To underscore the imbalance of this dynamic, technical language is employed and the service user remains largely passive (see Ludwig, 1975). This model fits well in a world where health care issues are seen as discrete problems of an individual, addressed case by case, and funded largely on a fee-for-service basis.

BIOPSYCHOSOCIAL MODEL

As the medical model flourished over time, a sizable number of commentaries and critiques surfaced. These argued that the model was unduly reductionist and that illness cannot be attributed solely to the deviations in biological or somatic variables. In an influential paper, American psychiatrist George Engel (1977) called for a new biomedical model based on a greater appreciation of the context of the individual's life. In Engel's view,

> To provide a basis for understanding the determinants of disease and arriving at rational treatments of patterns of health care, a medical model must also take into account the patient; the social context in which he [sic] lives; and the complementary system devised by society to deal with the disruptive effects of illness. (p. 132)

This was the inception of the *biopsychosocial model*, which asserts that health and illness are influenced by the interaction of biological, psychological, and social factors and that the content, organization, and delivery of health care services are more effective when they reflect this perspective. This model held great appeal, particularly for professions such as social work; it also moved the service user from passive obedience to active participation and affirmed the importance of the nontechnical aspects of the professional relationship. Additionally, those concerned with mental illness valued the challenge to mind–body dualism. This reminded people that health and illness are determined both individually and socially, underscoring the fact that elements outside the individual, such as the family or the surrounding environment, can contribute to the expression and trajectory of illness as well as the restoration and maintenance of health. As a result, this model extended care provision to a wider circle of professionals with various areas of expertise, including social workers. Additionally, placing mental illness and substance use disorders within a traditional medical framework actually seemed to reduce stigma. However, this expanded set of interventions did not fit neatly with existing patterns of service delivery, which were based solely on the medical model.

The biopsychosocial perspective also engendered a fair amount of debate. Searight (2015) suggested that this model encourages a form of eclecticism that does not advance the behavioral health field. Based on this multifaceted understanding of an illness process, the question became: How would this affect the work of a family practitioner or social worker in a community mental health center or primary care clinic? These concerns are understandable. Much work has been done to discover biophysical links to illnesses once considered outside the realm of medicine; indeed, many behavioral health conditions, ranging from severe mental illnesses to character traits, fall into this category. Given that such work can lead to more effective treatments, there is some fear that a biopsychosocial focus may divert attention away from promising areas of biomedical inquiry. However, Henningsen (2015) observed that the biopsychosocial model is inherently dynamic and can still account for new medical advances while steadfastly affirming the roles of individual and social forces in what we deem illness or health.

Some have argued that the impress of culture was ignored in the original articulation of the biopsychosocial model and that a more accurate terminology to capture the spirit of the model's intentions would be the *biopsychosociocultural model* (Henningsen, 2015). Setting aside any misgivings about the impact and practicality of the model to guide policy and practice, Engel's (1977) work was a vital step in redesigning the template for health care. It affirmed the importance of a collaborative helping alliance, the individual's response to illness and care, and the impact of a wider array of forces on illness and health. The model continues to guide new initiatives in health care to this day.

CHRONIC CARE MODEL

The Chronic Care Model (CCM) was first articulated more than 2 decades ago, but the conditions that gave rise to its eventual development are perhaps even more pressing now than at any other point in history (Wagner, Austin, & Von Korff, 1996). As elucidated at the beginning of this chapter, the combination of an ever-aging population and chronic conditions that persist across the lifespan (e.g., diabetes, asthma) places increased pressure on the health care system and on a host of ancillary services that provide additional medical and social support. Recognizing that the health care system was based on an acute care model, Wagner et al. (1996) understood that the entire infrastructure needed to be overhauled to effectively address chronic conditions. To this end, Coleman, Austin, Brach, and Wagner (2009) contended that the central aim of the CCM is to "transform the daily care for patients with chronic illnesses from acute and reactive to proactive, planned, and population-based" (p. 75). The CCM draws on the use of case and care management, utilizes the expertise of interdisciplinary teams, and promotes close partnership with individuals who are supported in self-care activities and behaviors to effectively monitor and manage long-term conditions.

As generally conceived, the CCM comprises several components: (a) self-management support, which underscores the role of individuals in managing their health and taking control over their care; (b) decision support, which involves integrating evidence-based guidelines into practice settings; (c) delivery system design, which includes the creation of practice teams and the establishment of a single point of care; (d) clinical information systems, which utilize service user registries and other management information tools that are useful for leaders, practitioners, and individuals; and (e) community linkages, resources, and policies, which affect the formal and informal relationships and partnerships that can sustain care and promote health (see Figure 2.1; see Barr et al., 2003; Bodenheimer, Wagner, & Grumbach, 2002; Wagner et al., 1996).

It is fair to suggest that the potential success of the CCM, and perhaps of all current health reform efforts, lies in activation of the service user. This refers to the extent

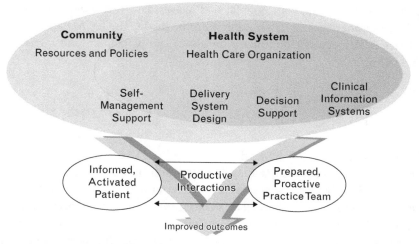

Chronic Care Model

Community
Resources and Policies

Health System
Health Care Organization

Self-Management Support

Delivery System Design

Decision Support

Clinical Information Systems

Informed, Activated Patient

Productive Interactions

Prepared, Proactive Practice Team

Improved outcomes

FIGURE 2.1: The Chronic Care Model. Reprinted with permission from "Chronic Disease Management: What Will It Take to Improve Care for Chronic Illness?" by E. H. Wagner, 1998, *Effective Clinical Practice, 1,* p. 3. Copyright 2002 by the American College of Physicians.

to which a person is willing and able to actively participate in the maintenance and improvement of his or her health (Hibbard & Greene, 2013). In 2002, Bodenheimer et al. detailed this problem and observed that, "too often, caring for chronic illness features an uninformed passive patient interacting with an unprepared practice team, resulting in frustrating, inadequate encounters" (p. 1775). The activation of the service user may ultimately have the greatest impact on health care because, regardless of whether systems are reconfigured, the core of the CCM is still self-management. For Koh et al. (2013), activation first requires health literacy, which they defined as the ability to "obtain, process, communicate, and understand basic health information and services" (p. 357). This is essential to comprehensive care for a wide range of medical disorders, including diabetes, cardiovascular disease, and asthma. Additionally, addressing these issues involves supporting individuals in making necessary lifestyle changes involving substance use, exercise, and diet, each of which can lessen the burden of chronic disorders.

The steps involved in providing services according to the CCM are wide ranging. First, chronic disorders must be recognized and assessed. From there, organizations must strive to implement evidence-based practices; help users learn and use self-management skills; and develop, manage, and effectively use clinical information tools as a collaborative system. When one adds to this list the necessity to form practice teams and enhance overall care management capability, it is obvious that major systems overhauls and cultural changes are required. This work cannot be done by a physician alone; it requires the active participation of social workers, dieticians, care managers, pharmacists, health educators, and peer support specialists (Milani & Lavie, 2015). Not surprisingly, the fiscal system that supports care must also be revised in order to reimburse interventions and reinforce the fact that these activities are central to care and not just supplementary.

Much has changed since the CCM was first introduced. What were once revolutionary ideas have become more commonplace. However, as with the biopsychosocial model presented earlier, there is still much progress to be made. The CCM can be expanded to fully embrace health promotion, incorporate wellness principles, and focus on population-level health.

PREVENTION AND WELLNESS MODEL

In 2010, the Patient Protection and Affordable Care Act (ACA) ushered in a new emphasis on prevention and wellness. By focusing attention on population-level care, models of prevention and wellness have drawn heavily from the public health model. As Power (2009) stated, the public health model is "a community approach to preventing and treating illnesses and promoting well-being" (pp. 581–582). Here, attention is devoted to the social determinants of health (SDH), and the health status and risks of a population are monitored. Even when illness is viewed from an exclusively medical perspective, it seems clear that genetic predispositions can become active or remain dormant in different contexts. Sederer (2016) asserted that the lion's share of health (both physical and mental) is determined by one's physical and social environments, which can over burden our stress response system.

Through its focus on population-level health and efforts to ameliorate threats to physical health, the prevention and wellness model also promotes mental health. The list of conditions of concern is lengthy and includes adverse childhood experiences, trauma in all its forms, poverty, food insecurity, and lack of access to care (Barr et al., 2003; Beardslee, Chien, & Bell, 2011; Fisher & Baum, 2010). Thomas et al. (2016) strongly believed that activities that promote mental health can be inserted into general medical practice. They highlighted the importance of mapping risk factors and resources in the surrounding community and of identifying individuals at risk for a disorder by instituting screening procedures. Practice should not focus exclusively on immediate problems but should strive to promote early intervention for all people when initial signs and symptoms arise.

Beyond the micro-level work, the prevention and wellness model emphasizes that attention should also be devoted to boosting community resilience through the promotion of good health, family education, the fostering of formal and informal support networks, and the creation of green spaces in urban environments. Certainly, many of these concerns are outside of the normal purview of primary care physicians and behavioral health professionals and fall into the area of public policy. However, prevention activities hold great potential for contributing to a comprehensive and integrated health care system.

THE RECOVERY MODEL

In many ways, the recovery model connects the other health care models presented earlier. Like the CCM, the recovery model focuses on self-management of long-term health disorders that have often been assessed and treated via the medical model. However, the term *chronically mentally ill* did not exactly inspire a great deal of hope for those with severe mental illnesses; it emerged during an era when people were cared for in poorly funded hospitals and segregated from the community. In the mid-1970s, more specialized community-based services were developed for those who were most in need, in part due to increased funding. In spite of an underlying pessimism both inside and outside the mental health care system, longitudinal research began to paint a different picture of the prognosis for people diagnosed with severe mental illnesses (see Bellack & Draplaski, 2012).

By the early 1990s, one of the founders of the psychiatric rehabilitation movement, William Anthony, published an influential article (1993) in which he suggested that not only is it possible to recover from mental illness but recovery should serve as the overall mission for all services. He proposed that "recovery, as we currently understand it, involves the development of new meaning and purposes in one's life as one grows beyond the catastrophic effects of mental illness" (p. 20). This message comforted many service providers who knew fully well that such outcomes could be achieved, as well as those individuals and families who were directly affected by mental illness.

For many current and former service users, the idea that one could surmount the impact of mental illness was well known; however, some felt that this was best accomplished outside the health care system. Judi Chamberlin's *On Our Own* (1978) asserted the rights of those who had been treated in the mental health system, labeled and rejected by society, and coerced and patronized by professional helpers. Through her work, Chamberlin introduced many to the term *psychiatric survivor*, a label adopted by some former service users to signify their rejection of and survival after coercive mental health services.

This model views mental health recovery not as a simple one-step task but instead as a multifaceted journey that has intrapersonal, interpersonal, and socioenvironmental dimensions. It is a response to those aspects in which the health care system has fallen short under the reign of the medical model, and in some cases it is a rebellion against a system that is considered demeaning and disempowering. The recovery model is predicated on strengths and empowerment approaches to practice that grant service users primary control over their own care. The adoption of recovery principles in mental health practice reflects a renewed hope that individuals with the most severe forms of mental illness can improve their circumstances and enjoy satisfying lives.

While the research and clinical experiences of professionals have been important in articulating the vision of recovery in mental health, the ideas that truly sustain this concept have come from the personal narratives of people with lived experience. Although these narratives mention that services and medications may help, they emphasize the professional relationship and the attitude of the helper, as opposed to any particular intervention. These individuals speak of recovery as a personal process, one in which important change is sometimes almost imperceptible to others, and one that involves rebuilding an identity and enhancing a sense of self-efficacy. Words like "hope" and "empowerment" are omnipresent in narratives, and the assessment of recovery is in many ways left to the individual (see Andersen, Oades, & Caputi, 2003; Deegan, 1988; Onken, Craig, Ridgway, Ralph, & Cook, 2007; Sullivan, 1994). However, one problem with the term *recovery* is that it is often assumed that what individuals must be recovering from is mental illness, whereas sometimes they are actually recovering from a society that labels and rejects them. This is why the ultimate mission of services should be full citizenship for all those whom they serve.

Davidson, O'Connell, Tondora, Lawless, and Evans (2005) delineated the differences between mental health and substance use disorders, stating that the latter involves remaining vigilant and engaging in health-promoting practices, including self-help, because of individuals' continuing vulnerability to relapse. As with mental health disorders, recovery from substance use disorders has social and communal aspects. Once a reasonable level of sobriety has been maintained, work must commence to reclaim one's life and strive toward successful performance as a productive member of society. Recovery from mental health disorders and from substance use disorders, therefore, are similar in that they underscore the roles of health maintenance and illness management, view hope for the future as critical, and consider a renewed sense of self to be a key outcome.

From this perspective, recovery is indeed a process as opposed to an endpoint, and many are quick to note that recovery does not simply mean the absence of symptoms. According to Braslow (2013), it can be thought of as a "mélange of beliefs and values" (p. 94). The working definition of recovery articulated by the U.S. Substance Abuse and Mental Health Services Administration (SAMHSA) in 2012 included four major dimensions: (a) health, which acknowledges the need to manage illness; (b) home, which means having a safe place to live; (c) purpose, which includes meaningful activities such as work and education; and (d) community, which involves relationships, social support, and love.

Like SAMHSA, the Betty Ford Institute Consensus Panel struggled to provide a useful definition of substance misuse recovery, ultimately considering it to be "a voluntarily maintained lifestyle comprised of sobriety, personal health, and citizenship" (McLellan, 2010, p. 109). This view shares some common ground with mental health recovery despite the important distinction that sobriety indicates complete abstinence, whereas mental health recovery cannot be reduced to a specific cure or symptom eradication.

Further obscuring the development of a standard operational definition, Tickle, Brown, and Hayward (2014) wondered whether the personally unique nature of recovery inherently defies general definition. For some, this imprecision is problematic and makes it difficult to translate such principles into a model of care that can predict outcomes and guide the development of effective policies and services (Liberman & Kopelowicz, 2005). The fact remains, however, that recovery is increasingly being used as a guide to develop and assess services. This was reflected in the efforts of the President's New Freedom Commission, which asserted that "recovery should become a defining expectation of future mental health care" (Hogan, 2003, p. 1469).

On closer inspection, elements of the previous frameworks can be found in the recovery model, in part because its quest is to successfully manage conditions that can portend difficulties in all life spheres. Whereas the CCM is built on a medical perspective and therefore is primarily concerned with illnesses and deficits, the recovery model is built on a person-centered perspective and is primarily concerned with individual and environmental strengths (Rapp & Goscha, 2006). The recovery model goes one step beyond the notion of the activated individual by not only emphasizing collaboration but also valuing user-centered services, user-operated programs, and peer support. Community linkages also take on a different shape, given that social rejection and stigma must be countered; for assisting professionals, this means that particular attention must be paid to advocacy.

The recovery model can inform strengths-based practice by affirming the service user as director of the helping process, reiterating the importance of the helping alliance, and emphasizing the role of community supports and resources. Strengths-based practice begins with an assessment of individual and environmental strengths, and care planning involves the development of a person-centered plan that is anchored by measurable goals. Strengths-based case management has been used extensively in mental health and substance abuse services, and users' goal-attainment rates have achieved noteworthy heights (Rapp & Goscha, 2006).

In mental health settings, illness management encompasses a wide range of approaches, including monitoring stress, coping with hallucinations, and managing medication. Salyers et al. (2009) underscored the centrality of this process by suggesting that "recovery can be thought of as managing one's illness in order to develop or regain a sense of self and place in society" (p. 483). Success here is essential to the individual, but it is also crucial for society in that it is necessary for reducing the superfluous use of expensive and specialized community health care services. The good news, according to Cook et al. (2009), is that it has been well documented for more than 2 decades that those with mental health challenges are extraordinarily capable of managing their own illnesses. In their assessment of the efficacy of Wellness Recovery Action Planning (WRAP), a model that is based on the development of an individual recovery plan, improvements were found for a wide range of illness conditions, and other important outcome areas also increased, such as levels of confidence and hopefulness. In a related study that involved a 10-module illness management and recovery model and six community mental health centers, positive results were found in the areas of illness management and hope; however, there was no change in users' overall satisfaction with services (Salyers et al., 2009). These two studies have added to earlier data suggesting that, as with other long-term health concerns, self-management techniques can be fruitfully employed in behavioral health care.

CONCLUSION

The medical model should never be thought of as the sole organizing framework in which integrated health care can flourish. Although the model does exert considerable influence in both physical and behavioral health care—and in many ways, this is appropriate—it is unduly reductionist. The assessment procedures and the interventions that follow from its principles focus solely on illnesses, disregarding individuals' social contexts and actual experiences. This failure to account for beliefs and attitudes can leave physicians and psychiatrists bewildered as to why service users refuse to take medication or follow through on additional recommendations.

The biopsychosocial model can be considered a critique of the medical model in its assertions that illness is also a social and cultural event and that it is imperative to consider the context of illness. The impress of this approach can be found in assessment processes that have been broadened and in the use of complementary practitioners, such as social workers, to attend to various aspects of a person's care.

The CCM (which emerged in medicine) and the recovery model (which emerged in behavioral health) have common aspects and can both be fruitfully extended by adopting tenets of the public health and prevention and wellness approaches. These two models are similar in that they recognize the importance of managing long-term disorders, depend on the active participation of service users, and thrive in contexts that support person-centered care. With increased concern about the quality, accessibility, and cost of health care, the CCM has now become the template for integrated health care initiatives. Likewise, the recovery model has much to contribute to the integration of care; however, because mental illnesses are heavily stigmatized, advocacy and a focus on individual rights and choice have held more prominent roles in the recovery model. The models are further distinguished in that the essence of the CCM is a tendency toward a medical focus and a departure from a system based on acute care, whereas the core of the recovery model is an emphasis on the strengths and abilities of individuals and environments.

Broadening our knowledge of health care relies on the decision by citizens, policy makers, organizations, and funders, whether governmental or private, to devote more attention to SDH and acknowledge them as valid health concerns. If these values are upheld, the ongoing evolution of health care may very well lead to a truly holistic focus on health and wellness.

RESOURCES

The Center for the Human Rights of Users and Survivors of Psychiatry (CHRUSP) http://www.chrusp.org/home/index

Center for Integrated Health Solutions (CIHS), Substance Abuse and Mental Health Services Administration (SAMHSA) http://www.integration.samhsa.gov/about-us/about-cihs

The National Mental Health Consumers' Self-Help Clearinghouse http://www.mhselfhelp.org/

Recovery to Practice (RTP) Initiative, Council on Social Work Education (CSWE) https://www.cswe.org/Centers-Initiatives/Initiatives/Recovery-to-Practice-Initiative

Recovery to Practice (RTP) Program, Substance Abuse and Mental Health Services Administration (SAMHSA) http://www.samhsa.gov/recovery-to-practice

REFERENCES

Andersen, R., Oades, L., & Caputi. P. (2003). The experience of recovery in schizophrenia: Towards an empirically validated stage model. *Australian and New Zealand Journal of Psychiatry, 37*(5), 586–594. doi: 10.1046/j.1440-1614.2003.01234.x

Anthony, W. A. (1993). Recovery from mental illness: The guiding vision of the mental health service system in the 1990s. *Psychosocial Rehabilitation Journal, 16*(4), 11–23. doi: 10.1037/h0095655

Barr, V. J., Robinson, S., Marin-Link, B., Underhill, L., Dotts, A., Ravensdale, D., & Salivaras, S. (2003). The expanded Chronic Care Model: An integration of concepts and strategies from population health promotion and the Chronic Care Model. *Healthcare Quarterly, 7*(1), 73–82. doi: 10.12927/hcq.2003.16763

Beardslee, W. R., Chien, P. L., & Bell, C. C. (2011). Prevention of mental disorders, substance abuse, and problem behaviors: A developmental perspective. *Psychiatric Services, 62*, 247–254. doi: 10.1176/appi.ps.62.3.247

Bellack, A. S., & Drapalski, A. (2012). Issues and developments on the consumer recovery construct. *World Psychiatry, 11*, 156–160. doi: 10.1002/j.2051-5545.2012.tb00117.x

Bodenheimer, T., Wagner, E. H., & Grumbach, K. (2002). Improving primary care for patients with chronic illness. *The Journal of the American Medical Association, 288*, 1775–1779. doi: 10.1001/jama.288.14.1775

Braslow, J. T. (2013). The manufacture of recovery. *Annual Review of Clinical Psychology, 9*, 781–809. doi: 10.1146/annurev-clinpsy-050212-185642

Chamberlin, J. (1978). *On our own: Patient-controlled alternatives to the mental health system.* New York, NY: McGraw-Hill.

Chapman, C. B. (1974). "The Flexner Report" by Abraham Flexner. *Daedalus, 103*(1), 105–117. Available from http://www.jstor.org/?redirected=true

Clare, A. W. (1980). *Psychiatry in dissent* (2nd ed.). London, England: Routledge.

Coleman, K., Austin, B. T., Brach, C., & Wagner, E. H. (2009). Evidence on the Chronic Care Model in the new millennium. *Health Affairs, 28*, 75–85. doi: 10.1377/hlthaff.28.1.75

Cook, J. A., Copeland, M. E., Hamilton, M. M., Jonikas, J. A., Razzano, L. A., Floyd, C. B., . . . Grey, D. D. (2009). Initial outcomes of a mental illness self-management program based on wellness recovery action planning. *Psychiatric Services, 60*, 246–249. doi: 10.1176/appi.ps.60.2.246

Davidson, L., O'Connell, M. J., Tondora, J., Lawless, M., & Evans, A. C. (2005). Recovery in serious mental illness: A new wine or just a new bottle? *Professional Psychology: Research and Practice, 36*, 480–487. doi: 10.1037/0735-7028.36.5.480

Deegan, P. E. (1988). Recovery: The lived experience of rehabilitation. *Psychosocial Rehabilitation Journal, 11*(4), 11–19. doi: 10.1037/h0099565

Engel, G. L. (1977). The need for a new medical model: A challenge for biomedicine. *Science, 196*, 129–136. doi: 10.1126/science.847460

Fisher, M., & Baum, F. (2010). The social determinants of mental health: Implications for research and health promotion. *Australian and New Zealand Journal of Psychiatry, 44*, 1057–1063. doi: 10.3109/00048674.2010.50931

French, M. (2009, April). *Shifting the course of our nation's health: Prevention and wellness as national policy* [Issue Brief]. Washington, DC: American Public Health Association. Retrieved from https://www.apha.org/~/media/files/pdf/factsheets/finalpreventionpolicy.ashx

Henningsen, P. (2015). Still modern? Developing the biopsychosocial model for the 21st century. *Journal of Psychosomatic Research, 79*, 362–363. doi: 10.1016/j.jpsychores.2015.09.003

Hibbard, J. H., & Greene, J. (2013). What the evidence shows about patient activation: Better health outcomes and care experiences; Fewer data on costs. *Health Affairs, 32*, 207–214. doi: 10.1377/hlthaff.2012.1061

Hogan, M. F. (2003). The President's New Freedom Commission: Recommendations to transform mental health care in America. *Psychiatric Services, 54*, 1467–1474. doi: 10.1176/appi.ps.54.11.1467

Kodner, D. L., & Spreeuwenberg, C. (2002). Integrated care: Meaning, logic, applications, and implications—A discussion paper. *International Journal of Integrated Care, 2*(14), 1–6. Available from http://doi.org/10.5334/ijic.67

Koh, H. K., Brach, C., Harris, L. M., & Parchman, M. L. (2013). A proposed "health literate care model" would constitute a systems approach to improving patients' engagement in care. *Health Affairs, 32*, 357–367. doi: 10.1377/hlthaff.2012.1205

Kuhn, T. S. (1970). *The structure of scientific revolutions* (2nd ed.). Chicago, IL: University of Chicago Press.

Liberman, R. P., & Kopelowicz, A. (2005). Recovery from schizophrenia: A concept in search of research. *Psychiatric Services, 56,* 735–742. doi: 10.1176/appi.ps.56.6.735

Ludwig, A. M. (1975). The psychiatrist as physician. *The Journal of the American Medical Association, 234,* 603–604. doi: 10.1001/jama.1975.03260190031016

McLellan, A. T. (2010). What is recovery? Revisiting the Betty Ford Institute Consensus Panel definition. *Journal of Social Work Practice in the Addictions, 10,* 109–113. doi: 10.1080/15332560903540052

Milani, R. V., & Lavie, C. J. (2015). Health care 2020: Reengineering health care delivery to combat chronic disease. *The American Journal of Medicine, 128,* 337–343. doi: 10.1016/j.amjmed.2014.10.047

Onken, S. J., Craig, C. M., Ridgway, P., Ralph, R. O., & Cook, J. A. (2007). An analysis of the definitions and elements of recovery: A review of the literature. *Psychiatric Rehabilitation Journal, 31,* 9–22. doi: 10.2975/31.1.2007.9.22

Power, A. K. (2009). A public health model of mental health for the 21st century. *Psychiatric Services, 60,* 580–584. doi: 10.1176/ps.2009.60.5.580

Rapp, C. A., & Goscha, R. J. (2006). *The strengths model: Case management with people with psychiatric disabilities.* New York, NY: Oxford University Press.

Salyers, M. P., Godfrey, J. L., McGuire, A. B., Gearhart, T., Rollins, A. L., & Boyle, C. (2009). Implementing the illness management and recovery program for consumers with severe mental illness. *Psychiatric Services, 60,* 483–490. doi: 10.1176/appi.ps.60.4.483

Searight, H. R. (2015). The biopsychosocial model: "Reports of my death have been greatly exaggerated." *Culture, Medicine, and Psychiatry, 40,* 289–298. doi: 10.1007/s11013-015-9471-6

Sederer, L. I. (2016). The social determinants of mental health. *Psychiatric Services, 67,* 234–235. doi: 10.1176/appi.ps.201500232

Shah, P., & Mountain, D. (2007). The medical model is dead—Long live the medical model. *The British Journal of Psychiatry, 191,* 375–377. doi: 10.1192/bjp.bp.107.037242

Substance Abuse and Mental Health Services Administration. (2012). *SAMHSA's working definition of recovery, updated* [Brochure]. Retrieved from http://store.samhsa.gov/shin/content//PEP12-RECDEF/PEP12-RECDEF.pdf

Sullivan, W. P. (1994). A long and winding road: The process of recovery from severe mental illness. *Innovations and Research, 3*(3), 19–27. Available from https://www.researchgate.net/

Thomas, S., Jenkins, R., Burch, T., Calamos Nasir, L., Fisher, B., Giotaki, G., ... Wright, F. (2016). Promoting mental health and preventing mental illness in general practice. *London Journal of Primary Care, 8,* 3–9. doi: 10.1080/17571472.2015.1135659

Tickle, A., Brown, D., & Hayward, M. (2014). Can we risk recovery? A grounded theory of clinical psychologists' perceptions of risk and recovery-oriented mental health services. *Psychology and Psychotherapy: Theory, Research and Practice, 87,* 96–110. doi: 10.1111/j.2044-8341.2012.02079.x

Wagner, E. H. (1998). Chronic disease management: What will it take to improve care for chronic illness? *Effective Clinical Practice, 1,* 2–4. Available from http://ecp.acponline.org/

Wagner, E. H., Austin, B. T., & Von Korff, M. (1996). Organizing care for patients with chronic illness. *The Milbank Quarterly, 74,* 511–544. doi: 10.2307/3350391

CHAPTER 3

POPULATION HEALTH

Heather Klusaritz, Julie A. Cederbaum, and Max D. Krauss

Social work is fundamentally grounded in the person-in-environment perspective (Pardeck, 1988), but many of the research, clinical, and policy practices that social workers engage in are focused on individual-level changes. Although social workers are taught how individual health is impacted by environmental contraints such as urban blight (Garvin, Branas, Keddem, Sellman, & Cannuscio, 2013), policy constraints such as a tax on soda to reduce obesity (Powell, Chriqui, Khan, Wada, & Chaloupka, 2013), and institutional constraints such as the school-to-prison pipeline (González, 2012), social work education focuses less on the systems-level changes that influence the wellbeing of individuals, families, and communities.

This chapter introduces the concept of population health, which offers a unique appreciation of the many determinants of health, the drivers of inequality, and the opportunities to influence health outcomes. It discusses the ways in which social workers can contribute to the continued adaptations that are needed to increase the efficiency and effectiveness of various environments, policies, and systems. Knowledge of these concepts is necessary to successfully navigate the evolving practice environment because health and behavioral health care teams are being increasingly called on to intervene at the community and population level to achieve the goals of health care reform.

WHAT IS POPULATION HEALTH?

A fundamental innovation of modern health care is the development of methodologies that go beyond the provision of individualized services within a provider-patient relationship to improve health outcomes on a societal level. These efforts take the form of public health initiatives and population health approaches. Although the concepts are interrelated and interdependent, these terms are often used interchangeably, contributing to confusion about their definitions and blurring the nuances that distinguish them.

Public health consists of "all organized measures (whether public or private) to prevent illness, promote health, and prolong life among the population as a whole. Its activities aim to provide conditions in which people can be healthy and focus on entire populations, not on individual patients or diseases," according to the World Health Organization (WHO) (Gurbutt, 2016, p. 3). Public health initiatives influence health outcomes by monitoring population health concerns, enacting policy solutions, and ensuring access to services. Organizations that seek to fulfill the objectives of this mission include the WHO, the Centers for Disease Control and Prevention (CDC), local departments of health, university research centers, nonprofit agencies, and advocacy groups. The agents of public health vary greatly in size and scope, and they can operate on a global, national, state, or community level. Examples of public health initiatives include the following:

- Food pantry programs, which exist to provide healthy food to individuals and families who cannot afford groceries
- Motor vehicle laws, which are designed to prevent accidents and injuries through measures such as requiring seatbelts and airbags and penalizing motorists for excessive speed or intoxicated driving
- Public information campaigns such as the "Learn the signs, act early" campaign, which aims to help parents identify the early warning signs of developmental delay (CDC, 2016)
- Regulation of potentially harmful products, including alcohol, drugs, tobacco, foods, and the materials used in consumer goods
- Vaccination requirements, which have helped to eradicate whooping cough, measles, and polio—illnesses that were formerly responsible for the deaths of children on an epidemic level
- Universal screening for elevated blood lead levels in young children and lead abatement programs to eliminate existing lead-based paint hazards in homes
- Medicare and Medicaid, which are federally sponsored programs that provide health insurance coverage to individuals affected by poverty or disability

Population health is a broadly cited term without a universally accepted definition. It has been used to describe a field, a methodology, and a goal in and of itself (Stoto, 2013). The modern concept of population health was developed in Canada and the United Kingdom in the late 20th century as a way of understanding why certain groups of people were healthier than others (Evans, Barer, & Marmor, 1994; Kindig & Stoddart, 2003). Its fundamental purpose has remained relatively the same over the years, and the term is now employed in the language of official agencies and initiatives, including the CDC, the WHO, the Institute of Medicine (IOM), and the Patient Protection and Affordable Care Act of 2010 (ACA).

In recent decades, a population health approach has emerged that emphasizes the ways in which society as a whole and communities within a society are affected by health issues (Fabrus, Pracilio, Nash, & Clarke, 2015). It expands the more traditional public health approaches, which have emphasized individual behavior change. It focuses on "the health outcomes of a group of individuals, including the distribution of such outcomes within the group. These groups are often geographic populations, such as nations or communities, but can also be other groups such as employees, ethnic groups, disabled persons" (Fabrus et al., 2015), or any other clearly defined groups. The subdivision of individuals aids population health in its goal to understand the roles of a wide range of determinants in the creation and perpetuation of health disparities.

Use of a population-based approach facilitates understanding of systems that affect individuals and how entities influence these efforts. In particular, the approach can be used to understand how different constituent groups might influence health. For example, whereas a county department of health bears responsibility for the total population of residents within its specified geopolitical jurisdiction, an advocacy group may concern itself with a subpopulation defined by circumstances, such as women who have experienced domestic violence or families of children with special needs (Jacobson & Teutsch, 2012). Likewise, a hospital is likely to define its subpopulation by its catchment area and other factors such as whether it accepts Medicaid or specializes exclusively in pediatric care. However, a health care delivery organization may take a system-within-systems approach by identifying a subpopulation within its total population; an example is the Centers for Medicare & Medicaid Services' Everyone With Diabetes Counts program (2016), which tracks people with diabetes. Understanding the many applications of a population health perspective helps social workers identify areas for advocacy and intervention to strengthen these efforts.

HEALTH DISPARITIES

The first step in designing population health approaches to address inequities is to define the denominator: the group of individuals at risk for the negative outcome. In the United States, great disparities exist between the health outcomes of white populations and those of racial and ethnic minorities, as well as between Americans at different levels of income, education, and employment (Woolf & Braveman, 2011). For example, non-Hispanic African-American women experience infant mortality rates 2.4 times greater than those of non-Hispanic white women (MacDorman & Mathews, 2011). Life expectancies for men and women in poverty are almost 7 years shorter than those for people with incomes four times above the poverty level, and failure to complete high school is associated with a 5-year reduction in life expectancy compared with college graduation (Braveman & Egerter, 2008). Poor Americans are more than two times as likely as Americans at twice the poverty level to have chronic illnesses such as diabetes and coronary heart disease, disorders that not only affect their mortality but also limit their ability to participate as productive members of society (Bravemen & Egerter, 2008). It can be argued that social programs that help people pay for college, find jobs, and secure housing in desegregated communities are just as influential for health care outcomes as laws governing health insurance and medical practices.

Although the goal of improving health outcomes across populations has existed for centuries, it has been pursued with increasing determination in recent decades. This is partially a result of technological advances; as society has ventured further into the information age, the potential that data-driven strategies hold for identifying and addressing disparities has been recognized. A growing body of research has documented that the

United States has poorer outcomes than other wealthy countries in domains such as life expectancy, teen pregnancy, HIV and AIDS, chronic illness, infant mortality, and deaths related to drugs, violence, and motor vehicle accidents (National Research Council and Institute of Medicine, 2013). At the same time, our country spends vastly more money per capita on health care than any other country in the world. This points to gross inefficiencies in the existing systems that underlie the nation's population health and a need to address these inequities to allow progress toward health and economic stability.

DETERMINANTS OF POPULATION HEALTH

Population health recognizes the multidimensionality of the determinants of health, particularly the nonmedical influences. A *determinant* is any factor that influences health outcomes. Several models with various levels of complexity exist to conceptualize the interrelationships among the determinants of health. Five commonly cited determinants are health care, individual behaviors, genetics, social environment, and physical environment (Kindig, 2012). Individual behaviors and genetics are considered *individual factors*, meaning that they are unique to each person (Jacobson & Teutsch, 2012). Social and physical environments are sometimes referred to as *upstream factors* because they originate outside of the individual and have obvious but indirect effects on the other determinants.

Underlying the interactions between determinants are the policies and programs created to address societal health concerns, which can take place at the organizational, municipal, county, state, or federal level. Kindig, Asada, and Booske (2008) developed a framework for understanding the relationships among social determinants of health, policies, and programmatic interventions; the framework can also be used to guide federal and state planning to improve the health of populations (see Figure 3.1).

Health care refers to access to and quality of health care services. Population health care access can be impeded by a scarcity of doctors serving a given area or accepting certain types of health insurance or by a temporal mismatch between when health care services are available (i.e., office hours) and when service users can seek care. People who are not able to receive regular preventive care due to access or cost often miss valuable opportunities to diagnose and treat disorders that can eventually become complex and life-threatening (Kaiser Family Foundation, 2015). Quality of health care depends on practitioners' having the resources and the competencies to provide effective treatments.

The ACA represents a federal policy attempt to address what Berwick, Nolan, and Whittington (2008) identified as the U.S. health care system's Triple Aim: improving the experience of care (i.e., quality), enhancing the health of populations, and reducing per capita costs of health care (see Chapter 1). The Triple Aim posits that these three components are interdependent: We cannot reduce health care costs without also improving population health, nor can we improve population health without also addressing the experience of care to ensure that individuals receive the right care, at the right time, and in the right setting. The ACA (2010) aims to address these barriers by mandating that all citizens be insured and requiring that insurance plans cover evidence-based preventive services, such as immunizations and screenings for many illnesses, at no cost to the

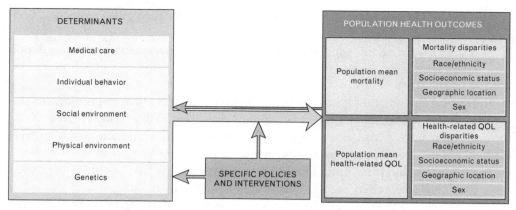

FIGURE 3.1: Schematic framework for population health planning. Broad population health outcomes are conceptualized on the *right*, and determinants of population health outcomes are represented on the *left*. The quadrants in the outcomes component are arbitrarily sized equally, as are the disparity domains within outcomes and the determinant categories. QOL, quality of life. From "A Population Health Framework for Setting National and State Health Goals," by D. A. Kindig, Y. Asada, and B. Booske, 2008, *Journal of the American Medical Association, 299,* p. 2082. Copyright 2008 by the American Medical Association.

service user. This policy initiative affects the determining factor of health care on a total population level across the United States.

Population management. The ACA created several drivers forcing health care systems and the providers or practitioners within those systems to think more broadly about their roles in population health. Before the inception of the ACA and the Triple Aim, population management tended to focus on populations defined only by an illness group (e.g., people with congestive heart failure discharged from the hospital) or an insurance category (e.g., people with diabetes who are insured by Medicaid HMO). Although interventions to address populations defined in this way still account for a large proportion of population management actions, health care systems are also defining populations by social determinant categories of risk, such as marginalized or vulnerable communities. This updated conception of population management "orients payment and the delivery of healthcare services toward the achievement of specific healthcare-related metrics and outcomes for a defined population" (Loehrer, Lewis, & Bogan, 2016, p. 82). It also harnesses the power of electronic health records to enable care teams to match populations to the most appropriate, targeted, and evidence-based interventions.

The Substance Abuse and Mental Health Services Administration–Health Resources and Services Administration's (SAMHSA-HRSA) Center for Integrated Health Solutions (CIHS) (2001) has identified four overarching key principles for population management:

1. Population-based care: focusing on caring for the whole population you are serving, not just the individuals actively seeking care
2. Data-driven care: using data and analytics to make informed decisions to serve those in your population who most need care

3. Evidence-based care: using the best available evidence to guide treatment decisions and delivery of care
4. Care management: engaging in actionable care management for the population you serve

In summary, population-based health care delivery requires a team of providers engaging in a data-driven approach to identify populations in need of intervention and utilizing the most up-to-date evidence to design and implement care interventions and to provide comprehensive, coordinated care management.

Individual behaviors. Individual behaviors are actions that people take in their daily lives that affect their health. Diet, physical activity, smoking, use of alcohol or other substances, and sexual activity carry various levels of risk and benefit for overall health outcomes (Sanchez & Burg, 2015). The population impact of just one individual behavior is evidenced by the estimated 480,000 deaths caused by smoking each year in the United States (U.S. Department of Health and Human Services, 2014). Regulations that curb sales and advertising of tobacco products to minors reflect policy efforts to prevent this harmful and avoidable habit from being adopted by people in the first place.

Individual behaviors are also influenced by the organizational contexts in which service users seek care. Driven by policy changes under the ACA, health care systems are accelerating their work in the area of team-based care, including patient-centered medical homes (PCMHs). The PCMH model recognizes that the design of the current health care system may inherently create barriers to achieving optimal health outcomes (see Chapter 5). Although primary care providers have historically been the main adopters of PCMH, other specialists have also begun to implement similar care models (CIHS, 2001). These health home models employ a team-based approach to better coordinate care delivery across providers in a health care system or network of care delivery sites. The team includes behavioral health care providers, medical specialists, hospitals, community-based social service agencies, and health home care providers (National Committee for Quality Assurance, 2011). Section 1945(h)(4) of the ACA (2010) defines health home services as "comprehensive and timely high quality services," and it includes the following health home services to be provided by designated health home providers or health teams:

- Comprehensive care management
- Care coordination and health promotion
- Transitional care from inpatient to other settings, including appropriate follow-up
- Individual and family support, including authorized representatives
- Referral to community and social support services, if relevant
- Use of health information technology to link services, as feasible and appropriate

Genetics. Genetics and biology describe the physiologic templates that underlie individual bodies and minds. The architecture is passed down from parents but is unique to each person. The genome determines specific traits that make up a human being, including skin color, susceptibility to certain illnesses, and developmental disorders such as

Down syndrome. Completion of the Human Genome Project led to scientific advancements that have increased understanding of the role played by genetics, enabled precise screening measures, and helped the development of effective treatments for illnesses (Belsky, Moffitt, & Caspi, 2013). For example, because of reduced genetic diversity, the Ashkenazi Jewish population has a distinct genome structure that increases susceptibility for disorders such as cystic fibrosis and Crohn disease (Guha et al., 2012). In this case, targeted screening has resulted in a greater than 90% decrease in Tay-Sachs disease within the Ashkenazi population (Shao, Liu, & Grinzaid, 2015).

However, examples of population-specific genetic traits are rare. It is difficult to make generalized statements about the health vulnerabilities of an entire population due to the normal genetic diversity contained within populations. Geographic groups have experienced generations of reproductive intermixing, and race and ethnicity are not so much measurable genomic states as they are social and ideological constructs (Fine, Ibrahim, & Thomas, 2005). Furthermore, genetic risk alone does not ensure the development of future pathology. In the case of alcoholism heritability, expression of this risk largely depends on exposure to childhood trauma (Enoch, 2013). Although targeted screening, gene therapies, and precision medicine represent cutting-edge innovations with an almost infinite capacity, the medical communities developing these technologies have been slow to embrace the potentials of population-level interventions (Khoury & Evans, 2015). Purveyors of the population health approach usually conceptualize genetics as a fixed condition and sometimes leave it out of models entirely (Jacobson & Teutsch, 2012; Remington, Catlin, & Gennuso, 2015). They assert that time and money may be wasted on developing genetic interventions if proportionate resources are not directed toward other determinants (Kindig, 2012).

Social environment. Social environment factors include socioeconomic status, employment, education, social support, and family network. These factors affect individual behavior by providing models of what is socially acceptable and what goals one should strive for in life. Through families and peers, people are taught eating habits (Cruwys, Bevelander, & Hermans, 2015), academic expectations (Oyserman, 2012), and maladaptive coping strategies such as smoking and drinking (Huang, Soto, Fujimoto, & Valente, 2014). Socioeconomic circumstances have a tremendous impact on individual and population health outcomes, often estimated to be larger than that of any other determinant (Marmot & Allen, 2014; Remington et al., 2015). Lower-income families may be unable to provide their children with essential components of early development such as nutritious food, quality education, and a safe environment in which to grow. Lower socioeconomic status is also linked to higher levels of toxic stress, which disrupts the development of neurological, metabolic, and regulatory systems (Shonkoff et al., 2012). These developmental insults often persist throughout the lifespan, leading to an array of later-stage health problems ranging from cardiovascular disease and liver cancer to anxiety and depression.

Physical environment. Physical environment characteristics include the neighborhoods in which people live and the other settings in which they work, play, travel, and go to school. This determinant's impact is demonstrated by the fact that children who have access to green spaces and healthy food tend to be healthier than children who live near fast food restaurants (Carroll-Scott et al., 2013). The health of individuals is threatened or undermined by physical environments that contain polluted air or water, roads that are unsafe for pedestrians or motorists, or crumbling infrastructure and no green spaces.

The water crisis in Flint, Michigan, serves as a tragic example of the effects of environmental health determinants. Thousands of children were exposed to lead, a chemical known to harm the developing central nervous system (Bellinger, 2016). Emergency cost-cutting measures led to a change in the source of the city's water supply, but alternative recommendations that could have prevented lead contamination were ignored. Flint's hardship highlights the vulnerability of low-income populations to physical environment determinants when policy interventions fail to protect them.

CASE VIGNETTE

Sage (a hypothetical city modeled after an actual town in the northeastern United States) is a midsized town located just outside a large metropolitan city. Although surrounded by productive farmland, Sage has a large number of fast food restaurants, a climbing obesity rate, and limited access to fresh fruits and vegetables except those purchased in national chain supermarkets. Community leaders, health providers, public health social workers, and community members congregated with the intention of improving the health and wellbeing of Sage residents. The population health problem was identified using a three-pronged lens—individual, systems, and policy. From the individual perspective, the group observed that the issue was food consumption behaviors, particularly the limited intake by Sage residents of fresh fruits and vegetables. From the systems perspective, the group highlighted the issue of access; the community was a *food desert*, lacking access to fresh fruits and vegetables. The problem from a policy perspective was twofold: the area lacked an ordinance to cap the number of fast food restaurants, and there were no established areas within the community to access fresh fruits and vegetables (e.g., a farmer's market). The coalition's collective action in these areas improved health and wellness among Sage community members, stimulated fruit and vegetable intake, generated income for local farmers, and established a permanent farmer's market. Improvements in the health of Sage individuals and the community in turn improved health at the population level through changes to systems and policies. The roles of social workers in this process are discussed in the following sections.

Individual-level changes. The goal at the individual level for Sage was to modify the eating behaviors of its community members. Barriers to achieving this goal included unfamiliarity with certain vegetables, discomfort with preparing the vegetables, and reluctance to try new foods. Social workers focused their individual-level behavior goals on educating residents about locally sourced vegetables and increasing their comfort with preparing these foods through cooking demonstrations. The coalition also created a Sage community cookbook, which they provided for free to patrons of the community's new farmer's market.

Systems-level changes. To increase access to healthy fruits and vegetables, the group collaborated with a local health facility and placed the farmer's market across the street from the clinic where residents were accessing health services. This strategy diminished issues of access by placing the market adjacent to a commonly used community resource. They further incentivized Sage residents by providing clinic patients with vouchers to purchase fruits and vegetables at the farmer's market. Because Sage was surrounded by lush farmland, the coalition also recruited local farmers to sell their produce at the market, thereby stimulating the community's economy.

Evaluation. Although the coalition had addressed the individual and systems-level needs of Sage residents, they also needed to evaluate the implementation of the farmer's market. They collected data from residents and market vendors (i.e., local farmers). Residents were asked about their eating habits, changes in diet since the introduction of the market, types of items purchased, and which items were most valued. Farmers provided information on their weekly sales (i.e., amount of each type of produce sold). Using these data, the coalition was able to make an assessment of behavior changes at the individual level and assess the economic influence of sales of locally grown foods on the income of local farmers.

IMPLICATIONS FOR SOCIAL WORK PRACTICE

Health has been identified as the second most common practice area among licensed personnel with a master's degree in social work (MSW) (Center for Health Workforce Studies, 2006), and educators and researchers have been calling for improved training in health care social work (Lynch, Greeno, Teich, & Delany, 2016; Ruth, Marshall, Velásquez, & Bachman, 2015; Ruth, Velásquez, Marshall, & Ziperstein, 2015). The ACA has answered this call by providing an opportunity for social work training programs to adopt curriculum that includes ways in which social workers can implement an integrated health care approach in direct practice. This has occurred at the individual school level in more than 30 institutions and through widespread efforts by the Council on Social Work Education (CSWE, n.d.) (see Chapter 7). For example, in 2012, CSWE launched the Social Work and Integrated Behavioral Healthcare Project to "infuse integrated behavioral health and primary care in master's level social work education" (CSWE, n.d., p. 1).

These endeavors consider the person within the environment and the ways in which the environment influences physical and mental health and substance use behaviors. Building on recent curricular advances, social work programs must include health-specific practice and policy courses to ensure content on the ACA, health care systems, insurance policy, and prevention. Social work education must develop health-specific educational tracks to meet the demographic and ambulatory care provision challenges to our nation's health.

Traditionally, field education in social work has placed health-focused students in hospitals. This typical arrangement has been driven by field educators (i.e., social work departments in hospitals have been relatively stable) and by students who are eager to gain this experience because they recognize that hospital-based social workers have usually received higher salaries than community-based social workers in nonprofit organizations. However, social work instructors can expand the range of locations where students are trained. Although the placements have often served those who already have health issues, more opportunities are expected to emerge for students to become involved in health education or health promotion and prevention. Creating new ways for social work students to integrate into nontraditional field placements will allow for more breadth and depth within the discipline. In addition, field education has historically underutilized placements in governmental organizations (i.e., local and federal health departments) and in national health policy and practice organizations (Jarman-Rohde, McFall, Kolar, & Strom, 1997). Partnering with these types of organizations can position social work trainees to fill future workforce needs, which are becoming increasingly based in the community and focused on prevention and maintenance of health.

CONCLUSIONS

Social work has a long professional history of helping to eliminate or minimize barriers to service access. Social workers need to know how to navigate the insurance market landscape, how to advocate within the patchwork system to meet individual service users' insurance coverage needs, and how to evaluate the impact on service user populations to inform future policy development. Although some of this material can be learned in the field, policy-specific courses can provide a framework for social work trainees to understand legislation and translate it into practice. Policy courses that incorporate ACA information help to prepare students to meet the needs of an ambulatory-based care environment that is focused on prevention and illness management.

Taking a population health approach to understanding individual-, family-, and community-level health behaviors is important for social workers, medical practitioners, and policy makers. Training in population health allows current and future social workers to keep pace with population needs.

RESOURCES

The Affordable Care Act (ACA) https://www.healthcare.gov/

The Association of State and Territorial Health Officials (ASTHO) http://www.astho.org/

County Health Rankings http://www.countyhealthrankings.org/

Division of Population Health, Centers for Disease Control and Prevention (CDC) http://www.cdc.gov/nccdphp/dph/

Health Affairs http://www.healthaffairs.org/

Healthy People 2020 https://www.healthypeople.gov/

The Institute for Healthcare Improvement (IHI) http://www.ihi.org/Pages/default.aspx

The Kaiser Family Foundation http://kff.org/

The National Association of City and County Health Officials (NACCHO) http://www.naccho.org/

The Partnership for a Healthier America http://ahealthieramerica.org/about/about-the-partnership/

The World Health Organization (WHO) http://www.who.int/en/

REFERENCES

Bellinger, D. C. (2016). Lead contamination in Flint—An abject failure to protect public health. *New England Journal of Medicine, 374,* 1101–1103. doi: 10.1056/NEJMp1601013

Belsky, D. W., Moffitt, T. E., & Caspi, A. (2013). Genetics in population health science: Strategies and opportunities. *American Journal of Public Health, 103*(S1), S73–S83. doi: 10.2105/AJPH.2012.301139

Berwick, D. M., Nolan, T. W., & Whittington, J. (2008). The Triple Aim: Care, health, and cost. *Health Affairs, 27,* 759–769. doi: 10.1377/hlthaff.27.3.759

Braveman, P., & Egerter, S. (2008). Overcoming obstacles to health: Report from the Robert Wood Johnson Foundation to the Commission to Build a Healthier America. Princeton, NJ: Robert Wood Johnson Foundation. Retrieved from http://www.rwjf.org/content/dam/farm/reports/reports/2008/rwjf22441

Carroll-Scott, A., Gilstad-Hayden, K., Rosenthal, L., Peters, S. M., McCaslin, C., Joyce, R., & Ickovics, J. R. (2013). Disentangling neighborhood contextual associations with child body mass index, diet, and physical activity: The role of built, socioeconomic, and social environments. *Social Science & Medicine, 95,* 106–114. doi: 10.1016/j.socscimed.2013.04.003

Center for Health Workforce Studies. (2006). *Licensed social workers in health, 2004.* Rensselaer, NY: Center for Health Workforce Studies. Retrieved from http://workforce.socialworkers.org/studies/health/health_chap1.pdf

Center for Integrated Health Solutions, Substance Abuse and Mental Health Services Administration-Health Resources and Services Administration. (2001). *Population management in community mental health center-based health homes.* Washington, DC: National Council for Behavioral Health. Retrieved from http://www.integration.samhsa.gov/integrated-care-models/14_Population_Management_v3.pdf

Centers for Disease Control and Prevention (CDC). (2016, April 4). Learn the signs: Act early. Retrieved from http://www.cdc.gov/ncbddd/actearly/

Centers for Medicare & Medicaid Services. (2016). *CMS quality strategy 2016.* Retrieved from https://www.cms.gov/Medicare/Quality-Initiatives-Patient-Assessment-Instruments/QualityInitiativesGenInfo/Downloads/CMS-Quality-Strategy.pdf

Council on Social Work Education. (n.d.). Social work and integrated behavioral health care project. Retrieved from https://www.cswe.org/Centers-Initiatives/Initiatives/Social-Work-and-Integrated-Behavioral-Healthcare-P

Cruwys, T., Bevelander, K. E., & Hermans, R. C. (2015). Social modeling of eating: A review of when and why social influence affects food intake and choice. *Appetite, 86,* 3–18. doi: 10.1016/j.appet.2014.08.035

Enoch, M.-A. (2013). Genetic influences on the development of alcoholism. *Current Psychiatry Reports, 15,* 412. doi: 10.1007/s11920-013-0412-1

Evans, R. G., Barer, M. L., & Marmor, T. R. R. (Eds.). (1994). *Why are some people healthy and others not? The determinants of health populations (social institutions and social change).* New York, NY: Aldine de Gruyter.

Fabrus, R. J., Pracilio, V. P., Nash, D. B., & Clarke, J. L. (2015). The population health promise. In D. B. Nash, R. J. Fabius, A. Skoufalos, J. L. Clarke, & M. R. Horowitz (Eds.), *Population health: Creating a culture of wellness* (2nd ed., pp. 1–17). Burlington, MA: Jones & Bartlett.

Fine, M. J., Ibrahim, S. A., & Thomas, S. B. (2005). The role of race and genetics in health disparities research. *American Journal of Public Health, 95,* 2125–2128. doi: 10.2105/AJPH.2005.076588

Garvin, E., Branas, C., Keddem, S., Sellman, J., & Cannuscio, C. (2013). More than just an eyesore: Local insights and solutions on vacant land and urban health. *Journal of Urban Health: Bulletin of the New York Academy of Medicine, 90,* 412–426. doi: 10.1007/s11524-012-9782-7

González, T. (2012). Keeping kids in schools: Restorative justice, punitive discipline, and the school to prison pipeline. *Journal of Law & Education, 41*(2), 281–335. Retrieved from https://papers.ssrn.com/sol3/papers.cfm?abstract_id=2658513

Guha, S., Rosenfeld, J. A., Malhotra, A. K., Lee, A. T., Gregersen, P. K., Kane, J. M., . . . Lencz, T. (2012). Implications for health and disease in the genetic signature of the Ashkenazi Jewish population. *Genome Biology, 13*, R2. doi: 10.1186/gb-2012-13-1-r2

Gurbutt, D. (Ed.). (2016). *Collaborative practice for public health.* Boca Raton, FL: CRC Press.

Huang, G. C., Soto, D., Fujimoto, K., & Valente, T. W. (2014). The interplay of friendship networks and social networking sites: Longitudinal analysis of selection and influence effects on adolescent smoking and alcohol use. *American Journal of Public Health, 104*(8), e51–e59. doi: 10.2105/AJPH.2014.302038

Jacobson, D. M., & Teutsch, S. (2012). *An environmental scan of integrated approaches for defining and measuring total population health by the clinical care system, the government public health system, and stakeholder organizations.* Washington, DC: National Quality Forum. Retrieved from http://www.improvingpopulationhealth.org/PopHealthPhaseIICommissionedPaper.pdf

Jarman-Rohde, L., McFall, J., Kolar, P., & Strom, G. (1997). The changing context of social work practice: Implications and recommendations for social work educators. *Journal of Social Work Education, 33*, 29–46. doi: 10.1080/10437797.1997.10778851

Kaiser Family Foundation. (2015). Preventive services covered by private health plans under the Affordable Care Act [Fact sheet]. Retrieved from http://files.kff.org/attachment/preventive-services-covered-by-private-health-plans-under-the-affordable-care-act-fact-sheet

Khoury, M. J., & Evans, J. P. (2015). A public health perspective on a national precision medicine cohort: Balancing long-term knowledge generation with early health benefit. *The Journal of the American Medical Association, 313*, 2117–2118. doi: 10.1001/jama.2015.3382

Kindig, D. A. (2012, September 4). If not genetics, then what? [Blog post]. Retrieved from http://www.improvingpopulationhealth.org/blog/2012/09/if-not-genetics-then-what.html

Kindig, D. A., Asada, Y., & Booske, B. (2008). A population health framework for setting national and state health goals. *Journal of the American Medical Association, 299*, 2081–2083. doi:10.1001/jama.299.17.2081

Kindig, D. A., & Stoddart, G. (2003). What is population health? *American Journal of Public Health, 93*, 380–383. doi: 10.2105/AJPH.93.3.380

Loehrer, S., Lewis, N., & Bogan, M. (2016). Improving the health of populations: A common language is key. *Healthcare Executive. 31*, 82–83. Available from http://www.ihi.org/Pages/default.aspx

Lynch, S., Greeno, C., Teich, J., & Delany, P. (2016). Opportunities for social work under the Affordable Care Act: A call for action. *Social Work in Health Care, 55*, 651–674. doi: 10.1080/00981389.2016.1221871

MacDorman, M. F., & Mathews, T. J. (2011). *Understanding racial and ethnic disparities in U.S. infant mortality rates* (NCHS data brief no. 74). Hyattsville, MD: National Center for Health Statistics. Retrieved from http://www.cdc.gov/nchs/data/databriefs/db74.pdf

Marmot, M., & Allen, J. J. (2014). Social determinants of health equity. *American Journal of Public Health, 104*(S4), S517–S519. doi: 10.2105/AJPH.2014.302200

National Committee for Quality Assurance. (2011). *NCQA patient-centered medical home 2011: Health care that revolves around you.* Retrieved from http://www.ncqa.org/portals/0/PCMH2011%20withCAHPSInsert.pdf

National Research Council and Institute of Medicine, Division of Behavioral and Social Sciences and Education, Board on Population Health and Public Health Practice; S. H. Woolf & L. Aron (Eds.). (2013). *U.S. health in international perspective: Shorter lives, poorer health.* Washington, DC: National Academies Press. Retrieved from http://www.nap.edu/read/13497/chapter/1

Oyserman, D. (2012). Not just any path: Implications of identity-based motivation for disparities in school outcomes. *Economics of Education Review, 33*, 179–190. doi: 10.1016/j.econedurev.2012.09.002

Pardeck, J. T. (1988). An ecological approach for social work practice. *Journal of Sociology and Social Welfare, 15*(2), 133–142. Retrieved from http://scholarworks.wmich.edu/jssw/vol15/iss2/11/

Powell, L. M., Chriqui, J. F., Khan, T., Wada, R., & Chaloupka, F. J. (2013). Assessing the potential effectiveness of food and beverage taxes and subsidies for improving public health: A systematic review of prices, demand and body weight outcomes. *Obesity Reviews, 14*, 110–128. doi: 10.1111/obr.12002

Remington, P. L., Catlin, B. B., & Gennuso, K. P. (2015). The county health rankings: Rationale and methods. *Population Health Metrics, 13*, 11. doi: 10.1186/s12963-015-0044-2

Ruth, B. J., Marshall, J. W., Velásquez, E. E. M., & Bachman, S. S. (2015). Teaching note—Educating public health social work professionals: Results from an MSW/MPH program outcomes study. *Journal of Social Work Education, 51*, 186–194. doi: 10.1080/10437797.2015.979096

Ruth, B. J., Velásquez, E. E., Marshall, J. W., & Ziperstein, D. (2015). Shaping the future of prevention in social work: An analysis of the professional literature from 2000 through 2010. *Social Work, 60*, 126–134. doi: 10.1093/sw/swu060

Sanchez, K., & Burg, M. A. (2015). Theories of health behavior and brief behavioral practice models. In M. A. Burg and O. Oyama (Eds.), *The behavioral health specialist in primary care: Skills for integrated practice* (pp. 41–72). Springer Publishing Company.

Shao, Y., Liu, S., & Grinzaid, K. (2015). Evaluation of two-year Jewish genetic disease screening program in Atlanta: Insight into community genetic screening approaches. *Journal of Community Genetics, 6*, 137–145. doi: 10.1007/s12687-014-0208-y

Shonkoff, J. P., Garner, A. S., Siegel, B. S., Dobbins, M. I., Earls, M. F., McGuinn, L., . . . Wood, D. L. (2012). The lifelong effects of early childhood adversity and toxic stress. *Pediatrics, 129*, e232–e246. doi: 10.1542/peds.2011-2663

Stoto, M. A. (2013, February 21). Population health in the Affordable Care Act era (Academy Health Issue Brief). Retrieved from http://www.academyhealth.org/publications/2013-02/population-health-affordable-care-act-era

U.S. Department of Health and Human Services, Centers for Disease Control and Prevention, National Center for Chronic Disease Prevention and Health Promotion, Office on Smoking and Health; J. M. Samet, T. F. Pechacek, L. A. Norman, & P. L. Taylor (Eds.). (2014). *The health consequences of smoking—50 years of progress: A report of the Surgeon General*. Atlanta, GA: U.S. Department of Health and Human Services. Retrieved from http://www.surgeongeneral.gov/library/reports/50-years-of-progress/full-report.pdf

Woolf, S. H., & Braveman, P. (2011). Where health disparities begin: The role of social and economic determinants—and why current policies may make matters worse. *Health Affairs, 30*, 1852–1859. doi: 10.1377/hlthaff.2011.0685

PART II

HEALTH AND MENTAL HEALTH POLICY

CHAPTER 4

THE EVOLUTION OF HEALTH CARE POLICY

Jennifer I. Manuel and Stacey L. Barrenger

Private and public health insurance originated in the 1800s, but the government was not involved in financing health care for the general population until the 1930s, beginning with state-enacted workers' compensation laws. By the 1960s, the federal government had become a significant payor of health care expenses with the establishment of Medicare and Medicaid, the two largest public health insurance programs.

The U.S. health care system is largely decentralized. Multiple state and local agencies have assumed primary responsibility for financing and regulating health care, which has contributed to a complex and fragmented system that is often difficult to navigate and lacks coordination and communication across the spectrum of health care providers. Until recently, efforts at health care reform have been ineffective in addressing the complex needs of an increasingly diverse population. The Patient Protection and Affordable Care Act (ACA) of 2010 represents a significant shift away from a system that is fragmented and uncoordinated toward a system that offers person-centered care, is clinically integrated, and is accountable for maximizing outcomes.

This chapter provides an overview of the current U.S. health care system and places it within its historical context. It traces the history of private and public sources of health insurance and health care reform initiatives. Next, the emergence of behavioral health care services for individuals with a mental health or substance use disorder is discussed. Disparities in behavioral health care access and use are examined, along with the parity policies that have evolved to address these disparities. The chapter concludes with various prospects for health care reform and implications for future social work policy and practice.

PRIVATE INSURANCE

Unlike most developed countries, the United States does not have a national health insurance program or a national health care system that provides universal access to basic and routine health services for all. Instead, multiple insurance systems have been developed through private and public industries and government-sponsored programs. Private health insurance is the predominant financing mechanism for health services in the United States (Smith & Medalia, 2015).

Private health insurance originated in the mid-1800s, when the Franklin Health Assurance Company of Massachusetts began reimbursing injuries related to steamboat and railway accidents (Scofea, 1994). The system was further developed when the Travelers Insurance Company of Hartford introduced the first health plan covering medical expenses in 1863, and by the late 1860s more than 60 competing companies were offering similar policies (Scofea, 1994). Although these early plans provided limited financial coverage and benefits only for automobile and other accidents, by the turn of the century they had expanded to include a number of disabilities and surgical procedures.

A major factor contributing to the slow uptake of private health insurance was the poor quality of health care, which deterred people from using these services. Medical technology was limited, hospitals were unreliable, and the medical profession was unlicensed and unregulated until the late 1800s (Zinner & Loughlin, 2009). By 1900, however, the public's sharp aversion to health care had been lessened by significant medical advances, including the development of vaccines and the advancement of relevant technologies. This progress, along with the establishment of standards for medical training and licensure, improved the quality of health care and helped to legitimize the medical profession. Although the supply of doctors and hospitals was limited, innovations in medicine contributed to a greater demand for medical services and increased costs. At the same time, the labor force became increasingly industrialized. Concerns about better wages, reasonable work hours, and safer working conditions prompted the development of organized labor unions, which converged with mounting economic distress to precipitate the development of modern health insurance (Zinner & Loughlin, 2009).

The first private health insurance group plan originated in 1929, when Baylor University Hospital in Dallas contracted with local schoolteachers who were struggling to pay their medical bills. To ease the teachers' struggles and ensure consistent payments, hospital administrators created the Baylor Plan. The teachers paid a predetermined fee of 50 cents per month in exchange for room, board, and medical services for up to 21 days per year (Scofea, 1994). With the Great Depression in full swing in the 1930s, many hospitals were struggling financially and developed single-hospital health insurance plans similar to the Baylor Plan to create a steady flow of income (Holman & Cooley, 1950).

In 1932, the American Hospital Association (AHA), the main hospital trade association, began promoting the concept of group hospital plans, later known as Blue Cross plans (Holman & Cooley, 1950; Zinner & Loughlin, 2009). The plans offered subscribers a choice among a variety of hospitals and were considered nonprofit organizations that cooperated in prepayment models with hospitals for patient care. By 1940, there were 39 Blue Cross plans with more than 6 million subscribers (Star, 1982). By 1955, these plans made up about 45% of all private health insurance (Shonick, 1995).

Blue Shield prepaid plans emerged during this time to cover physician and surgeon expenses. Because of their nonprofit status, the early Blue Cross and Blue Shield plans were exempt from paying taxes and were able to keep monthly premiums low (Zinner

& Loughlin, 2009). This gave them a competitive edge when private, commercial health insurance companies began offering group plans to cover hospital expenses in 1934 and physician and surgical bills in 1938 (Star, 1982).

Employer-sponsored insurance. Private health insurance was not offered as a standard employment benefit until the 1930s. Nonprofit and for-profit private health insurance companies marketed group health plans to employees of large businesses and their dependents to gain many customers en masse. Obtaining health insurance was more difficult for employees of small businesses and for those who were self-employed or unemployed (Shonick, 1995). Employer-sponsored insurance (ESI) grew rapidly during World War II as a result of strict wage and price controls, which meant that, by law, employers could not increase wages. Employers created competitive benefit packages, including health care insurance, as an alternative means of attracting desirable workers (Zinner & Louglin, 2009).

In the years that followed, union organizations such as the American Federation of Labor (AFL) and the Congress of Industrial Organizations (CIO) successfully negotiated health benefits for their members through collective bargaining agreements, thereby increasing the number of Americans covered by private health insurance (Hoffman, 2003). Since then, ESI has been the predominant financing mechanism for health services in the United States (Smith & Medalia, 2015). Today, most ESI plans also cover the employee's spouse and dependents. They are mutually funded by monthly fees from employees, whose contributions are taken from their wages before taxes, and from employers, whose contributions are typically larger and are not taxed (Askin & Moore, 2014).

ESI has evolved over time into two markets: large group market insurance, which covers more than 50 employees in a company, and small group market insurance, which covers 2 to 50 employees in a company. Most large companies provide self-funded coverage, in which the employer acts as the payor and assumes the risk for the employees' claims costs; these arrangements are typically handled through a third-party private insurance company. Other large employers opt for fully insured coverage. The employer purchases private insurance, and the insurance company acts as the payor. In these cases, the employer and insurance company negotiate different insurance options from which employees choose.

Although employees are restricted to employer-approved insurance plans, thereby diminishing choice, the premiums for these plans are typically lower. From the perspective of insurance companies, contracting with employers typically means that they can insure a large group of people who are in relatively good health compared with those who are unemployed. The larger a company is, the less the employer is required to pay in premiums for each employee. Small companies are therefore unlikely to offer benefits that are as comprehensive as those provided by large companies. However, this may change under the ACA because many small businesses need to increase their minimum level of benefits to comply with the policy requirements (Askin & Moore, 2014).

Direct purchase or individual insurance. People who are unemployed or self-employed, early retirees, and employees of companies that do not offer ESI must rely on the individual insurance market for coverage. Historically, the number of people covered by the individual market has been low due to high premiums and the refusal of insurance companies to cover people with preexisting illnesses. Under the ACA, the individual market is expected to be easier to access (Askin & Moore, 2014). For example, the ACA stipulates that new insurance plans must cover people with preexisting disorders; health care exchanges are required to provide low-income individuals with affordable and equitable options; expanded coverage of preventive services is mandated; and gender rating is strictly prohibited, meaning that the companies are forbidden to charge women more than men for the same health plan (see Chapters 5).

PUBLIC GOVERNMENT-SPONSORED INSURANCE

Whereas private health insurance focuses primarily on the labor force and to a lesser extent on unemployed, self-employed, and retired individuals, government-sponsored or public health insurance is designed to support vulnerable populations, including the elderly and low-income children and their parents. Other government programs are provided for people on active duty in the military and veterans.

Until the early 20th century, federal involvement in health care was limited to a few select populations, primarily people in the military and their families, veterans with disabilities, and Native Americans residing in tribal communities. Federal laws that established this minimal scope of health care included the U.S. Marine Hospital Service Act of 1798, which provided health benefits to merchant marines and the navy; the 1914 War Risk Insurance Act and related expansions in 1917, which provided medical benefits and life insurance to active-duty soldiers, veterans with disabilities, and families of soldiers who died in service; and the Snyder Act of 1921, which increased access to health care for Native Americans (Almgren, 2013).

The first federal legislation that provided financial support to populations outside these groups was the Sheppard-Towner Act of 1921. It pledged matching funds to states for prenatal and child health centers, with the primary goal of reducing mortality rates among native-born, white infants and children (Almgren, Kemp, & Eisinger, 2000). Although this statute expired in 1929 and was never reauthorized, it remains historical in several ways.

The Sheppard-Towner Act was firmly supported by women reformers, including prominent social workers of the time, who provided a compelling case through research findings from community studies for the need to remedy the widespread lack of child and maternal health services (Almgren et al., 2000). On the heels of women's suffrage in 1920, men in Congress recognized the political gravity of securing and retaining women's votes, which prompted them to pass the legislation.

Despite a progressive attitude about women's rights, the Sheppard-Towner Act funded only programs that targeted primarily maternal and child health issues of white families living in rural communities while ignoring poor African-American and other families living in urban communities (Almgren, 2013). The legislation was met with great resistance from social conservatives and members of the American Medical Association (AMA), who feared that health care would become federalized and that the government would then monopolize the market (Almgren et al., 2000). Funding for child and maternal health issues was then placed on the back burner until passage of the Social Security Act (SSA) of 1935, which provided grants to states to restore the child and maternal health programs and other child welfare services (Kaiser Commission, 2013).

The Sheppard-Towner Act served as the precursor for future policies that expanded federal involvement in regulating health care for vulnerable populations after World War II. In the 1940s and 1950s, the capacities of the U.S. health care system significantly increased with the introduction of new facilities, modern technologies, enhanced staff training, and additional resources. The Hill-Burton Act, which was signed into law by President Truman in 1946, facilitated these advancements by providing funds to reform hospital infrastructure and boost patient capacity (Zinner & Loughlin, 2009). By the 1960s, the nation's overall life expectancy had risen, and access to hospitals and competent medical providers had improved.

The primary barrier to health care at that point was the availability of health insurance, although this problem had been partially alleviated by the adoption of health insurance as a standard employment benefit and the increase in wages after World War II (Starr, 1982). However, a significant number of people, particularly the elderly, remained uninsured. Before 1965, an estimated 50% of older adults did not have insurance (Cubanski et al., 2015). This situation prompted a further expansion in federal legislation for health care, including the 1960 Kerr-Mills Act, which funded an entitlement program for low-income older adults who could not afford medical care. This act was the forerunner to Medicare and Medicaid, which were signed into law by President Johnson in 1965 (Zinner & Loughlin, 2009).

MEDICARE

Title XVIII of the SSA marked the inception of Medicare. Originally known as Health Insurance for the Aged and Disabled, the program was established to provide health and financial security to address the medical needs of people 65 years of age or older and those with permanent disabilities regardless of age. This program complemented the insurance benefits for retirement and disability that had already been granted by Title II of the SSA.

Medicare benefits were initially divided into two parts: Part A, also known as the Hospital Insurance (HI) program; and Part B, also known as the Supplementary Medical Insurance (SMI) program. Part A helps cover inpatient hospital stays, skilled nursing care, home health visits, and hospice care, and it does not involve monthly premiums. Part B covers physician, outpatient, home health care, and preventive services but requires beneficiaries to pay monthly premiums based on their income. In 1997, Part C (i.e., the Medicare Advantage program) was established to offer greater options for beneficiaries who prefer a private plan instead of traditional Medicare coverage.

The Medicare Prescription Drug, Improvement, and Modernization Act, also referred to as the Medicare Modernization Act (MMA), established Part D in 2003. It was designed to expand access to prescription drugs and initially provided prescription drug benefit cards to all beneficiaries on a voluntary basis at a reduced cost. However, in 2006, Part D began subsidizing access to prescription drug benefits on a voluntary basis through private plans contracting with Medicare.

An estimated 19 million people received Medicare benefits when the program was first implemented in 1966 (Klees, Wolfe, & Curtis, 2010). By 2015, more than 55 million people had enrolled in Medicare, including 46.3 million older members and 9 million members younger than 65 years of age with permanent disabilities (Cubanski et al., 2015). A person must meet the following requirements to be eligible for coverage:

- Be 65 years or older, be a U.S. citizen or permanent resident with at least 5 years of continuous residence, and have (or have a spouse who has) worked for 10 years and paid Medicare taxes
- Be younger than 65 years of age with a permanent disability and have received Social Security Disability Income (SSDI) payments for the past 2 years
- Be younger than 65 years of age with end-stage renal disease or amyotrophic lateral sclerosis and currently receive SSDI payments (people in this category can receive Medicare benefits as soon as they start receiving SSDI payments because there is no waiting period)
- Be younger than 65 years of age and have developed medical disorders as the result of exposure to environmental health hazards in an emergency declared area (Cubanski et al., 2015; Klees et al., 2010)

MEDICAID

Medicaid, Title XIX of the SSA, was established to provide supplemental medical care coverage for people already receiving public assistance: low-income families with children, low-income older adults, and individuals with disabilities. Over the years, the program was expanded to include more uninsured people at risk for (or currently experiencing) poverty (Cubanski et al., 2015). Jointly run by federal and state governments, Medicaid is required to cover members of these populations if their income level falls below established thresholds based on the federal poverty level (FPL), although eligibility and reimbursement policies vary by state. Because enrollment is unlimited, meaning that there is no cap on the number of eligible people who can receive benefits, Medicaid has become the primary safety net program for low-income people in the United States. The program covers the following categorically needy eligibility groups:

- Infants born to Medicaid-eligible women
- Children younger than 6 years of age whose family income does not exceed 138% of the FPL
- Children younger than 19 years of age whose family income is equal to or below the FPL
- Pregnant women
- Parents with dependent children

- Low-income elderly people with disabilities (who also receive Medicare) and people with severe physical and mental disabilities

As of 2015, Medicaid covered more than 62 million people (U.S. Department of Health and Human Services, 2016). Of these beneficiaries, approximately 31 million were children, 16 million were adults in low-income families, and 16 million were elderly individuals and people with disabilities. Historically, Medicaid has neglected many poor and near-poor individuals due to its strict exclusions of low-income adults without dependent children and those who hover just above the FPL threshold. However, the ACA includes opportunities for states (at their individual discretion) to expand Medicaid eligibility to adults with income at or below 138% of the FPL (see Chapter 5). Medicaid provisions currently exclude coverage for adults in the age bracket of 22 to 64 years who live in institutions for mental diseases (IMDs), defined as nursing facilities or psychiatric institutions with more than 16 beds dedicated for people with mental illnesses. IMDs are categorized as custodial institutions and are therefore considered to be the responsibility of individual states, a position that has been rationalized by the need to control costs (Shirk, 2008). Medicaid does, however, provide coverage for children younger than 21 years of age and adults 65 years or older who live in IMDs.

THE CHILDREN'S HEALTH INSURANCE PROGRAM

The Children's Health Insurance Program (CHIP), formerly known as the State Children's Insurance Program, was established in 1997 and expanded in 2009 to insure children who are not eligible for Medicaid. As of 2015, CHIP covered approximately 9 million children who could not receive Medicaid benefits (U.S. Department of Health and Human Services, 2016).

Similar to Medicaid, CHIP is jointly run by federal and state governments, and states have flexibility in eligibility and coverage policies. One of the goals of this legislation is to support states in creating strategies to identify and enroll children who do not receive Medicaid or CHIP benefits but are eligible to do so. To further encourage this objective, states also receive performance incentives for increasing the enrollment of children through Medicaid.

HEALTH CARE FOR MILITARY PERSONNEL

TRICARE, formerly known as the Civilian Health and Medical Program of the Uniformed Services, is a Department of Defense health insurance program that covers active duty military members and military retirees and their dependents. TRICARE is the scion of two earlier government-supported programs: the Emergency Maternal and Infant Care Program of 1943, which provided benefits to spouses of active duty military personnel; and the Military Dependents Acts of 1956 and 1966, which provided obstetrical services, outpatient and ambulatory care, and benefits for dependents of active duty military personnel. The Veterans Health Administration, a self-contained health care system that serves over 5 million people, provides medical care to veterans and their families at low or no cost.

THE FAILURE OF NATIONAL HEALTH CARE REFORM: A BRIEF HISTORY

Although the United States has always had a mix of private and public health insurance programs, there have been numerous proposals to establish universal health insurance since the early 1900s. For example, in 1912, President Roosevelt called for a national health insurance program as an alternative to the dominant fee-based model of medical care, which excluded many low-income people who were unable to afford medical services. As the number of uninsured individuals grew significantly in the 1930s and 1940s, President Truman called for a federally sponsored national health insurance program that would be open to all Americans but would be optional and would require monthly fees to participate. In the 1970s, Senator Edward Kennedy co-sponsored legislation that would ensure comprehensive health care for all U.S. residents. In 1993, President Clinton and First Lady Hillary Rodham Clinton proposed a national health care program called the Clinton Plan; however, it never received Congressional approval.

These reform efforts were resisted due to political partisan issues and a preoccupying interest in containing costs rather than expanding coverage (Zinner & Loughlin, 2009). In early reform efforts, the AMA was most vocal against national health insurance for two major reasons. First, it was thought that government-supported insurance would undermine the expertise and authority of medical providers. Second, the AMA thought that health care financed by the government would put an end to the significant profits of fee-based medical services (Almgren, 2013). Much resistance also came from other interest groups, including the AHA and, more recently, pharmaceutical companies.

The next attempt at national health care reform occurred in 2009, when the United States was in a deep recession and almost 50 million people were uninsured, many of whom were former members of the middle class who had lost their jobs (Almgren, 2013). Concerned about potential resistance and a repeat of the Clinton Plan's fate, President Obama proposed a compromise health care reform package that used a mixed public and private approach to near universal health coverage. This was the inception of the ACA, which was successfully signed into law on March 23, 2010, and represented the most dramatic change to the health care system since the establishment of Medicare and Medicaid.

The legislative focus on health care reform continues, with President Trump and the Republicans running successful election campaigns in 2016 that included a pledge to repeal Obamacare. Characterizing the health care legislation as a "disaster" and as an example of government overreach, President Trump and the 115th Congress have created the expectation that they will roll back the provisions of the ACA. Republican proposals to repeal and replace the ACA have included removing the mandate and premium subsidies for individuals, using high deductible plans to cover people with costly health care needs, giving states greater latitude in decisions about coverage, and block granting

Medicaid. The most contested issue remains whether and how to cover people with pre-existing conditions.

While these issues are debated in Congress, President Trump has considerable executive power over the ongoing implementation of the ACA. His appointment of Tom Price as Secretary of Health and Human Services, a firm opponent of the ACA, is a strong indication that the administration may impede ACA operations through regulatory means (Park & Sanger-Katz, 2017). One strategy the Administration can take to destabilize the ACA is withholding federal subsidies from the health exchanges. However, as more people receive coverage and the health care system invests in ACA reforms, repealing it becomes more difficult and politically risky for legislators. The increasing threat to the ACA has been accompanied by a rise in its popularity, with many constituencies rallying to defend the legislation (Fingerhut, 2017). Current and future administrations will undoubtedly continue the battle over health care reform and reflect the profound and persistent divisions about the role of government in promoting our health and wellbeing.

BEHAVIORAL HEALTH CARE

The term *behavioral health care* encompasses treatment for mental illnesses and substance use disorders. These services were not explicitly acknowledged in most health care policies until the middle of the 20th century. Disabled individuals can receive care through Medicaid or Medicare. Although this stipulation has obvious benefits, it is not without fault. Eligibility based on disability and the limited range of services available for these populations have contributed to the fragmentation of the current U.S. system of behavioral health care. However, similar to the shift in the funding landscape that followed the ACA, there is hope that the legislation will increase access to behavioral health care and that these needs will be met regardless of disability status. Passage of the ACA and mental health and substance abuse parity laws (discussed later) helps to ensure that mental health and substance abuse services are insured equitably. Despite a patchwork system of behavioral health care in the United States, these important measures will expand behavioral health care services and grant access to many who were previously uninsured.

THE COMMUNITY MENTAL HEALTH ACT

At the start of the 20th century, most people with mental illnesses lived in state-run asylums or hospitals, which had come to be responsible for this population. This practice began to change in the mid-20th century due to the convergence of several ideological, economic, and political factors (Mechanic & Rochefort, 1990). People had become increasingly concerned about the inhumane treatment that was notoriously rampant in state psychiatric hospitals, the costs of maintaining these institutions, and the increasing burden of care placed on states to provide for this population. The advent of psychotropic medications and legal challenges to denying people a life in the community also contributed to the beginning of deinstitutionalization (Schnapp, 2006). From 1955 to 1963, state hospital populations decreased by 3% each year (Gronfein, 1985).

Although ideological shifts initiated the movement for deinstitutionalization as early as the mid-1950s, this practice did not become official policy until the 1960s. In 1963, President Kennedy signed the Community Mental Health Act (CMHA), which formalized the policy of deinstitutionalization through an emphasis on community care for mental illness and the creation of Community Mental Health Centers (CMHCs) (Kennedy, 1964). Each CMHC was responsible for a particular geographic or catchment area and for providing inpatient care, outpatient care, partial hospitalization, emergency services, education, and consultation (Gronfein, 1985). The CMHA also signaled the federal government's increasing involvement in caring for people with mental illnesses, a responsibility that had previously been shouldered by the states. Populations in state hospitals then decreased more rapidly; the steepest declines occurred between 1965 and 1975 (Gronfein, 1985). By 1976, there were fewer than 200,000 people left in state hospitals—a significant difference from the all-time high of 560,000 in 1955 (Clarke, 1979).

BENEFITS FOR PEOPLE WITH BEHAVIORAL HEALTH NEEDS

After the CMHA, few other policies directly addressed behavioral health care; instead, expansion of other benefits for people with behavioral health care needs became more common. For example, although SSDI was not initially intended for those with mental illnesses, a broadening of the disability definition in 1984 allowed for this population to receive benefits (Autor & Duggan, 2006). Supplemental Security Income (SSI) was legislated in 1972 (U.S. Social Security Administration, 2000). Although the program was initially intended to provide basic income to older adults, those deemed to be disabled, including many people with mental illnesses, came to represent the majority of SSI caseloads by 1994 (Clarke, 1979). People with substance use disorders who were unable to work were also eligible for SSI benefits, although their eligibility was contingent on engagement in mandated drug treatment and acquisition of a representative payee (Hogan, Unick, Speiglman, & Norris, 2008). However, these benefits were quite short-lived for individuals with substance use disorders because the 1996 Contract with America Advancement Act (CAAA) eliminated disability due to a substance use disorder as a valid criterion for SSI and SSDI (Davies, Iams, & Rupp, 2000). Thirty-five percent of those who lost their benefits were reinstated based on another disability (Bachman, Drainoni, & Tobias, 2004), but an estimated 110,000 low-income people with substance use disorders remained uninsured. Their hardship was further augmented by the revocation of health care benefits because removal from SSI resulted in the loss of Medicaid benefits (Hogan et al., 2008).

Community care for those with mental illnesses was emphasized again in 1999 with the Supreme Court case *Olmstead v. L.C. and E.W.* This ruling declared that it was discriminatory under the Americans with Disabilities Act (ADA) to keep individuals in institutions without the option of community-based treatment—provided that community-based care was appropriate for the individual, the individual expressed a desire to live in the community, and community placement was possible with *reasonable accommodations* (Fishman, 2000). States have attempted to cover the costs of community care through Medicaid and other state resources (Frank & Glied, 2006), but they are limited by what Medicaid considers reasonable accommodation under the Supreme Court ruling (Teitelbaum, Burke, & Rosenbaum, 2004). This approach has produced a medley of funding sources for community-based care that often varies by state according to each one's unique interpretation of the court's ruling.

PRESIDENT'S NEW FREEDOM COMMISSION ON MENTAL HEALTH

At the turn of the 21st century, the federal government again focused on severe mental illnesses. President George W. Bush convened the President's New Freedom Commission on Mental Health in 2002 to address a wide range of mental health issues, including the limits on involuntary institutionalization, the factors contributing to criminalization of people with mental illnesses, and the scientific advances in knowledge and treatment of mental illnesses (Hogan, 2004). The Commission acknowledged the fragmentation of mental health care resulting from the variety of funding streams for services and the equally partitioned social welfare system (e.g., SSDI, SSI, Medicaid, Medicare, housing services) that is not specifically designed for people with mental illnesses (Frank & Glied, 2006). Several recommendations were made in an effort to improve overall mental health care in the United States, such as adopting a family- and individual-driven focus, addressing health disparities, expanding early screening and assessment, and improving research and delivery of mental health care (Hogan, 2004).

Despite efforts for reform, many people with mental health or substance use disorders continue to have unmet treatment needs. They receive inadequate care or do not receive care at all. Among people with mental health disorders, between 22% and 28% reported an unmet need for mental health care within the previous 12 months (Chen et al., 2013; Urbanoski, Cairney, Bassani, & Rush, 2008). An estimated 8.5% of people with substance use disorders reported unmet treatment needs (Mojtabai & Crum, 2013).

High costs and difficulty obtaining health insurance are among the most common barriers to behavioral health services (Chen et al., 2013; Mojtabai, 2009; Mojtabai, Chen, Kaufmann, & Crum, 2014). Health insurance plans still routinely discriminate against people with mental health and substance use disorders. Coverage tends to be far more restricted for behavioral health services than for medical services, a routine injustice that began in the post-WWII era, when insurance policies first began providing benefits for certain psychiatric hospital stays (Goldman, Sharfstein, & Frank, 1983). For most workers with ESIs, psychiatric inpatient stays were shorter than medical inpatient stays (30 to 60 days vs. 120 days or unrestricted per year, respectively). Almost one fourth had higher copayments (copays) for mental health compared with medical services (50% vs. 20%, respectively) (Barry et al., 2003).

MENTAL HEALTH AND SUBSTANCE ABUSE PARITY

The Mental Health Parity Act (MHPA) was passed in 1996. It was introduced by Senators Pete Domenici and Paul Wellstone as the nation's first federal mental health parity law. The MHPA required that large group plans provide equitable annual and lifetime monetary limits for mental health and medical benefits (Barry, Huskamp, & Goldman, 2010). However, because the equity requirement did not specifically apply to other types of benefits, such as annual day or visit limits, insurance companies were able to circumvent the law by restricting them. The MHPA also did not apply to coverage for substance abuse treatment (Barry et al., 2010).

Dissatisfied with the excessive limitations of the federal parity law, many states resorted to drafting stricter mental health parity laws of their own. Thirty-three states and the District of Columbia created such legislation by 2001 (Morton & Aleman, 2005); all but one state had done so by 2011 (National Conference of State Legislatures, n.d.). However, states struggled to implement and enforce these laws, and many insurance companies found loopholes in the mandates. Contrary to advocates' expectations, the movement for mental health parity was less than successful, and significant disparities remained for many benefits such as inpatient days and outpatient visits (Mechanic, McAlpine, & Rochefort, 2014).

Informed by the failure of the MHPA, the 2008 Mental Health Parity and Addiction Equity Act (MHPAEA) represented an attempt to renew the cause. Implemented in 2010, the law improved on the original MHPA legislation through its inclusion of substance use and its expansion to eliminate *all* disparities between behavioral health and medical services. However, the MHPAEA did have some limitations. For example, the law applied only to large businesses and addressed coverage disparities only for insurance plans that already offered behavioral health services—it fell short of mandating such coverage in the first place. An additional challenge facing the MHPAEA and all parity efforts is defining the nonquantifiable parts of coverage. Quantitative measures such as deductibles, copays, and number of coverage days and visits readily lend themselves to standardization. It is much more difficult to develop stable criteria for the nonquantifiable aspects, such as medical necessity, due to their vulnerability to interpretation (Mechanic et al., 2014). This ambiguity requires ongoing monitoring to confirm that insurance companies adhere to established parity provisions.

CONCLUSIONS

Financing, structure, and delivery of health and behavioral health care services have significantly evolved over the past century. Most Americans agree that access to health care should be a prominent goal of federal policy (Roberts, 2007), but there is still ongoing public concern about structural reform leading to universal health care. This lingering resistance is fueled by fears about associated costs, increased involvement or overinvolvement of the government, and public health programs that cannot be sustained (Almgren, 2013). Partisan politics and lobby groups invested in maintaining the status quo continue to cloud serious discourse on policy alternatives, despite the examples in other industrialized countries of policies that have achieved simultaneous cost savings and national health insurance coverage.

Although universal health care has not been attained, recent legislation has had important implications for increased access to and improved quality of health and behavioral health services. This topic is explored further in subsequent chapters.

RESOURCES

Centers for Medicare & Medicaid Services (CMS) https://www.cms.gov/

The Kaiser Family Foundation (KFF) http://kff.org/

NASW Health Care Reform—Member Resources, National Association of Social Workers (NASW) http://www.socialworkers.org/advocacy/healthcarereform/default.asp

Social Work Education Principles for Health Care Reform, Council on Social Work Education (CSWE) http://www.cswe.org/CentersInitiatives/PublicPolicyInitiative13785/Campaigns/23163.aspx

Substance Abuse and Mental Health Services Administration (SAMHSA) http://www.samhsa.gov/

Upcoming Webinars, U.S. Department of Health and Human Services (DHHS) http://www.hhs.gov/about/agencies/iea/partnerships/webinars/index.html

REFERENCES

Almgren, G. (2013). *Health care politics, policy, and services. A social justice analysis* (2nd ed.). New York, NY: Springer.

Almgren, G., Kemp, S. P., & Eisinger, A. (2000). The legacy of Hull House and the Children's Bureau in the American mortality transition. *Social Service Review, 74*, 1–27. doi: 10.1086/514458

Askin, E., & Moore, N. (2014). *The health care handbook: A clear and concise guide to the United States health care system* (Vol. 2). St. Louis, MO: Washington University in St. Louis.

Autor, D., & Duggan, M. (2006). The growth in social security disability rolls: A fiscal crisis unfolding. *Massachusetts Institute of Technology Department of Economics Working Paper Series* (Working Paper 06-23). doi: 10.2139/ssrn.921123

Bachman, S. S., Drainoni, M. L., & Tobias, C. (2004). Medicaid managed care, substance abuse treatment, and people with disabilities: Review of the literature. *Health and Social Work, 29*, 189–196. doi: 10.1093/hsw/29.3.189

Barry, C. L., Gabel, J. R., Frank, R. G., Hawkins, S., Whitmore, H. H., & Pickreign, J. D. (2003). Design of mental health insurance coverage: Still unequal after all these years. *Health Affairs, 22*, 127–137. doi: 10.1377/hlthaff.22.5.127

Barry, C. L., Huskamp, H. A., & Goldman, H. H. (2010). A political history of federal mental health and addiction insurance parity. *The Milbank Quarterly, 88*, 404–433. doi: 10.1111/j.1468-0009.2010.00605.x

Chen, L. Y., Crum, R. M., Martins, S. S., Kaufmann, C. N., Strain, E. C., & Mojtabai, R. (2013). Service use and barriers to mental health care among adults with major depression and comorbid substance dependence. *Psychiatric Services, 64*, 863–870. doi: 10.1176/appi.ps.201200289

Clarke, G. J. (1979). In defense of deinstitutionalization. *The Milbank Memorial Fund Quarterly. Health and Society, 57,* 461–479. doi: 10.2307/3349722

Cubanski, J., Swoope, C., Boccuti, C., Jacobson, G., Casillas, G., Griffin, S., & Neuman, T. (2015). *A primer on Medicare: Key facts about the Medicare program and the people it covers* (Report no. 7615-04). Menlo Park, CA: Kaiser Family Foundation's Program on Medicare Policy. Retrieved from http://files.kff.org/attachment/report-a-primer-on-medicare-key-facts-about-the-medicare-program-and-the-people-it-covers

Davies, P., Iams, H., & Rupp, K. (2000). The effect of welfare reform on SSA's disability programs: Design of policy evaluation and early evidence. *Social Security Bulletin, 63*(1), 3–11. Retrieved from https://www.ssa.gov/policy/docs/ssb/v63n1/v63n1p3.pdf

Fingerhut, H. (February 23, 2017). Support for 2010 health care law reaches new high. Retrieved from http://www.pewresearch.org/fact-tank/2017/02/23/support-for-2010-health-care-law-reaches-new-high/

Fishman, S. (2000). *Olmstead v. Zimring:* Unnecessary institutionalization constitutes discrimination under the Americans with Disabilities Act. *Journal of Health Care Law and Policy, 3,* 430–451. Retrieved from http://www.law.umaryland.edu/academics/journals/jhclp/

Frank, R. G., & Glied, S. A. (2006). *Better but not well: Mental health policy in the United States since 1950.* Baltimore, MD: Johns Hopkins University Press.

Goldman, H. H., Sharfstein, S. S., & Frank, R. G. (1983). Equity and parity in psychiatric care. *Psychiatric Annals, 13,* 488–491. doi: 10.3928/0048-5713-19830601-09

Gronfein, W. (1985). Incentives and intention in mental health policy: A comparison of the Medicaid and community mental health programs. *Journal of Health and Social Behavior, 26,* 192–206. Retrieved from http://www.jstor.org

Hoffman, B. (2003). Health care reform and social movements in the United States. *American Journal of Public Health, 93,* 75–85. doi: 10.2105/AJPH.93.1.75

Hogan, M. F. (2004). The President's New Freedom Commission on mental health: Transforming mental health care. *Capital University Law Review, 32,* 907–923. Retrieved from http://law.capital.edu/LawReview/

Hogan, S. R., Unick, G. J., Speiglman, R., & Norris, J. C. (2008). Social welfare policy and public assistance for low-income substance abusers: The impact of 1996 welfare reform legislation on the economic security of former Supplemental Security Income drug addiction and alcoholism beneficiaries. *Journal of Sociology & Social Welfare, 35,* 221–245. Retrieved from http://scholarworks.wmich.edu/jssw/

Holman, E. J., & Cooley, G. W. (1950). Voluntary health insurance in the United States. *Iowa Law Review, 35,* 183–208. Retrieved from http://heinonline.org/

Kaiser Commission on Medicaid and the Uninsured. (2013). *Medicaid: A primer: Key information on the nation's health coverage program for low-income people* (Report no. 7334-05). Retrieved from https://kaiserfamilyfoundation.files.wordpress.com/2010/06/7334-05.pdf

Kennedy, J. F. (1964). Message from the President of the United States relative to mental illness and mental retardation. *The American Journal of Psychiatry, 120,* 729–737. doi: 10.1176/ajp.120.8.729

Klees, B. S., Wolfe, C. J., & Curtis, C. A. (2010). *Brief summaries of Medicaid & Medicare: Title XVIII and Title XIX of the Social Security Act.* Washington, DC: U.S. Department of Health and Human Services, Centers for Medicare and Medicaid Services. Retrieved from https://www.cms.gov/Research-Statistics-Data-and-Systems/Statistics-Trends-and-Reports/MedicareProgramRatesStats/Downloads/MedicareMedicaidSummaries2010.pdf

Mechanic, D., McAlpine, D. D., & Rochefort, D. A. (2014). *Mental health and social policy. Beyond managed care* (6th ed.). New York, NY: Pearson.

Mechanic, D., & Rochefort, D. A. (1990). Deinstitutionalization: An appraisal of reform. *Annual Review of Sociology, 16,* 301–327. doi: 10.1146/annurev.so.16.080190.001505

Mojtabai, R. (2009). Unmet need for treatment of major depression in the United States. *Psychiatric Services, 60,* 297–305. doi: 10.1176/appi.ps.60.3.297

Mojtabai, R., Chen, L. Y., Kaufmann, C. N., & Crum, R. M. (2014). Comparing barriers to mental health treatment and substance use disorder treatment among individuals with comorbid major depression and substance use disorders. *Journal of Substance Abuse Treatment, 46,* 268–273. doi: 10.1016/j.jsat.2013.07.012

Mojtabai, R., & Crum, R. M. (2013). Perceived unmet need for alcohol and drug use treatments and future use of services: Results from a longitudinal study. *Drug and Alcohol Dependence, 127,* 59–64. doi: 10.1016/j.drugalcdep.2012.06.012

Morton, J. D., & Aleman, P. (2005). Trends in employer-provided mental health and substance abuse benefits. *Monthly Labor Review, 128*(4), 25–35. Retrieved from http://www.jstor.org

National Conference of State Legislatures. (n.d.). State laws mandating or regulating mental health benefits. Last update December 30, 2015. Retrieved from http://www.ncsl.org/research/health/mental-health-benefits-state-mandates.aspx

Park, H., & Sanger-Katz, M. (April 12, 2017). What Trump can do without Congress to dismantle Obamacare. Retrieved from https://www.nytimes.com/interactive/2017/04/12/us/what-trump-can-do-to-dismantle-obamacare.html

Roberts, J. (2007, March 1). Poll: The politics of health care. *CBS News.* Retrieved from http://www.cbsnews.com/2100-500160_162-2528357.html

Schnapp, W. B. (2006). The c's in community mental health. *Administration and Policy in Mental Health and Mental Health Services Research, 33,* 737–739. doi: 10.1007/s10488-005-0005-3

Scofea, L. A. (1994). The development and growth of employer-provided health insurance. *Monthly Labor Review, 117*(3), 3–10. Retrieved from http://www.jstor.org

Shirk, C. (2008). *Medicaid and mental health services* (Background Paper No. 66). Washington, DC: The George Washington University National Health Policy Forum. Retrieved from https://www.nhpf.org/library/background-papers/BP66_MedicaidMentalHealth_10-23-08.pdf

Shonick, W. (1995). *Government and health services: Government's role in the development of U.S. health services, 1930-1980.* New York, NY: Oxford University Press.

Smith, J. C., & Medalia, C. (2015). *Health insurance coverage in the United States: 2014* (Current Population Report No. P60-253). Washington, DC: U.S. Government Printing Office.

Starr, P. (1982). Transformation of defeat: The changing objectives of national health insurance, 1915-1980. *American Journal of Public Health, 72,* 78–88. doi: 10.2105/AJPH.72.1.78

Teitelbaum, J., Burke, T., & Rosenbaum, S. (2004). Law and the public's health. *Public Health Reports, 119,* 371–374. Retrieved from http://www.publichealthreports.org/issueopen.cfm?articleID=1385

Urbanoski, K. A., Cairney, J., Bassani, D. G., & Rush, B. R. (2008). *Psychiatric Services, 59,* 283–289. doi: 10.1176/appi.ps.59.3.283

U.S. Department of Health and Human Services, Centers for Medicare & Medicaid Services. (2016). Medicaid & CHIP: May 2015 monthly applications, eligibility determinations and enrollment report. Retrieved from https://www.medicaid.gov/medicaid-chip-program-information/program-information/downloads/december-2015-enrollment-report.pdf

U.S. Social Security Administration. (2000, July 13). Statement before the subcommittee on social security of the Committee on Ways and Means. Retrieved from https://www.ssa.gov/history/edberkdib.html

Zinner, M. J., & Loughlin, K. R. (2009). The evolution of health care in America. *Urologic Clinics of North America, 36,* 1–10. doi: 10.1016/j.ucl.2008.08.005

THE PATIENT PROTECTION AND AFFORDABLE CARE ACT OF 2010

Victoria Stanhope and Meredith Doherty

Passage of the Patient Protection and Affordable Care Act (ACA) of 2010 was a historical event that marked a significant shift in the federal government's approach to health care. However, passage of the legislation championed by President Barack Obama was fraught and continues to be subject to intense legal and political challenges. These tensions reflect a century of political battles over the extent to which government should be involved in the delivery of health care services.

Franklin D. Roosevelt, in the New Deal era, first contemplated providing universal health care—ensuring that all people have access to health care but it was soon concluded that this was not politically feasible. Since then, the federal government has passed health care reforms incrementally, focusing on particular groups rather than seeking universal access to health care. Gaining political support to provide benefits to groups that have been perceived as deserving has been a far more successful strategy historically and has enabled federal legislation to target groups such as veterans, the elderly, the poor, and children. Most notable among these policies have been the Social Security Amendments of 1965, which created Medicaid for low-income people and Medicare for the elderly and disabled, and the 1997 Children's Health Insurance Program (CHIP).

This chapter provides an overview of the ACA while focusing on how the landmark health care policy is designed to initiate, expand, and sustain the integration of primary care and behavioral health care. By the time of its passage in 2010, the crisis in health care had already driven innovations in the area of integrated health care at the state and local levels. The ACA drew on much of this innovative thinking and what had been happening in the field with the aim of promoting reforms at the national level. Although the legislation may still be in jeopardy, many of the strategies used to integrate care will most likely continue in one form or another as systems strive to improve quality of care and control costs.

This chapter provides a broad understanding of how the ACA shapes health care delivery and encourages social workers and health care service users to further explore policies that may affect them. The legislation is 2700 pages long and has promulgated more than that in regulations, reflecting its complexity and broad reach.

Overall, the purpose of the ACA is to expand existing public and private health insurance while controlling costs through innovative approaches and financial incentives. Much of the innovation lies in its integrated health care approach, which seeks to both prevent and treat chronic illnesses more effectively. Given the enormity of this task and the ongoing resistance to the legislation, the ACA used an incremental strategy that phases in regulations over an 8-year period and encourages rather than mandates much of the innovation. The main areas of reform in the ACA are expansion of insurance coverage, delivery system reform, and payment reform. This chapter addresses the first two areas, and Chapter 6 covers payment reform in detail.

THE HEALTH CARE CRISIS

Passage of the ACA reflected concerns about the lack of health coverage and the rising costs of health care. During the Nixon (1969–1974), Carter (1977–1981), and Reagan (1981–1989) administrations, the dominant concern was the escalating costs associated with both publicly and privately funded health care; this precipitated cost control measures including managed care (Almgren, 2012). Presidents Clinton (1993–2001) and Obama (2008–2016) first framed the health care crisis in terms of a lack of coverage. By the time Obama became president, 43.3 million people (16.6% of the population) were without coverage (Cohen, Makuc, Bernstein, Bilheimer, & Powell-Griner, 2009). Clinton made universal health care a major priority in his first administration, placing First Lady Hillary Rodham Clinton at the head of the task force to develop a health care reform proposal. With a plan called *managed competition*, Clinton attempted to overhaul both private and public health care insurance but failed to win the support of major vested interests, most notably the health care insurance and pharmaceutical industries, and the plan was ultimately unsuccessful.

Obama learned from the failures of the Clinton efforts and instead crafted a plan that sought to expand coverage not by changing the health care benefits that people already had but by expanding existing public and private health care programs to include everyone. In the spirit of the Triple Aim, Obama simultaneously addressed the issue of cost control, seeking to offset the cost of expanding health care coverage by making health care more effective and efficient. This approach rested heavily on the promotion of integrated health care, a less publicized aspect of the ACA but one that is key to delivering improved health care quality while reducing costs.

The ACA was essentially an exercise in pragmatism. Obama was well aware that he needed to maintain public support for his proposal while keeping the major stakeholders at the negotiation table. Most Americans support the idea of universal coverage in theory, but they quickly become ambivalent when reform entails changes to their own health care plans. Obama did not seek to overhaul the whole health care system but instead to build on the existing mix of private and public health care systems to expand coverage and improve quality. In this respect, Obama did not fundamentally change the health care model of the United States, which is significantly different from those in other industrialized countries.

Despite claims by political opponents, the ACA is not socialized medicine, which involves a nationalized health service such as those seen in Great Britain, Spain, the Scandinavian countries, and Cuba. Although there are variations among these countries, all provide a national health care system that is funded directly by taxes, with most hospitals and clinics being owned by the government. Health care is funded through individuals' tax contributions rather than through insurers, making the system less expensive to administer. However, there can also be a private tier of care, in which people choose to have private insurance and access to private doctors; this supplements the care they receive from the nationalized system.

Another model is social insurance, in which employers and employees pay into *sickness funds*, and these plans reimburse care at what are largely private hospitals and clinics (Saltman, Busse, & Figueras, 2004). Although this resembles the U.S. system, the insurers are all nonprofit, and the government plays a strong regulatory role in ensuring cost control. Countries that have adopted this model include Germany, France, and Japan.

Canada's health care model, often a point of comparison for the United States, is referred to as a *single-payor system*, with the government acting as the sole insurer for health care services. People pay into the government-run system, which reimburses private hospitals and clinics for care. With only one payor, the system is more efficient to administer, and the government is in a strong position to keep costs down by negotiating the prices of pharmaceutical drugs and medical services.

The key features of health care models are whether they are tax funded or insurance based, whether health care facilities are private or nonprofit, and the extent of the government's role in regulating, delivering, and paying for services.

PASSAGE OF THE AFFORDABLE CARE ACT

Passage of the ACA was a roller-coaster affair, often coming close to failure, which presaged the continuing opposition this legislation has faced in the years since. Obama took office in 2008, vowing to provide universal health care with a strategy first proposed by Republicans in the 1990s. This strategy involved achieving coverage through an *individual mandate*, which requires all people to have health care coverage, with tax penalties administered to those who do not have health care insurance plans. Because health insurance companies were required to cover everyone regardless of health condition (previously they had been able to deny coverage according to pre-existing conditions), they needed to have both healthy and sick people in their insurance pools to spread the risk. This arrangement was key to gaining support from the insurance companies, and in the same way, the promise that the policy would not demand lower drug prices persuaded the pharmaceutical industry to support the bill.

In March 2009, Obama convened a Health Care Summit with major stakeholders and declared that the status quo was no longer acceptable. By July, the House of Representatives had produced a 1000-page bill, which was the first step in the legislative process. However, during the summer recess, elected representatives were met with intense opposition from their constituents to what they dubbed *Obamacare* (see Figure 5.1).

The bill passed the House with only one Republican supporter and passed the Senate by 60 votes, the minimum needed to overcome a Republican filibuster. Then, in the Senate, the death of Democrat Edward Kennedy from Massachusetts led to the election of Republican Scott Brown, who was a fervent opponent of health care reform. The irony of this setback was that Massachusetts, under Governor Mitt Romney, had implemented a health care model at the state level similar to what Obama was proposing. With the loss of this vital vote, it seemed as if there would not be enough votes to pass the final bill. However, an increase in premiums of 39% by a California health care insurer brought another wave of public support and pushed Democrats to rally around the bill once more (Helfand, 2010).

In a televised White House meeting of Republican and Democratic leaders, Obama again demanded action. Speaker of the House Nancy Pelosi, a Democrat from California, worked tirelessly to shore up support among Democrats who feared for their reelection prospects, and in the end, the House passed the Senate version of the bill by a 219 to 212 vote. The Senate then passed the final measure as part of a budget reconciliation bill, thus

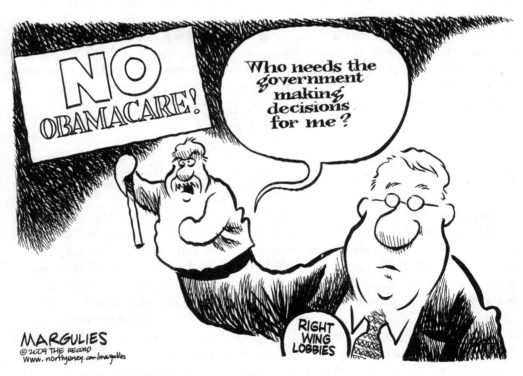

FIGURE 5.1: Health reform protests. Reprinted with permission from "Health Reform Protests," by Jimmy Margulies, 2009 (https://www.politicalcartoons.com/cartoon/fd0ff244-7527-4971-add7-e5c68df4ac04.html). Copyright 2009 by *The Record* of Hackensack, NJ.

avoiding the necessity of having a two-thirds majority to stop a filibuster. Obama signed the bill into law on March 23, 2010. The contentious legislative history of the ACA that culminated in passage of the bill using a procedural technicality rather than gaining broad Congressional support meant that the resistance to health care reform was not over and would continue to play out in the courts and at the ballot box.

After passage of the ACA, its opponents quickly transferred their energies to challenging it in the courts. The third branch of government, the legal system, plays a major role in enforcing or impeding policies by judging whether they are constitutional. In the case of the ACA, many court challenges have been brought with the intent of overturning key parts of the policy, and several have been appealed to the level of the Supreme Court.

The most substantive case to reach the Supreme Court came in 2012 in the case of *The National Federation of Independent Business v. Sebelius*, which challenged the individual mandate to purchase health insurance and the requirement that states expand Medicaid to all people younger than 65 years of age whose income is less than 133% of the federal poverty level (FPL) (Musumeci, 2012). In a 5 to 4 decision, the Supreme Court upheld the individual mandate by claiming that although it was not referred to as a tax in the bill, it essentially functioned as a tax, with enforcement being the responsibility of the Internal Revenue Service. However, by a 7 to 2 vote, the court concurred with the prosecution in regard to Medicaid expansion, stating that the requirement was coercive because the federal government did not provide adequate notice for the states to voluntarily consent. Three of the judges ruled that this finding invalidated the entire ACA, but the majority stated that the ACA could stand without the federal government's right to withhold current Medicaid funds if a state chose not to expand its system (Musumeci, 2012). This decision undercut the potential for the ACA to offer universal coverage because the decision by some states not to expand Medicaid resulted in some individuals' being both ineligible for Medicaid and unable to afford private insurance. The following sections address how this decision has affected implementation of the ACA.

EXPANDING INSURANCE COVERAGE

Perhaps the most publicly debated sections of the ACA are those regulating the public and private insurance markets. To address the vast disparities in insurance coverage that hit a critical peak in 2010, the ACA proposed several reforms to the health insurance system. The primary aim of insurance reform has been to provide comprehensive health coverage to all Americans. To accomplish this, the ACA mandated a variety of changes in how health insurance is delivered and regulated, including the establishment of Health Benefit Exchanges with income-sensitive subsidies for middle-income individuals, the expansion of Medicaid, protections that prevent insurance companies from denying coverage to individuals due to preexisting conditions, and allowing dependent adults younger than 26 years of age to remain on their parents' insurance plan (Blumenthal, Abrams, & Nuzum, 2015).

The first American health exchanges were established in 2014. State and federal exchanges, also known as marketplaces, help individuals understand their health insurance options under the new law, choose one of the plans available in their state, and purchase the plan that fits their needs. States have the option of using a federally run exchange or developing their own. Only 16 states and the District of Columbia initially chose to establish their own exchange; the remaining states used the infrastructure provided by the federal government (Collins, Rasmussen, Doty, & Beutel, 2014). The exchanges are charged with determining whether individuals qualify for payment assistance and tax credits to cover out-of-pocket costs and with tracking the relative affordability of health exchange plans based on collected individual income data (Families USA, 2010). Similar small business exchanges have been developed to help business owners purchase affordable group plans for their employees (Kaiser Family Foundation, 2011).

Plans purchased on the exchanges are required to cover basic essential services such as preventive and chronic illness care, ambulatory clinic and emergency department visits, maternal and newborn care, mental health and substance misuse treatment, prescription drugs, and rehabilitation services. As long as they meet the essential benefits requirement, plans sold on the health exchange can offer a tiered system of coverage, typically described as bronze, silver, gold, and platinum plans. Each level indicates the percentage of the cost of care covered by the insurance plan. The lowest-level (bronze) plans cover 60% of the cost of care, silver plans cover 70%, gold plans cover 80%, and platinum plans cover 90% (Families USA, 2010). The federal exchange website endured some highly publicized technical difficulties during the program's initial enrollment period, but these problems diminished, and in the 2015 enrollment period, 11.7 million people purchased insurance on the state and federal marketplaces (Blumenthal, Abrams, & Nuzum, 2015).

To ensure affordability, the law allows various forms of payment assistance to middle-income individuals and families who purchase plans on the exchanges. People whose income falls between 133% and 400% of the FPL are eligible for tax credits and other subsidies to contain the out-of-pocket costs of premiums, deductibles, and copayments (Kaiser Family Foundation, 2011). Assistance with premiums is means tested (i.e., based on a sliding scale according to income); people may be required to pay as little as 2% or up to 9.5% of their taxable income for the cost of premiums. Premium assistance is also provided directly to service users through individual tax credits. After the tax credits, 80% of individuals who purchased plans on the marketplace in 2015 reported paying less than $100 per month (Misra & Tsai, 2015).

The other form of payment assistance available to lower- and middle-income families reduces their total health care costs by increasing the percentage of health care costs paid by insurers. Subsidies to insurers allow them to reduce the deductibles and copays the individuals and families are responsible for. The law also proposes a cap on total out-of-pocket costs for all plans purchased on the exchanges, regardless of income. The cap is significantly lower for those earning less than 400% of the FPL.

INDIVIDUAL AND EMPLOYER MANDATES

The ACA promotes maximal participation in the insurance market through individual and employer mandates. Individuals who can afford insurance are required to either carry a basic plan or pay a penalty of $695 per year or 2.5% of their taxable income, whichever is greater. Individuals who cannot find an affordable plan (i.e., one with premiums lower than 8% of taxable income), who have low incomes, or who are exempt for religious reasons do not have to purchase insurance.

Under the ACA's employer mandate, businesses with 50 or more employees must offer an insurance plan to full-time employees and their dependent children. These plans must cover at least 60% of health care costs and require the employee to contribute no more than 9.66% of his or her household income toward premiums. Employers who fail to offer coverage that meets these minimum requirements may be subject to penalties of up to $3240 each year per employee (Snyder, Rudowitz, Dadayan, & Boyd, 2015). Although they are exempt from the mandate rule, small businesses with fewer than 25 full-time employees are encouraged to offer similar coverage and may be eligible for tax credits to help purchase affordable group plans on the small business health insurance exchanges.

MEDICAID EXPANSION

The ACA made groundbreaking changes to Medicaid and CHIP, the public health insurance programs for low-income Americans. These programs are jointly financed by state and federal funds, but leadership and administration are primarily managed independently by the states. This arrangement has led to much variation in Medicaid coverage among states. The ACA initially intended to expand access to Medicaid to any U.S. citizen or legal resident whose income was lower than 138% of the FPL, but a June 2012 Supreme Court ruling (discussed earlier) amended that policy, making state participation in the program optional (Snyder et al., 2015). To incentivize states to expand Medicaid enrollment in accordance with ACA recommendations, the federal government offered to fund 100% of the total cost of providing Medicaid to each state's newly eligible population through 2016 and then reduce the federal share to 90% by 2020. By the start of 2016, 31 states and the District of Columbia had implemented the new regulations.

Medicaid expansion has been extremely successful in reducing the number of uninsured Americans, particularly the so-called working poor, whose incomes are too low to afford insurance but slightly too high to qualify for Medicaid. Before enactment, Medicaid eligibility requirements varied widely across states, but the mean income threshold for eligibility was 64% of the FPL for a family of three, and only 11 states allowed individuals without dependent children to participate in Medicaid (Families USA, 2010). Since its inception in 2013, an additional 11.2 million children and adults who would have been too poor to afford health insurance have been provided with coverage through the ACA's Medicaid expansion initiative (Executive Office of the President, 2015). Most individuals who are still uninsured live in states that opted not to expand Medicaid (Collins et al., 2014).

CHIP provides insurance to children whose parents make less than 200% of the FPL. The ACA mandated protections for this program by including provisions for funding and administration through 2019. Federal contributions to state funding of the program were increased by 23%. The rate of uninsured children and adults has fallen steadily and significantly each year since implementation (Alker & Chester, 2014; Blumenthal et al., 2015).

HOME AND COMMUNITY-BASED SERVICES

The ACA proposed strong guidelines and incentives that encourage states to invest in improving their home and community-based services (HCBS). HCBS programs comprise a variety of health and social care services that assist individuals with functional care needs to live independently in the community. These services include case management, family support, wellness activities, and personally directed care. They are part of a larger set of services encompassed by the term *long-term services and supports* (LTSS), which also includes care provided in institutional settings. Historically, institutional care made up the greatest share of LTSS expenditures funded by public dollars, but social and political movements in recent decades have begun to tip the balance in favor of HCBS (Long-term care policy, 2013).

In the *Olmstead v. L.C. and E.W.* decision of 1999, the Supreme Court acted to strengthen the Americans with Disabilities Act by requiring states to provide services to people with disabilities in the most integrated and least restrictive environments. This decision reflected a growing national commitment to moving away from institutional care for people with long-term care needs and establishing HCBS that allow people to continue to participate meaningfully in their community for as long as possible.

To incentivize further investment by states in home and community-based care, the ACA developed two new HCBS funding mechanisms. The first was Community First Choice, which was launched on October 1, 2011, as a new HCBS financial incentive plan under Medicaid. This option increases federal matching of Medicaid spending on HCBS programs by 6% for states that choose to participate. The ACA also expanded two programs that had been established under the Deficit Reduction Act (DRA) of 2005. Money Follows the Person, a time-limited demonstration project, incentivized states to allow individuals to transfer out of institutional settings and into community-integrated settings by increasing the rate of federal matching by up to 90% for the HCBS they would need to live more independently. The other DRA program, known as the 1915(i) State Plan, was revised in the ACA to be more flexible, allowing states to acquire federal funding to develop tailored HCBS programs for targeted populations. Before the ACA, the 1915(i) benefit allowed states to use Medicaid funds to deliver HCBS to individuals who met state-defined skilled care needs and whose income fell below 150% of the FPL (Damler & Howard, 2015).

Under the new legislation, states could define target populations and tailor HCBS packages to their needs. To access this mechanism under the ACA, states had to expand eligibility criteria to include individuals earning up to 300% of the federal Supplemental

Security Income (SSI) benefit rate who also meet the state-defined criteria for medically necessary HCBS or institutional care. The ACA eliminated states' ability to cap the number of people who can receive HCBS through the 1915(i) state plan.

CONSUMER PROTECTIONS

Several ACA provisions intervene in the private insurance market, setting regulations that protect consumers and make the market fairer and more accessible to certain social groups previously underserved. Two provisions in particular have made substantial contributions to reducing the number of uninsured Americans. First, beginning in 2014, plans could no longer deny coverage or charge higher premiums to people with pre-existing conditions. This provision kicked in earlier for children: Beginning in 2010, children with pre-existing conditions could not be denied coverage in the individual insurance markets (Families USA, 2010). Up to 129 million Americans have had health concerns that qualified as pre-existing conditions, meaning that before this legislation, one half of the population could have been denied coverage (Office of the Assistant Secretary for Planning and Evaluation [ASPE], 2011). The second provision extended the age limits on insurance for dependents and allowed adult children to remain on their parents' insurance plans until age 26. Collectively, these two provisions have increased the number of insured Americans by 11 to 16 million people (Blumenthal et al., 2015).

In addition to increasing access to health insurance, protections focus on guaranteeing insurance of decent and consistent quality. Under the ACA, insurers in the individual and small group markets are obligated to cover 10 categories of essential health benefits. Although the federal law sets forth a basic guideline for the medical service domains that must be covered (see Figure 5.2), states and individual insurers are allowed some flexibility in exactly how essential benefit coverage is delivered through private insurance plans.

To ensure a degree of consistency, states were encouraged to select a sample benchmark plan to illustrate their standards for essential benefit coverage or to allow the federal government to select a default plan for them. These benchmark plans are the kinds of items and services that would be covered within each essential health benefit category (Giovannelli, Lucia, & Corlette, 2014).

Before the ACA, the Mental Health Parity and Addiction Equity Act (MHPAEA) prevented private insurers from restricting mental health and substance misuse treatment benefits any more than physical health coverage. However, the legislation did not mandate that the insurers cover mental health or substance abuse treatment at all, which left many people without needed care. Acknowledging this, the ACA's essential health benefit provision required all new small group and individual plans to cover mental health and substance abuse services (Aggarwal & Rowe, 2013; Frank, Beronio, & Glied, 2014).

It is known that the burden of chronic and serious illnesses can be lessened with adequate preventive services and early intervention. However, people who are uninsured or

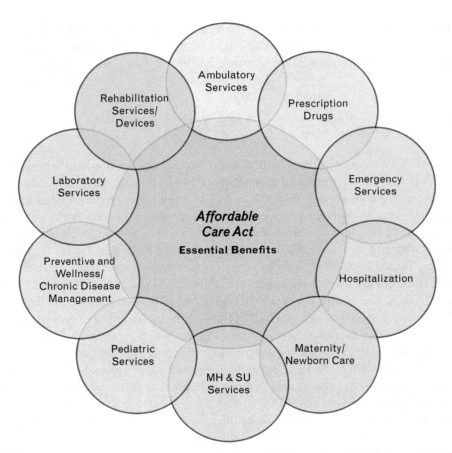

FIGURE 5.2: The Affordable Care Act's 10 essential health benefits categories. MH, mental health; SU, substance use. Adapted from *Implementing the Affordable Care Act: Revisiting the ACA's Essential Health Benefits Requirements* (p. 2), by J. Giovannelli, K. W. Lucia, and S. Corlette, 2014, New York, NY: The Commonwealth Fund. Copyright 2014 by The Commonwealth Fund.

underinsured tend to avoid cancer screenings and non-emergent medical visits because of concerns about cost (Collins et al., 2014). For this reason, the ACA takes a robust stance regarding preventive services that includes eliminating cost sharing for preventive services in non-grandfathered private and public insurance plans. Preventive services that are rated as A (i.e., strongly recommended) or B (i.e., recommended) by the U.S. Preventive Services Task Force are exempt from cost sharing. Examples of these services include cancer screenings and immunizations (Koh & Sebelius, 2010).

In addition to preventive services, the ACA's insurance reform provisions address disparities in women's health coverage that existed under the previous system. For instance, the ACA prohibits charging women more than men for the same plan or denying coverage due to a pre-existing but common condition such as high-risk pregnancy. Under the essential health benefit provisions, insurers must provide adequate coverage for maternity and newborn care. Women are also entitled to one "well-woman visit" per year exempt from cost sharing to discuss prevention, screening, and family planning (Lee & Woods, 2013).

DELIVERY SYSTEM REFORM

The ACA's strategy was intended to encourage innovation among providers rather than mandate wholesale change in the provision of care. The delivery system envisaged by health care reform was on such a scale that sudden change would likely encounter resistance and also place systems at risk. Instead, the ACA makes resources available for providers who propose new delivery system models and financial incentives for cost-efficient provider organizations. Many of these innovations are driven by payment reform, which incentivizes different types of care delivery. The federal hub for delivery system reform is the Center for Medicare and Medicaid Innovation, which is designed to test, evaluate, and disseminate new delivery models and payment structures using Medicare, Medicaid, and CHIP funds. Innovation is assessed according to the Triple Aim, and new models need to demonstrate their ability to improve quality of care and promote population health while reducing costs.

The ACA allocates $10 billion to the Innovation Center for 10 years, which is a significant investment but represents only 0.1% of the total budget for Medicare and Medicaid. The intent of the legislation was to allow the Innovation Center much latitude to make investments in promising programs, evaluate and disseminate findings, and scale-up successful programs to a national level. If a model can demonstrate quality improvement and cost savings, the Secretary of the U.S. Department of Health and Human Services has the authority to expand that model without Congressional approval. The Innovation Center oversees the implementation of required demonstration programs, such as accountable care organizations (ACOs) and primary care redesign, but it also solicits new ideas by working closely with the private sector.

COORDINATED CARE

At the heart of delivery system reform is the creation of the structural conditions (i.e., physical configuration and resources) and financial conditions (i.e., reimbursement for care delivered) that are necessary for a system to provide coordinated care. Coordinated care is "the deliberate organization of patient care activities between two or more participants (including the patient) involved in a patient's care to facilitate the appropriate delivery of services. Organizing care involves the marshalling of personnel and other resources to carry out the required patient care activities and is often managed by the exchange of information among participants responsible for different aspects of care" (McDonald et al., 2010, p. 4). Coordinated care has specific tasks:

1. To determine and update care coordination needs
2. To create and update a proactive plan of care
3. To communicate and exchange information, preferences, goals, and experiences among participants in an individual's care
4. To facilitate transitions by sharing information among providers and service users

5. To connect with community resources
6. To align resources with population needs (Meyers et al., 2010)

Models aimed at achieving coordinated care vary in terms of their target population, scope, and funding streams, but they share some common features. In terms of organization, all innovations propose some level of integration, from the co-location of services to provider networks that facilitate the coordination between primary care, mental health, and substance abuse services. Financing strategies change the incentives to reward quality over volume, which means tying payment to outcomes rather than using fee-for-service models.

ACCOUNTABLE CARE ORGANIZATIONS

The ACA created voluntary programs through the Centers for Medicare and Medicaid Services (CMS) for providers to create ACOs for Medicare recipients. These programs support providers already experienced in integrated health care in moving to a population-based model of care using patient-centered primary care, payment reform, and performance measurement to provide care to an assigned population. By meeting certain quality standards—including delivering coordinated care and evidence-based practices, tracking outcomes on quality and cost, and including primary care physicians—providers can meet the designation of an ACO and qualify for the Medicaid Shared Savings Program (MSSP). The MSSP, also enacted by the ACA, incentivizes coordinated care by ensuring that all providers contributing to more efficient care benefit from the savings generated from reform. ACOs, by demonstrating cost savings and quality improvement, receive payments known as shared savings.

An example is the Mount Sinai Care ACO in New York City, which must show a 2.5% cost savings annually for their Medicare recipients and hit benchmarks indicating patient satisfaction, care coordination, patient safety, prevention, and chronic disease management. If the organization is successful, CMS returns 50% of the savings, which can be reinvested in the Mount Sinai Care ACO and paid to primary care physicians (Xenakis, 2015).

ACOs bring together a broad array of providers—including hospitals, physician groups, home health agencies, specialty care providers, and nursing homes—with the aim of providing a seamless care experience for the individual. Although much of the care is delivered in the primary care setting, there remains a need for specialty care, resulting in the creation by ACOs of *medical neighborhoods* that can include community-based organizations such as behavioral health clinics (Collins, 2011a). These networks assume responsibility for all of a person's care across facilities and therefore must possess the necessary infrastructure to coordinate care, including managing electronic health records, delivering interprofessional team–based care, using internal metrics to measure performance, and aligning financial incentives.

A key part of service delivery is managing care for people with chronic illnesses and preventive care, including the integration of behavioral health care, because this has the most potential to shift the cost curve and reap quality improvements. Part of the shift is moving from individually based care to population health management (see Chapter 3). For instance, people with diagnoses such as diabetes may be assigned to high-, medium-, or low-risk categories, resulting in different levels of tracking and intervention. Integral to population health management is the use of the electronic health record, which allows care coordination staff to create patient registries, track people in the system for health events, and alert providers to appropriate interventions.

Given the broad range of activities within ACOs, there are many potential roles for social workers, including care coordinators, case managers, and patient educators (see Chapter 14). They can bring their expertise as behavioral health care providers into primary care settings and community-based clinics that form part of the medical neighborhood. Linkage with community-based agencies can be challenging for ACOs because this is a new initiative for many hospital-based systems. As a result, ACOs are employing community health workers who share the culture of the people they are serving and help people manage their wellness through home visits. Supervising these community health workers is another role that social workers can play in ACOs.

While the ACA had initially invested in ACOs for Medicare, the model has already gained much traction in the private sector, and many think that it may become the dominant model of health care delivery in the future. Although many managed care companies are involved in ACOs, the fundamental difference is that an ACO is a health care delivery system rather than an insurer that contracts with providers to deliver services. Another important difference is that people are assigned to an ACO based on where they receive most of their care, but they are allowed to receive care wherever they choose without network restrictions. By tying payment to outcomes, the hope is that people will see an improvement in their care and choose ACOs over more traditional forms of services.

PATIENT-CENTERED MEDICAL HOMES

The patient-centered medical home (PCMH) has emerged from privately funded and Medicare- and Medicaid-funded systems. The model was not created by the ACA; it first appeared in pediatric medicine in the 1990s. The PCMH emphasizes the role of primary care, designating it as the hub for coordinating care across different provider types. A PCMH can stand alone or be a part of a larger integrated health care model such as an ACO.

In 2007, four primary care professional societies promulgated a set of joint principles for PCMHs to help insurers determine what constitutes a PCMH (American Academy of Family Physicians, American Academy of Pediatrics, American College of Physicians, & American Osteopathic Association, 2007). The principles focused on having a whole-person orientation, coordinating care across systems, enhancing access and quality improvement, and having a value-based payment system. Similarly, the National Committee for Quality Assurance developed standards that included 30 elements to determine if and at what level a group of providers is functioning as a PCMH.

The shared element of a PCMH is that all patients have a personal primary care physician who is the first point of contact. The physician works with a team, which can include specialist physicians, nurses, social workers, pharmacists, nurse practitioners, physician assistants, medical assistants, educators, behaviorists, and care coordinators. The team is designed to address primary and behavioral health needs within a single setting and to coordinate care across specialty settings, hospitals, home health agencies, and nursing homes. The PCMH team can also work with families and the community to ensure coordination beyond the formal care provision. A PCMH can vary in size from a physician practice to a larger health care system. Infrastructure enhancements such as electronic health records are used to ensure patient tracking, clinical monitoring, and population health management. Success of the PCMH structure depends on accessibility, which can be facilitated by having providers located in one facility, extending hours to evenings and weekends, and using telephone and email contact to ease communication (Cassidy, 2010). There are many opportunities for social workers in PCMHs, including care coordination, case management, health promotion and illness self-management, transitional care, family support, behavioral health, and community linkages (Collins, 2011b).

As with many of these new delivery models, PCMHs rely on payment mechanisms that provide compensation for the activities of care coordination not just face-to-face visits. Additional compensation is given if PCMHs demonstrate reduced hospitalization and improved quality of care and if they serve individuals with complex needs (Rittenhouse & Shortell, 2009). PCMHs are supported by ACA provisions that increase Medicaid reimbursement for primary care and providing 100% federal financing.

While encouraging a broad array of providers to propose PCMH models, the ACA particularly targets Federally Qualified Health Centers (FQHCs) as a natural setting for PCMHs. The health centers deliver primary care and prevention regardless of ability to pay, making them a key part of the social safety net for vulnerable populations. Some 1300 health centers are currently providing care to more than 20 million people throughout the United States, giving them a key role in implementing integrated health care. The ACA created the Community Health Center Fund to provide $11 billion over 5 years for infrastructure improvements such as health information technology, expanded capacity for primary and preventive care, and new centers in medically underserved areas (Health Resources and Services Administration, n.d.). Given the extensive funding that FQHCs have received through the ACA, community-based mental health clinics are also safety net providers with the potential to deliver integrated health care and have lobbied successfully to apply for FQHC "Look-Alike" status.

HEALTH HOMES

The health home model is closely related in design to the PCMH, but as the name suggests, it is not restricted to a medical setting. The ACA allowed states the option of enrolling Medicaid recipients with at least two chronic conditions or one severe mental illness in a health home. This has provided an important opportunity for states to extend primary care to people with severe mental illnesses who primarily seek services at community mental health clinics. By 2015, 20 states had had health home plans approved and many behavioral agencies were applying for this designation (Snyder et al., 2015). Among the payment approaches for funding health homes, the most common is payment to providers at a per-member per-month rate that varies according to the acuity of individuals' conditions and the type of intervention provided.

Unlike patient-centered medical homes, health home providers do not have to be based in a primary care setting and have the option to be in a community mental health agency, a health home agency, or a clinical/group practice. The level of integration can also vary with an in-house model; for example, an agency can provide all the primary care and behavioral health care through a co-located partnership model, or it can use a facilitated referral model in which the agency coordinates off-site services (Alexander & Druss, 2012). Unlike PCMHs, health homes do not have to provide the services; they can act primarily as coordinators of services across a network of providers, including medical providers, housing agencies, and community-based agencies.

The health home model adheres closely to the chronic care model and has a focus on delivery system redesign, self-management support, decision support, and clinical information support. These components enhance the delivery of comprehensive care management, care coordination, and health promotion and offer transitional care from inpatient to other settings, family support, linkage to community and social support services, and use of health technology. As in PCMHs, services are delivered by a interprofessional team and can include a care manager or care coordinator, a behavioral health clinician, a health navigator, a peer specialist, a nurse, a social worker, and a primary care physician, depending on the setting. Social workers can fulfill a number of these roles.

Care management is the key activity of a health home. It involves service user activation and education, developing a single care plan collaboratively with the individual and the family, care coordination, and monitoring service user progress in treatment (Alexander & Druss, 2012). The shift to a population-based care approach is key. Rather than delivering care in response to individual demand, population-based care demands that health homes track care for their entire population using data analytics to identify care gaps, target people with high use of avoidable services, and establish level of need.

THE IMPACT OF THE AFFORDABLE CARE ACT

The ACA's insurance reform and expansion initiatives have provided an estimated 11 to 16 million additional people with insurance coverage. These initiatives have reduced disparities in access to health care that had previously undermined the health and wellbeing of certain social groups. For example, studies indicate that the greatest improvements have been experienced by younger, low-income African-American and Hispanic individuals who now have affordable, adequate health insurance (ASPE, 2015; Blumenthal, et al., 2015). The rate of being uninsured fell by 9.2% for African Americans and 12.3% for Hispanics, numbers that constitute undeniable gains (ASPE, 2015). Another subpopulation that experienced dramatic increases in rates of insurance is people with pre-existing conditions, 80% of whom had never been able to purchase insurance in the private insurance market before this legislation (Doty, Collins, Nicholson, & Rustgi, 2009). By some calculations, 70% of individuals newly insured since the ACA was enacted are people with pre-existing conditions who were previously discriminated against (Blumenthal et al., 2015). However, there is still progress to be made because millions of Americans remain uninsured and many with employer-sponsored and individual plans continue to avoid needed medical care because of the high cost of their plans' deductibles and copays (Collins et al., 2014).

Medicare projections for spending in 2020 have been adjusted from $1038 million to $829 million, a 20% decrease since the ACA was enacted (Blumenthal, Abrams, & Nuzum, 2015). Most cost savings are attributed to new delivery system reforms, most notably the PCMHs and ACOs, which are becoming increasingly more widespread. As of January 2015, there were 744 private and public ACOs covering approximately 23.5 million people (Muhlestein, 2015).

IMPLICATIONS FOR SOCIAL WORK PRACTICE

Passage of the ACA has hastened a transformation of services that had already been occurring on the local level in response to escalating costs and poor quality of care. Many social workers in health care and community-based settings are experiencing a dramatic change in their practice as delivery system reform takes hold to integrate primary and behavioral health care. Each part of the ACA offers new opportunities for social work but also demands new skills and, for some, a shift into different settings (Stanhope, Videka, Thorning, & McKay, 2015). Through insurance reform, many service users have more access to care, which greatly enhances social workers' ability to improve lives. The increase in the number of insured means greater demand for services, particularly mental health and substance abuse services that are now designated as essential benefits (Cochran, Roll, Jackson, & Kennedy, 2014).

Delivery system reform also means that many more social workers will be working within models such as PCMHs and ACOs and providing coordinated care in interprofessional teams. Care integration may mark a shift away from social work's greater emphasis on behavioral health and toward more work in primary care settings, particularly FQHCs. Because hospitals are participating in these new models, hospital social workers can expand on their roles in coordinating care as people transition out of the hospital to another level of care.

As discussed in the following chapters on practice, social workers have the opportunity to bring their valuable skills in service user engagement and activation, shared decision making, and case management into these new spheres of practice. However, they also need to acquire more skills in health screening and prevention activities. The focus on community linkages in many of the new models offers social workers the greatest opportunities to apply a person-in-environment perspective. Because the ACA requires social workers and the entire workforce to develop new practices, it includes legislation focused on extensive training and capacity building implemented through the Health Resources and Services Administration. Social workers have been directly involved in these training initiatives, particularly those targeting the development of interdisciplinary behavioral health programs (see Chapter 7).

Payment reform means that providing a service is no longer sufficient for reimbursement; instead, funding is tied to outcomes. Provider organizations take on the financial risk for populations, placing the onus of cost saving on them (see Chapter 6). All providers, including social workers, must demonstrate their value-added benefit, particularly in relation to reducing emergency department visits and hospitalizations. The challenge for social workers is to identify their unique contributions to care coordination and teamwork and to measure those contributions in terms of the Triple Aim.

CONCLUSIONS

The ACA represents the most significant overhaul of the health care system since the enactment of Medicaid and Medicare in the 1960s. Amid intense political opposition, the legislation sought reform in the areas of insurance, delivery systems, and payment to meet the goals of the Triple Aim: improving quality of care, promoting population health, and reducing costs. Changes have resulted in some mandatory requirements such as the individual mandate to buy insurance. Enough time has elapsed to begin to evaluate the impact of the ACA in terms of the Triple Aim goals. Particularly important has been the reduction of health care expenditures during the first 4 years of the ACA (Schoen, 2016). However, health care reform still rests on a market-driven system, and market forces can always undermine these positive trends in order to maximize profits.

As the models are tested and evaluated, they will be refined further, but overall the common elements of coordinating care across systems, including the use of interprofessional teams and payment systems that reward quality over volume, will remain key. The future of health care across the private and public sectors may end up looking like ACOs, which use the PCMHs and create networks of coordinated providers. Whatever the future course of the ACA, health care systems will continue to evolve toward integration as the only way to provide effective and efficient care to people with complex health needs.

RESOURCES

AMA Comments on ACA Implementation Regulations, American Medical Association (AMA) https://www.ama-assn.org/delivering-care/efforts-improve-aca-implementation

The Children's Health Insurance Program (CHIP), U.S. Centers for Medicare & Medicaid Services https://www.healthcare.gov/medicaid-chip/childrens-health-insurance-program/

The Commonwealth Fund http://www.commonwealthfund.org/

Employee Benefits Security Administration—Affordable Care Act, U.S. Department of Labor (DOL) https://www.dol.gov/agencies/ebsa/laws-and-regulations/laws/affordable-care-act/for-employers-and-advisers

Home & Community Based Services (HCBS) Clearinghouse, National Association of States United for Aging and Disabilities (NASUAD) http://www.nasuad.org/hcbs/

The Innovation Center, U.S. Centers for Medicare & Medicaid Services https://innovation.cms.gov

The Kaiser Family Foundation (KFF) http://kff.org/

ObamaCare Facts http://obamacarefacts.com/

Obama's Deal, PBS http://www.pbs.org/video/1468710007/

Patient-Centered Medical Home (PCMH) Recognition, The National Committee for Quality Assurance (NCQA) http://www.ncqa.org/Programs/Recognition/Practices/PatientCenteredMedicalHomePCMH.aspx

The Patient-Centered Primary Care Collaborative (PCPCC) https://www.pcpcc.org/

Read the Law, U.S. Department of Health & Human Services (HHS) http://www.hhs.gov/healthcare/about-the-law/read-the-law/index.html

REFERENCES

Aggarwal, N. K., & Rowe, M. (2013). The individual mandate, mental health parity, and the Obama health plan. *Administration and Policy in Mental Health and Mental Health Services Research, 40,* 255–257. doi: 10.1007/s10488-011-0395-3

Alexander, L., & Druss, B. (2012). *Behavioral health homes for people with mental health & substance use conditions: The core clinical features.* Washington, DC: Center for Integrated Health Solutions, Substance Abuse and Mental Health Services Administration-Health Resources and Services Administration. Retrieved from http://www.integration.samhsa.gov/clinical-practice/cihs_health_homes_core_clinical_features.pdf

Alker, J., & Chester, A. (2014). *Children's coverage at a crossroads: Progress slows.* Washington, DC: Center for Children and Families, Health Policy Institute.

Almgren, G. R. (2012). *Health care politics, policy, and services: A social justice analysis* (2nd ed.). New York, NY: Springer.

American Academy of Family Physicians, American Academy of Pediatrics, American College of Physicians, & American Osteopathic Association. (2007, March 7). Joint principles of the patient-centered medical home. Retrieved from http://www.aafp.org/dam/AAFP/documents/practice_management/pcmh/initiatives/PCMHJoint.pdf

Blumenthal, D., Abrams, M., & Nuzum, R. (2015). The Affordable Care Act at 5 years. *New England Journal of Medicine, 372,* 2451–2458. doi: 10.1056/NEJMhpr1503614

Cassidy, A. (2010, September 14). Health policy briefs: Patient-centered medical home. Retrieved from http://www.healthaffairs.org/healthpolicybriefs/brief.php?brief_id=25

Cochran, G., Roll, J., Jackson, R., & Kennedy, J. (2014). Health care reform and the behavioral health workforce. *Journal of Social Work Practice in the Addictions, 14,* 127–140. doi: 10.1080/1533256X.2014.902244

Cohen, R. A., Makuc, D. M., Bernstein, A. B., Bilheimer, L. T., & Powell-Griner, E. (2009). *Health insurance coverage trends, 1959–2007: Estimates from the National Health Interview Survey* (National Health Statistics Rep. No. 17). Hyattsville, MD: National Center for Health Statistics. Retrieved from https://www.cdc.gov/nchs/data/nhsr/nhsr017.pdf

Collins, S. (2011a). *Accountable Care Organizations (ACOs): Opportunities for the social work profession.* Washington, DC: National Association of Social Workers. Retrieved from https://www.socialworkers.org/assets/secured/documents/practice/health/ACOs%20Opportunities%20for%20SWers.pdf

Collins, S. (2011b). *The medical home model: What is it and how do social workers fit in?* Washington, DC: National Association of Social Workers. Available from http://www.socialworkers.org/Practice/practice_tools/the_medical_home_model.asp

Collins, S. R., Rasmussen, P. W., Doty, M. M., & Beutel, S. (2014). *Too high a price: Out-of-pocket health care costs in the United States. Findings from the Commonwealth Fund Health Care Affordability Tracking Survey. September-October 2014* (Issue Brief Pub. No. 1784). New York, NY: The Commonwealth Fund. Retrieved from http://www.commonwealthfund.org/~/media/files/publications/issue-brief/2014/nov/1784_collins_too_high_a_price_out_of_pocket_tb_v2.pdf

Damler, R. M. & Howard, M. T. (2015). Medicaid and the ACA. *Contingencies, May/June 2015*, 40–43. Available from http://www.contingencies.org/past.asp

Doty, M. M., Collins, S. R., Nicholson, J. L., & Rustgi, S. D. (2009). *Failure to protect: Why the individual insurance market is not a viable option for most U.S. families: Findings from the Commonwealth Fund Biennial Health Insurance Survey, 2007* (Issue Brief Pub. No. 1300). New York, NY: The Commonwealth Fund. Retrieved from http://www.commonwealthfund.org/~/media/Files/Publications/Issue%20Brief/2009/Jul/Failure%20to%20Protect/1300_Doty_failure_to_protect_individual_ins_market_ib_v2.pdf

Executive Office of the President of the United States. (2015). *Accomplishments of the Affordable Care Act: A 5th year anniversary report.* Washington, DC: Executive Office of the President of the United States. Retrieved from https://www.whitehouse.gov/sites/default/files/docs/3-22-15_aca_anniversary_report.pdf

Families USA. (2010). *A summary of the health reform law.* Washington, DC: Families USA. Retrieved from http://familiesusa.org/sites/default/files/product_documents/summary-of-the-health-reform-law.pdf

Frank, R. G., Beronio, K., & Glied, S. A. (2014). Behavioral health parity and the Affordable Care Act. *Journal of Social Work in Disability & Rehabilitation, 13*, 31–43. doi: 10.1080/1536710X.2013.870512

Giovannelli, J., Lucia, K. W., & Corlette, S. (2014). *Implementing the Affordable Care Act: Revisiting the ACA's essential health benefits requirements* (Issue Brief Pub. No. 1783). New York, NY: The Commonwealth Fund. Retrieved from http://www.commonwealthfund.org/~/media/files/publications/issue-brief/2014/oct/1783_giovannelli_implementing_aca_essential_hlt_benefits_rb.pdf

Health Resources and Services Administration, U.S. Department of Health and Human Services (2012). The Affordable Care Act and health centers [Fact sheet]. Retrieved from http://www.hrsa.gov/about/news/2012tables/healthcentersacafactsheet.pdf

Helfand, D. (2010, February 9). Obama official "very disturbed" by Anthem Blue Cross rate hikes. *The Los Angeles Times.* Retrieved from http://articles.latimes.com/2010/feb/09/business/la-fi-anthem-obama9-2010feb09

Kaiser Family Foundation. (2011). Summary of new health reform law (Fact Sheet Pub. No. 8061-02). Retrieved from http://files.kff.org/attachment/fact-sheet-summary-of-the-affordable-care-act

Koh, H. K., & Sebelius, K. G. (2010). Promoting prevention through the Affordable Care Act. *New England Journal of Medicine, 363*, 1296–1299. doi: 10.1056/NEJMp1008560

Lee, N. C., & Woods, C. M. (2013). The Affordable Care Act: Addressing the unique health needs of women. *Journal of Women's Health, 22*, 803–806. doi: 10.1089/jwh.2013.4549

"Long-term care policy." (2013). In E. A. Capezuti, M. L. Malone, P. R. Katz, & M. D. Mezey (Eds.), *The encyclopedia of elder care: The comprehensive resources on geriatric health and social care* (3rd ed., pp. 439–441). New York, NY: Springer.

Margulies, J. (2009). Health reform protests [Illustration]. Retrieved from https://www.politicalcartoons.com/cartoon/fd0ff244-7527-4971-add7-e5c68df4ac04.html

McDonald, K. M., Schultz, E., Albin, L., Pineda, N., Lonhart, J., Sundaram, V., . . . Malcolm, E. (2010). *Care Coordination Measures Atlas* (Version 3, AHRQ Pub. No. 11-0023-EF). Rockville, MD: Agency for Health Care Research and Quality. Retrieved from https://pcmh.ahrq.gov/sites/default/files/attachments/Care%20Coordination%20Measures%20Atlas.pdf

Meyers, D., Peikes, D., Genevro, J., Peterson, G., Taylor, E. F., Lake, T., . . . Grumbach, K. (2010). *The roles of patient-centered medical homes and Accountable Care Organizations in coordinating patient care.* (AHRQ Pub. No. 11-M005-EF). Rockville, MD: Agency for Healthcare Research and Quality. Retrieved from https://pcmh.ahrq.gov/sites/default/files/attachments/Roles%20of%20PCMHs%20And%20 ACOs%20in%20Coordinating%20Patient%20Care.pdf

Misra, A. & Tsai, T. (2015, February 9). Health insurance marketplace 2015: Average premiums after advance premium tax credits through January 30 in 37 states using the healthcare.gov platform from the Office of the Assistant Secretary of Planning and Evaluation. Retrieved from https://aspe.hhs.gov/ report/health-insurance-marketplace-2015-average-premiums-after-advance-premium-tax-credits-through-january-30-37-states-using-healthcaregov-platform

Muhlestein, D. (2015, March 31). Growth and dispersion of Accountable Care Organizations in 2015 [Health Affairs Blog]. Retrieved from http://healthaffairs.org/blog/2015/03/31/growth-and-dispersion-of-accountable-care-organizations-in-2015-2/

Musumeci, M. (2012). A guide to the Supreme Court's Affordable Care Act decision (Issue Brief Pub. No. 8332). Retrieved from https://kaiserfamilyfoundation.files.wordpress.com/2013/01/8332.pdf

Office of the Assistant Secretary for Planning and Evaluation (ASPE), U.S. Department of Health and Human Services. (2011, November 1). At risk: Pre-existing conditions could affect 1 in 2 Americans. Retrieved from https://aspe.hhs.gov/basic-report/risk-pre-existing-conditions-could-affect-1-2-americans

Office of the Assistant Secretary for Planning and Evaluation (ASPE), U.S. Department of Health and Human Services. (2015, September 22). Health insurance coverage and the Affordable Care Act. Retrieved from https://aspe.hhs.gov/basic-report/health-insurance-coverage-and-affordable-care-act-september-2015

Rittenhouse, D. R., & Shortell, S. M. (2009). The patient-centered medical home: Will it stand the test of health reform? *The Journal of the American Medical Association, 301*, 2038–2040. doi: 10.1001/ jama.2009.691

Saltman, R. B., Busse, R., & Figueras, J. (Eds.). (2004). *Social health insurance systems in Western Europe.* Berkshire, England: Open University Press. Retrieved from http://www.who.int/health_financing/ documents/shi_w_europe.pdf

Schoen, C. (2016). *The Affordable Care Act and the U.S. Economy: A five-year perspective* (Pub. No. 1860). New York, NY: The Commonwealth Fund. Retrieved from http://www.commonwealthfund.org/~/ media/files/publications/fund-report/2016/feb/1860_schoen_aca_and_us_economy_v2.pdf

Snyder, L., Rudowitz, R., Dadayan, L., & Boyd, D. (2015). *Economic and fiscal trends in expansion and non-expansion states: What we know leading up to 2014* (Issue Brief). Menlo Park, CA: The Kaiser Commission on Medicaid and the Uninsured, The Kaiser Family Foundation. Retrieved from http:// files.kff.org/attachment/issue-brief-economic-and-fiscal-trends-in-expansion-and-non-expansion-states-what-we-know-leading-up-to-2014

Stanhope, V., Videka, L., Thorning, H., & McKay, M. (2015). Moving toward integrated health: An opportunity for social work. *Social Work in Health Care, 54*, 383–407. doi: 10.1080/00981389.2015.1025122

Xenakis, N. (2015). The role of social work leadership: Mount Sinai Care, the Accountable Care Organization, and population health management. *Social Work in Health Care, 54*, 782–809. doi: 10.1080/ 00981389.2015.1059399

CHAPTER 6

HEALTH CARE FINANCING

Peter C. Campanelli, Andrew F. Cleek, and Mary M. McKay

When President Barack Obama took office in 2008, he faced a number of formidable financial challenges, one of which was the escalating cost of health care. Health care expenses in the United States were $2.8 trillion per year, which amounted to 16% of the country's gross national product (Barr, 2011). The nation was spending more than any other industrialized country on an advanced health care system but still ranked 37th in terms of health outcomes. The president and many experts came to a similar conclusion: health care dollars were being spent in the wrong places on the wrong things, resulting in a system characterized by serious health and care disparities.

To understand how the country's health care system arrived at a place where the Patient Protection and Affordable Care Act (ACA) was critically needed, it is essential to understand the evolution of health care in the United States and the attendant power struggles that shaped the health care financing structure. For decades, the United States rejected the belief of the World Health Organization and many other industrialized nations that health care is a fundamental human right. Instead, with the exception of Medicare and Medicaid, the nation viewed health care as a marketplace commodity predicated on one's ability to pay (Barr, 2011). This commodity view is the reason millions of Americans remained uninsured or marginally insured.

This chapter reviews the evolution of fee-for-service (FFS) care in the United States and the range of forces that worked to maintain this financing strategy. The policy and public implications of the FFS system and the professional interests that may be gained from it are also discussed. A review of health care financing is not complete without considering the evolution and role of Medicare, the federally funded health insurance for elderly people, and Medicaid, the health insurance for indigent and disabled people that is funded by a combination of federal and state dollars. The chapter also considers the role of managed care within the commercial and government insurance marketplaces as one effort to control costs and redirect spending and explores the concept of value-based purchasing (VBP) as a set of incentives designed to encourage quality of care over quantity of care.

MEDICARE AND MEDICAID

Despite the many promises of the ACA, its passage and implementation have been controversial, as were Medicare and Medicaid. Although these programs differed in terms of their intent, structure, and the people they aimed to help, their 45-year history is instructive in understanding the government's current approach to health care and the backdrop for VBP structures.

President Lyndon B. Johnson, a Democrat who championed social justice issues under his Great Society mantra, enjoyed a cooperative Democratic majority in Congress. Political unity enabled President Johnson to develop and enact Medicare and Medicaid in 1965, using the legislative framework provided by the Social Security Act of 1935. Financial considerations also propelled these medical programs forward. Although the economy was prosperous, the health care system was expanding rapidly and required a large, stable funding stream to provide care to everyone in need. The medical profession was at first staunchly opposed to government interference. However, it soon realized that Medicare was likely the only program that could supply the funding needed to care for people who were elderly and disabled.

Medicare was originally composed of two parts. Part A paid for hospital costs and was derived entirely from employment tax revenues, and Part B paid for provider or practitioner costs and was copaid by the covered individual. This arranged formula stipulated that the federal government was accountable for all hospital-based costs (Part A) and 75% of doctor-allowable costs (Part B), whereas the service user was responsible for the remaining 25% of doctor-allowable costs (Part B). In 2003, prescription coverage (Part D) was added (Barr, 2011) (see Chapter 4).

The positive impact of Medicare on the health of elderly people was clearly demonstrable and resulted from significant increases in access to and affordability of services (Davis & Reynolds, 1976). From 1965 to 1998, hospital use expanded faster for this group than for any other age category; however, whether there was an improvement in the *quality* of care delivered remains less clear. Medicare also experienced steep spending increases during this period, but the high costs were largely attributed to the FFS environment, which pays for the volume of services provided and does not explicitly address individual outcomes. In this system, providers are incentivized to deliver as many services as possible rather than prioritize the improvement of individual health. For example, a primary care doctor makes more money from briefly seeing six patients than from spending more time with one or two to understand their unique needs. If a patient does not get better and has to return for additional services, the doctor is also paid for that visit.

Medicare and Medicaid are different in many respects. Medicare is a broad-based insurance program for elderly people, with age as its primary eligibility criterion. Medicaid is an entitlement program for people affected by poverty or disability, with the principal eligibility criteria being income level and health status. Medicaid initially grew out of a federal aid program legislated by the 1960 Kerr-Mills Act, which distributed federal funds to states to help pay for indigent health care. This Medicaid precursor had four principal characteristics, which have largely been retained in the current Medicaid program and continue to influence VBP financing:

1. State and federal funds were combined to pay for care to the poor.
2. Eligibility for the program was tied to eligibility for cash welfare grants.
3. Administration was carried out at the state level and was subject to each state's discretion under broad federal guidelines.
4. As long as the broad federal guidelines were followed, each state was free to set its own level of additional benefits (Barr, 2011).

As indicated by these characteristics, Medicaid is administered by the states with various sets of optional services and levels of access. Optional services by states may include the following:

- Prescriptions
- Institutional care for intellectual and developmental disabilities
- Home- and community-based care
- Dental and vision services

In an attempt to incentivize states to use the Medicaid program, federal subsidies were based on a complex formula that relied on the relative wealth (i.e., income level) of each state, with the federal government covering 50% to 75% of Medicaid costs. For a state Medicaid program to be eligible for federal funding participation, it must provide the following basic services:

- Hospital care (inpatient and outpatient)
- Nursing home care
- Physician services
- Laboratory and x-ray services
- Immunization and preventive medicine for children
- Family planning services
- Services provided at federally approved community clinics
- Nurse midwife and nurse practitioner services

In an additional effort to ensure participation by hospitals and other providers in Medicare and Medicaid, Congress mandated that hospitals and providers be reimbursed for the services rendered to Medicare and Medicaid recipients at "reasonable costs," which were usually interpreted by provider groups with considerable liberty (Weiner, 1977). It was quickly realized that this rate-setting method did not represent sound public policy, and rate setting was consequently shifted into the hands of the payors. Audit standards emerged to keep close track of provider expenses and emphasized efficiency, use, and planning. However, no mention was made of the expected outcome of a service or the measurement of its quality. Thus, a rate-setting method was established that many viewed as balanced but that nonetheless resulted in an inherent conflict between the government's need to control costs and its responsibility to fairly reimburse providers.

The costs of Medicaid grew even more rapidly than those of Medicare. Between 1975 and 1989, Medicaid costs increased an average of 11.9% per year, for a total net increase of approximately 166%; between 1989 and 1993, the average increase was 21.2% per year (Barr, 2011). Overall, these surges in spending added considerable cost burdens to federal and state budgets. The common misconception is that these escalations were caused only by an increase in the number of people living in poverty. However, a closer examination of spending across the nation reveals that the increase in service use was concentrated primarily among elderly and non-elderly disabled people who accessed Medicaid for long-term care services (e.g., nursing homes) that were not covered by Medicare. During those periods, states (to the extent permitted) shifted the cost of care for these populations from the local to the federal level via the Medicaid cost-sharing formulas.

Although the primary goal of Medicaid was to offer relief from the FFS system for those affected by poverty or disability, the program often failed to do so. Many people who earned above the federal poverty level (FPL) still earned too little to purchase health insurance privately, did not receive insurance as part of their employment benefits, or were excluded from the private insurance market due to preexisting health conditions regardless of their ability to pay. Financial eligibility for Medicaid was uniform across states before 2010, but tremendous disparities emerged nevertheless. For example, spending per beneficiary was $3168 in California and $3892 in Georgia but $8450 in New York and $8796 in Rhode Island (Barr, 2011).

There was an obvious and pervasive sense of apathy among states about providing medical care to people who were poor and indigent, as well as a paucity of financial resources. The fundamental national indifference was reflected in the Supreme Court's 2012 ruling that Medicaid expansion of the ACA—an essential component of the strategy to ensure that individuals impacted by poverty were uniformly eligible for health insurance—could not be mandated by the federal government to the states (see Chapter 5). At that time, 14 states announced that they would not expand their Medicaid programs to accommodate people above the FPL threshold, and as a result, 3.6 million people failed to obtain health care insurance (Price & Eibner, 2013).

EMERGENCE OF MANAGED CARE

An employee-based system of health care emerged during the post–World War II era. This period also gave rise to commercial insurance plans known as *indemnity plans*, which reimbursed individuals for the care that they arranged on their own after a modest copayment was given to the provider or a deductible was met for hospital expenses, or both. Unlike life insurance, which is profitable to the seller because it is betting that the individual will not die before he or she pays sufficient premiums to cover the insurance benefit, health insurance is used more frequently as the individual ages and is subject to cost escalation as medical technology and pharmacy advances occur. Commercial plans, which typically set aside 25% of the premiums collected for profit and overhead, found that their medical expenses exceeded 75% of the premiums collected from employers each year (i.e., >75% medical loss ratio). Consequently, they began the practice of adding the previous year's losses to the succeeding year's premiums.

Employers seeking relief from escalating premiums turned to contracting with health maintenance organizations (HMOs). This type of managed care organization (MCO) attempts to capture cost savings through a vertical integration model in which a single company is responsible for both the insurance risk of the individual and the provision of care. Put simply, the insurance company employs the doctors and also owns the hospital. An early example was Kaiser Permanente (Bodenheimer & Grumbach, 2012). HMOs accepted so-called *capitated contracts*, which limited payment for each recipient of care during an entire contractual period, regardless of how much or how little care was provided. These plans were the early versions of *profit and loss corridors* within capitated managed care contracts, in which an insurance company gets a set amount of money for each person whom it insures. This development also set the stage for VBP financing.

MCOs expanded during the 1980s, partly in response to the failure of HMOs to provide the kind of cost savings needed and partly because many were for-profit enterprises that saw a chance to wring out inefficiency and reap large profits. Most types of MCOs were practically integrated, in that managed care insurance companies contracted with disconnected community-based hospitals and provider groups while integrating their operations under service delivery rules, capitated rates, and service preauthorization rules. Managed care experienced an initial success and a one-time cost savings, mostly by restricting care through the denial of services that were not deemed to be medically necessary or by not providing payment for certain services regardless of their benefits. However, it was difficult for MCOs to maintain cost savings without cutting into necessary care to realize further savings (Barr, 2011). Gradually, MCOs became enormously unpopular with the general public, who saw themselves as being deprived of necessary care for the sake of corporate profits, and providers resented receiving inadequate rates at the same time that MCO executives earned large salaries and benefits.

In the meantime, federal and state government budgets continued to increase due to unsustainable cost overruns associated with FFS models of care and inefficiency, ineffectiveness, and abuse due to billing for inappropriate services or services that did not occur. Health care quality and outcomes continued to be separated from payment methods and service delivery and were misaligned with incentives that could have been used to improve the system. Providers were incentivized to perform the highest number of services so as to make the most amount of money; conversely, insurance companies made the most money by paying for the least number of services. There continued to be a lack of financial incentive for improved care or outcomes, and the result was a broken system that required a transformative overhaul.

TRANSFORMATIVE FINANCING

An analysis of the health care spending patterns in the United States in this era reveals several underlying problems, including lack of adequate insurance for a significant percentage of the population. This lack of insurance led to overuse of expensive emergency and hospital-based care. Additionally, private insurance companies were allowed to cherry-pick low-risk and healthy populations while leaving high-risk and chronically ill populations without insurance; they did this by setting rules that did not allow coverage for individuals with pre-existing conditions. A redesign of the U.S. health care system was required, and any redesign had to consider the nature of the interactions among cost, quality, and coverage (Bellin, 2015).

While managed care programs within the commercial marketplace continued to draw negative attention, states continued to move Medicaid populations into these managed care programs, most often within companies that were organized as for-profit corporations, in an effort to control costs. Medicaid managed care utilized strategies similar to those of commercial managed care to reduce costs. These included:

- Obtaining preauthorizations for care
- Using low-cost technologies and treatments before authorizing higher-cost approaches (especially for pharmacies)
- Establishing narrow networks of authorized providers based on their proven abilities to provide high-quality and low-cost services
- Lowering rates paid to providers based on the belief that revenue could be made up through volume (Bellin, 2015)

Most MCOs complained that the complexity of the population being served required flexibility, which was not permitted by Medicaid regulations. States petitioned the federal government to issue various Medicaid waivers, enabling more flexible use of funding by the MCOs. The federal government agreed but retained the right to conduct periodic reviews because the concern about for-profit managed care still loomed large, especially for people who were poor and/or disabled. In addition, payment bonus methods began to emerge to induce quality and create financial holdbacks for failure to meet expected quality outcome benchmarks. These changes formed the basis of a financial structure that would connect quality with outcome (Bellin, 2015).

ACCOUNTABLE CARE

Faced with considerable cost overruns on the Medicare side of government health care financing, Congress began to enact laws that permitted a fair amount of flexibility in what types of organizations could take insurance risks. The Centers for Medicare and Medicaid Services (CMS) Innovation Center, established by the ACA, authorized the creation of accountable care organizations (ACOs) as pilot projects designed to reduce the cost of care for elderly people. The ACA also provided financial incentives for ACOs through its Medicare Shared Savings Program, which established a mechanism for sharing the savings with ACOs that demonstrated improved quality and cost savings. ACO eligibility was limited to organizations that had the capacity to form networks, were able to manage large systems of care, and had sufficient technology and data infrastructure capacity. ACOs

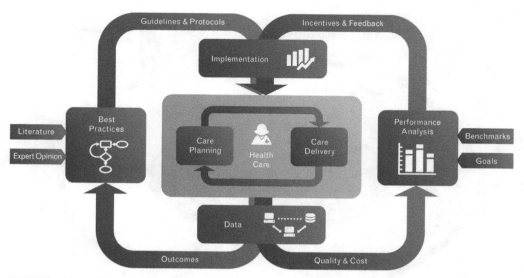

FIGURE 6.1: How accountable care organizations work. Reprinted with permission from "The Humunculus is a Metaphor for Clinical Process Improvement Frameworks," by R. E. Ward, 2011 (http://rewardhealth.com/archives/1975#more-1975). Copyright 2016 by Reward Health Sciences, Inc.

tend to be organized and led by hospitals, university medical centers, large independent practice associations (IPAs), and MCOs.

The first ACOs in Medicare were operated by IPAs and focused on elderly individuals, many of whom had chronic illnesses for which there were established therapeutic benchmark targets of care. Early ACOs were quite successful at improving outcomes and reducing costs. One of the reasons for the success of the predominantly Medicare ACOs was that they consolidated care, thereby limiting fragmentation and establishing continuity. Under an ACO system, providers faced reductions in future bonus payments for a portion of spending when they failed to meet clinical benchmarks or exceeded their budgets. In the fifth performance year of a 10-year pilot, all 10 of the physician groups achieved benchmark performance on at least 30 of the 32 measures established by Medicare (Kocot, Dang-Vu, White, & McClellan, 2013).

Based on the early successful results, Congress converted the ACO legislation from pilot to permanent status, and CMS permitted expansion of the program (Kocot et al., 2013). ACOs rely heavily on evidence-based practices, effective implementation and care planning on the input side and on outcome data and quality analysis on the output side (see Figure 6.1). ACOs also rely on the formation of effective community-based networks of care. Bonus payments in the form of shared savings are based on outcome-dependent data analysis. By mid-2013, Medicare included more than 250 ACOs that were serving more than 4 million traditional Medicare beneficiaries.

Medicaid has organized ACOs in terms of geographically proximate networks of service, most of which are clinically and functionally integrated (see Figure 6.2). Community-based providers with entire arrays of community-based social services are also included in this network as independent providers. In many states, the development of ACOs has

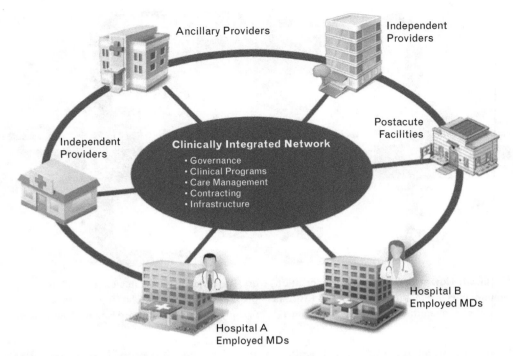

FIGURE 6.2: Accountable care organization networks in Medicaid. From "Clinically Integrated Networks: You Can't Stop Change, But You Can Control Your Momentum," by Daniel J. Marino, 2015 (http://blog.thecamdengroup.com/blog/bid/360171/Clinically-Integrated-Networks-You-Can-t-Stop-Change-But-You-Can-Control-Your-Momentum). Copyright 2015 by GE Healthcare Camden Group.

been encouraged financially by advanced funding from the federal government, with future funding predicated on savings to be realized as the ACO becomes fully functional.

VALUE-BASED PURCHASING IN HEALTH CARE

The financing system of health care in the United States has evolved over the past 50 years, gradually moving toward a more inclusive and integrated approach. However, much work needs to be done to eliminate health disparities and integrate care in a manner that is seamless for service users and providers. A largely unaddressed factor is the issue of quality. None of the major segments of insurance (i.e., Medicaid, Medicare, and commercial firms) have designed payment mechanisms to incentivize quality in a systemic way.

To address this issue, there has been a national movement to develop methods of VBP. VBP involves any model in which insurers and providers of care share in the risks for the costs of services and receive payments based on achieved outcomes. In this context, providers lose funding if they do not achieve certain outcome, and they receive extra payments for positive individual outcomes. VBP requires each part of the Triple Aim (i.e., reduced costs, improved population health, and enhanced service user experience) to be met for an arrangement to be successful. To achieve this, a set of metrics must be put into place that holds all parties accountable for quality of care. The Agency for Healthcare Research and Quality (2011) breaks quality measures into three broad categories:

1. Structural measures are those that identify processes, programs, or certifications that an organization has achieved. They can include use of an electronic health record or credentialing of a certain number of clinicians in a particular practice.

2. Process measures are the most common measurements of providers in value-based arrangements. They involve actions that a provider takes with a service user or a group of service users that have been shown to achieve better outcomes. Common process measures include outpatient follow-up after a hospitalization to ensure continuity of care, checking blood sugar levels in people with diabetes, and assessment of postpartum depression in new mothers.

3. Clinical measures address the actual impacts of provided services. A clinical measure indicates whether an individual's health has improved. Although clinical measures highlight the outcomes of interventions, pinpointing the causes of those outcomes may be more complicated. For example, if an individual's blood sugar level improves, is it because of the work of a primary care physician or because the individual began to eat healthier after nutrition counseling at a local social service agency? In this case, how should a bonus payment be assigned?

To determine any VBP arrangement, a shared savings agreement and quality indicators are combined to arrive at payment terms. For a provider to receive incentive payments or share in savings with the payor, both conditions must be met. This rule is designed to incentivize brief but effective interventions and to deter a move to achieve profit through high-volume low-quality services or to restrict care to reduce costs.

The concept of financial risk is key to the development of a VBP arrangement. A traditional FFS system assigns all risk to the payors and reimburses providers according to their volume of services, with no regard for quality. However, MCOs benefit most by reducing the number of services provided (i.e., restricting care). The ACA has worked to address this issue of restricting care by insisting on a minimum medical loss ratio that requires the plan to spend a specific percentage of its capitation on individual care. In a VBP arrangement, the incentives are further realigned to promote high-quality and cost-effective services that reduce the likelihood of higher-cost services in the future, such as hospitalization. In this model, savings are derived from avoiding expensive services; providers and plans then share in those savings. The Medicare Shared Savings Program, designed to incentivize ACOs, is one example of a value based purchasing strategy. As this movement continues, and payors experiment with different VBP models, we can expect to see a much closer relationship between health outcomes and payment.

IMPLICATIONS FOR SOCIAL WORK

The ACA and VBP have several implications for social workers, particularly those who are engaged in direct practice or in the administration of direct practice agencies. In past decades, there has been a trend in both private and agency-based work to increase the volume of services provided in order to increase revenue. A move toward VBPs may reduce some of the pressure to provide a high volume of services and increase the emphasis on providing services that produce the most benefit. Regardless of the specific form that VBP structures take, social workers will be required to demonstrate the effectiveness of these services at individual and systemic levels. Demonstration of outcomes will involve being able to show both clinical effectiveness and the way in which clinical improvement is connected to the cost of services. A practitioner or provider agency will need to gather and analyze data as evidence for the outcomes their services can be expected to achieve for certain populations at an acceptable cost. In addition to being able to demonstrate these outcomes to an MCO, providers must develop internal cost models to determine whether a particular contract is financially feasible.

With the transition to VBP arrangements, there may be more opportunity for provider specialization. The FFS model has not incentivized MCOs to seek specialized providers, but VBP will likely lead to increased opportunities for social workers who can demonstrate improved outcomes for particular populations. For example, if a provider is skilled at providing time-limited services shown to reduce anxiety, he or she will be more attractive to an MCO than a general practitioner who has demonstrated few similar outcomes. Social workers employed under VBP arrangements need to cultivate affiliations and partnerships with other entities. As ACOs and other arrangements emerge, practitioners and agencies must develop contractual relationships with them to ensure referrals and payments.

CONCLUSIONS

Use of a value-based approach to determine payment arrangements in health care holds much promise for progression toward the Triple Aim of more affordable and effective services that meet the expressed needs of service users. At this time, however, VBP arrangements are not widely used and are just beginning to achieve prominence in the health care system. Several examples of fully integrated systems have been operating successfully for many years, including Kaiser Permanente and the Cleveland Clinic, but little is known about whether these systems are scalable to the rest of the health care system or how individual care and provider organizations would be affected. Another concern is whether these systems can be fully integrated under one corporate entity, operate collectively through IPAs, or develop some other structure. It is also unclear what the impact will be on small community-based organizations that address the social determinants of health. It is uncertain whether VBP, when taken to scale, can ultimately lead to a health care system in which all members of society can expect access to high-quality services that meet their needs.

RESOURCES

Accountable Care Organizations (ACOs), Centers for Medicare & Medicaid Services (CMS) https://www.cms.gov/Medicare/Medicare-Fee-for-Service-Payment/ACO/index.html?redirect=/aco

Center for Value-Based Insurance Design (V-BID), University of Michigan http://vbidcenter.org/

The Commonwealth Fund http://www.commonwealthfund.org/

The Facts on Medicare Spending and Financing, The Kaiser Family Foundation (KFF) http://kff.org/medicare/fact-sheet/medicare-spending-and-financing-fact-sheet/

Families USA http://familiesusa.org/

Health Care Financing, Management Sciences for Health (MSH) https://www.msh.org/our-work/health-system/health-care-financing

Health Care Incentives Improvement Institute (HCI3) http://www.hci3.org/

Health Systems Financing, World Health Organization (WHO) http://www.who.int/healthsystems/topics/financing/en/

Institute for Healthcare Improvement (IHI) http://www.ihi.org

National Business Coalition on Health (NBCH) http://www.nbch.org

National Compendium on Payment Reform, Catalyst for Payment Reform (CPR) http://compendium.catalyzepaymentreform.org/

Payment Reform and ACOs, Massachusetts Medical Society (MMS) http://www.massmed.org/Advocacy/Key-Issues/Payment-Reform/Payment-Reform-and-ACOs/#.V6JiRGPcYto

REFERENCES

Agency for Healthcare Research and Quality (2011, July). Types of quality measures. Retrieved from http://www.ahrq.gov/professionals/quality-patient-safety/talkingquality/create/types.html

Barr, D. A. (2011). *Introduction to U.S. health policy: The organization, financing, and delivery of health care in America* (3rd ed.). Baltimore, MD: Johns Hopkins University.

Bodenheimer, T., & Grumbach, K. (2012). *Understanding health policy: A clinical approach* (6th ed.). New York, NY: McGraw-Hill Medical.

Bellin, E. (2015). *Riddles in accountable healthcare: A primer to develop analytic intuition for medical homes and population health.* North Charleston, SC: CreateSpace Independent Publishing Platform of Amazon.

Davis, K., & Reynolds, R. (1976). The impact of Medicare and Medicaid on access to medical care. In R. N. Rosett (Ed.) *The role of health insurance in the health services sector* (pp. 391–436). Cambridge, MA: The National Bureau of Economic Research.

Kocot, S. L., Dang-Vu C., White, R. & McClellan, M. (2013). Early experiences with accountable care in Medicaid: Special challenges, big opportunities. *Population Health Management, 16*(Suppl. 1), S4–S11. doi: 10.1089/pop.2013.0058

Marino, D. J. (2015, January 20). Clinically integrated networks: You can't stop change, but you can control your momentum [Blog post]. Retrieved from http://blog.thecamdengroup.com/blog/bid/360171/Clinically-Integrated-Networks-You-Can-t-Stop-Change-But-You-Can-Control-Your-Momentum

Price, C. C., & Eibner, C. (2013). For states that opt out of Medicaid expansion: 3.6 million fewer insured and $8.4 billion less in federal payments. *Health Affairs, 32,* 1030–1036. doi: 10.1377/hlthaff.2012.1019

Ward R.E. (2011, December 10). The humunculus is a metaphor for clinical process improvement frameworks [Blog post]. Retrieved from http://rewardhealth.com/archives/1975#more-1975

Weiner, S. M. (1977). "Reasonable cost" reimbursement for inpatient hospital services under Medicare and Medicaid: The emergence of public control. *American Journal of Law and Medicine, 3,* 1–47.

CHAPTER 7

WORKFORCE DEVELOPMENT

Anthony Salerno, Jeff Capobianco, and Larry Fricks

Three major factors will dramatically affect workforce needs in the near future: the aging of the population, the changing racial and ethnic composition of the United States, and the health reforms initiated by the 2010 Patient Protection and Affordable Care Act (ACA). The needs of the aging population, especially in behavioral health, will increasingly require specialized expertise. Unfortunately, the number of behavioral health practitioners focusing on the needs of elderly people is grossly insufficient (Institute of Medicine, 2012).

Minority populations in the United States comprise about 40% of the total population (Humes, Jones, & Ramirez, 2011). Changing demographics pose daunting challenges for service providers to ensure an adequate number of practitioners with culturally competent approaches to care. A federal report revealed that practitioners from nonwhite minority backgrounds accounted for only 19.2% of psychiatrists, 5.1% of psychologists, 17.5% of social workers, 10.3% of counselors, and 7.8% of marriage and family therapists (Substance Abuse and Mental Health Services Administration [SAMHSA], 2012). Because minority populations are more likely to struggle with poverty, unemployment, health disparities, homelessness, limited education, and language barriers that affect access to behavioral health services, the insufficient number of behavioral health practitioners with diverse backgrounds compared with the size of the minority population is likely to affect engagement and access to services (Clay, 2015).

The aging of the workforce contributes to the disparity between the demand for behavioral health services and the supply, particularly in rural communities. According to the Bureau of Labor Statistics, the median age of professionals who work in the mental health and substance abuse fields is 42 years for social workers and counselors, 50 years for psychologists, and 56 years for psychiatrists. Data reveal a looming crisis in the supply of psychiatrists because 46% of current practitioners are older than 65 years of age (SAMHSA, 2013). As the current workforce retires, there will be an insufficient number of new practitioners to meet the need for behavioral health services. The solution will require a multipronged approach involving higher salaries, improved working conditions, opportunities for advancement, elevation of the status of behavioral health practitioners, and incentives to attract individuals to underserved areas. Hoge, Morris, Laraia, Pomerantz, and Farley (2014) emphasized that the workforce must be sufficient in size, diversity, cultural awareness, and cultural competence to successfully apply core skills and knowledge when delivering services in organizational contexts that guide and reinforce the best practices within and between integrated teams.

This chapter describes the numerous forces influencing the development of a workforce that is sufficient in number, composition, and training to effectively function in an integrated system of behavioral and physical health care. Efforts to improve the quality of health care services require a workforce with the values, knowledge, and skills to collaborate, coordinate, and work in interprofessional teams. This chapter describes how to prepare such a workforce, with an emphasis on the unique contribution of the social work profession in a system that is based on a whole-health perspective, equity, multidisciplinary collaboration, system-wide coordination, and integration of care.

INVESTING IN THE HEALTH CARE WORKFORCE

Health care reform will have a significant impact on the capacities of state and local governments and service providers to meet the needs of an expanding number of recently insured individuals. Efforts are underway to invest in expansion and quality improvement of the workforce to meet the challenges raised by increased access to behavioral health care services as a result of the expansion of Medicaid under the ACA and the parity laws. A recent analysis projected that health care reform will expand substance abuse and mental health services to more than 60 million people (Uberoi, Finegold, & Gee, 2016). There are serious concerns and uncertainty regarding the ability of the ACA workforce development provisions to keep pace with the anticipated need.

At the federal level, the U.S. Department of Health and Human Services (DHHS) is responsible for oversight of all aspects of Medicaid and Medicare funding, including workforce improvement grants and system redesign waivers. Unlike grants, waivers allow states to use federal Medicaid and/or Medicare funding to redesign how health care is delivered. This has a direct impact on the behavior of the health care workforce because this group of professionals assists with the creation of new system design initiatives. Examples of waiver mechanisms that have had a significant direct impact on health care workers are the Medicaid Health Home waivers and Medicare Accountable Care Organization (ACO) waivers.

Medicaid Health Home waivers allow states to design health care delivery provider networks that treat Medicaid recipients who have multiple physical and behavioral health conditions. Health care staff working in states adopting this program are required to change their practice approaches to meet the new demands associated with a wellness and whole-health focused approach to care provision. ACO waivers are Medicare waivers that allow providers to develop provider networks that agree to work together to be accountable for all of the health care needs of a defined group of no fewer than 5000 service users in the network catchment area. In Health Homes and ACOs, providers are responsible for demonstrating quality metrics (i.e., indicators that demonstrate service user health improvement) in exchange for flexible funding arrangements (see Chapter 5). Health care workers in these waiver states are experiencing a shift toward interprofessional, team-based care within and across providers. All health care staff members are required to have at least functional knowledge of prevention and chronic care approaches for mental illnesses, substance use problems, and physical health conditions. One of the biggest workforce findings in the states where health care services are being redesigned in this way is the need for staff to learn how to manage and coordinate care among various health care disciplines.

The ACA recognizes and promotes significant investment in the workforce of the future to achieve the Triple Aim. The strategies for achieving this goal include increases in the supply of health care professionals through state grants, loan repayment programs, and scholarships (Institute for Healthcare Improvement, 2016). This approach has enabled the ACA to directly address projected shortages in areas such as nursing through the provision of grants to employ and provide training to family nurse practitioners who deliver primary care in Federally Qualified Health Centers (FQHCs) and nurse-managed health clinics (Redhead, Lister, Colello, Sarata, & Heisler, 2013). The ACA invests resources to increase graduate-level medical education training positions in primary care in the most underserved communities.

PRIMARY AND BEHAVIORAL HEALTH CARE INTEGRATION GRANTS

Since 2010, SAMHSA, in collaboration with the Health Resources and Services Administration (HRSA), has funded the Primary and Behavioral Health Care Integration (PBHCI) grants to support integration models designed to coordinate care for individuals with the most challenging behavioral and physical health problems. Support for these models will require a workforce guided by a new set of values, knowledge, and skills (SAMHSA, 2016). PBHCI grants have been awarded to more than 200 behavioral health agencies that have established their own health care services or partnerships with primary care providers, developed comprehensive care coordination supports, and offered wellness and illness prevention programs designed to promote highly accessible health services.

In addition to grants, the PBHCI initiative has established a technical assistance entity, the Center for Integrated Health Solutions (CIHS). CIHS provides an extensive array of resources and supports to grantees and to the general public and health care providers across the country who focus on the best practices in health-promoting services such as tobacco cessation, weight management, chronic disease self-management, and substance abuse treatment. Attention is also given to helping these parties build effective partnerships with primary care services. CIHS offers grantees access to national experts in integrated health care subject areas and state-specific information on the financing of integrated health care–related services (CIHS, 2016a). The PBHCI initiative continues to receive support from Congress and will disseminate information in communities throughout the nation. The bidirectionality of integration that expands the accessibility of behavioral health services in health centers has also gained momentum with grants and payment systems designed to make services accessible to underserved communities in settings such as FQHCs (Rural Health Information Hub, 2015).

HEALTH RESOURCES AND SERVICES ADMINISTRATION

HRSA is a federal agency that is an integral part of DHHS and is charged with ensuring that U.S. citizens who are geographically isolated and economically or medically vulnerable receive quality health care services. The ACA provided HRSA with workforce improvement funding opportunities in five areas: student loan repayment to health care providers who agree to work in federally designated health professional shortage areas; primary care provider training and training program enhancements; health professions training for diversity; programming of interdisciplinary, community-based linkages; and health professions and public health workforce improvements. Unfortunately, the U.S. Congress approved only a small portion of these ACA-appropriated discretionary funds.

Workforce funding to HRSA that was made mandatory for reauthorization by the ACA largely consisted of tax-free loan repayment programs designed to support qualified child, adult, and geriatric health care providers who choose to take their medical and behavioral health care skills to the most underserved communities. In 2012, Congress approved ten million dollars in discretionary funding for HRSA to fund behavioral health education and training grants. These grants recruited and educated students with training in social work and psychology and created internships and other field placement programs related to child and adolescent mental health. Special focus was devoted to recruiting from and placing graduates into areas with high-need and high-demand populations (Redhead et al., 2013). The following case is an example of one of the HRSA grants awarded to New York University's (NYU) Silver School of Social Work (SSSW) to train social work students in integrated health care.

CASE VIGNETTE

Funded by the HRSA training grant, SSSW partnered with the NYU Schools of Nursing and Dentistry and two large community-based organizations—the Institute for Community Living (ICL) and Community Access (CA)—to create the NYU Integrated Behavioral Health Project (NYU-IBH). NYU-IBH was developed to implement and examine the impact of a focused learning opportunity for students seeking a master's degree in social work (MSW); this consisted of an integrated and interdisciplinary curriculum bringing together classroom content and field education. Through this specialized training, NYU-IBH focused on preparing emerging social work professionals to provide interdisciplinary, integrated health care services to people who struggle with severe mental health challenges.

NYU-IBH trained participants from the NYU MSW program and the staff from the partnered community-based organizations (i.e., ICL and CA). As part of this program, selected students engaged in specialized training consisting of interdisciplinary, elective coursework at the SSSW, the NYU School of Nursing, and the NYU School of Dentistry. Social work students learned about community nursing and the importance of oral health. Students also joined agency staff in a class on collaboration with peers. In conjunction with this classroom instruction, students received real-world training and supervisory support while completing field placements at the partnering community-based agencies. This training focused on developing evidence-informed competencies related to integrated health, including management of mental and physical health challenges, crisis and trauma care, parenting, and overall economic empowerment. All classroom and field instructors were guided by a competency-based, interdisciplinary curriculum and faculty manuals developed by NYU-IBH. The long-term goal of NYU-IBH was to transform the behavioral health and health curriculum at SSSW, train the next generation of social workers, and enhance community-based social work staff competency in integrated health.

ROLES OF EDUCATIONAL INSTITUTIONS AND NONPROFITS

The role of higher education in the development of an educated workforce able to provide an integrated system of care is critical. Although progress in this area is slow, several promising efforts are trying to ensure that professional educational institutions train health care professionals to meet the needs of the changing health care environment. Several graduate certificate programs have been specifically created to train health care professionals in the theory and practice of integrated health care (McSilver Institute for Poverty Policy and Research, n.d.; University of Massachusetts Medical School, n.d.; University of Michigan School of Social Work, 2016).

Accreditation bodies play an important role, albeit indirectly, by influencing educational institutions, providers, and the health care workforce as a whole. These bodies are responsible for developing and monitoring standards specific to education and health care delivery. An example of an education accrediting body affecting the workforce is the Council on Social Work Education (CSWE), which is responsible for accrediting schools of social work. In collaboration with the National Council for Behavioral Health (the National Council) and with funding from the New York Community Trust, CSWE designed a program to provide social work graduate students with the critical knowledge and skills necessary to provide integrated health care (CSWE, n.d.).

CSWE's Social Work and Integrated Behavioral Healthcare Project connected 28 schools of social work in 19 states with local integrated primary and behavioral health care clinics to design, implement, and evaluate an educational experience for graduate social work students that combined classroom education with hands-on practice in integrated field placement settings. The project provided students with the critical knowledge and skills necessary to work effectively in the field of integrated health care. It also funded the creation of a graduate social work course curriculum that addressed policy and practice issues and was made available to any social work faculty member interested in expanding curriculum offerings for their students (CSWE, n.d.).

Other important resources for developing a workforce prepared for integrated health care are state and national provider associations. A provider association is an organization that represents a constituency of health care providers. One example of this is the National Council, which works with more than 2500 health care provider organizations across the United States. The National Council represents these providers by advocating for state and federal legislation to improve health care services while providing workforce training and technical assistance. The National Council has received DHHS funding, for example, to provide workforce training specific to integrated health through CIHS.

In addition to national organizations with investments in workforce development, many provider organizations, including hospitals, substance use disorder clinics, mental health centers, and primary care practices, are aggressively working to train their staff to deliver health care differently. This urgency comes from rapid changes in the health care marketplace created by the ACA and the increasing expectations of payors demanding value-based outcomes linked to the competencies of the workforce. Providers understand that they will lose funding and eventually go out of business if their staff does not begin delivering care in a whole-health, wellness-focused, and integrated way.

Individuals and their family members are also creating significant incentives for workforce care delivery changes. They are achieving this through their associations with advocacy groups such as the National Alliance on Mental Illness (NAMI) (Diehl et al., 2015). NAMI provides report cards that rate states based on how well providers deliver mental health services. Many internet-based rating services are available for individuals and family members to compare the performance of providers across several domains, including clinical outcomes and satisfaction. More than ever, the health care workforce is aware that people will not choose to receive their care unless they provide excellent customer service and value in the form of good clinical outcomes.

CHANGING THE FACE OF THE WORKFORCE

Recognition of the importance of engagement and outreach into communities has led to the emergence of new roles within the workforce. These practice roles are focused on spanning cultural and resource boundaries by connecting health care to the lives of people in the community. As a result, the understanding of *interdisciplinary practice* must broaden to include collaboration with and supervision of people in these new roles, and this requires an understanding and appreciation of their unique contributions to the health care field.

CIHS defines a *peer provider* as "a person who uses his or her lived experience of recovery from mental illness and/or addiction plus skills learned in formal training to deliver services in behavioral health settings to promote mind-body recovery and resiliency" (CIHS, 2016b, para. 1). In her 2010 book entitled *Within Our Reach*, former First Lady Rosalynn Carter argues that stigma, prejudice, and discrimination are still the biggest challenges in the field of behavioral health (Carter, Golant, & Cade, 2010). Mrs. Carter credits the new workforce of peer providers—many of whom have had experiences that include long-term hospitalization, trauma, social exclusion, and poverty—as major catalysts who have helped transform stigmatizing, stereotypical beliefs about individuals living with severe behavioral health conditions through their new and empowering roles that promote outcomes of recovery and resiliency (Carter et al., 2010). There is mounting evidence demonstrating the positive impact of peer services, including improved mental health and reduced hospitalization (Eiken and Campbell, 2008).

The services offered by peer providers are reimbursed by Medicaid. A rapidly growing workforce of peer providers are activating self-management to address chronic conditions by using their lived experiences and skills gained in training and by focusing on "what's strong" rather than "what's wrong." These new-wave providers are also proving to be powerful change agents for health integration by supporting those they serve to set person-centered, whole-health goals and by engaging in peer support to create new health behaviors. For example, the state of Georgia pioneered Medicaid-billable peer support services in 2001 under a new rehabilitative services state plan option. In evaluating the first 3 years of this new program compared with the standard day treatment, the Georgia Department of Behavioral Health and Developmental Disabilities found that service recipients who were teamed up with certified peer specialists experienced reductions in symptoms and increases in self-management skills and abilities. The peer service cost Georgia $997 per year on average, compared with $6491 in day treatment, a savings of $5494 per person (Purington, 2016).

Because peer services are Medicaid billable in most states, the practice has experienced huge growth and acceptance, particularly in the wake of the 2007 guidance sent to state Medicaid directors from CMS. The CMS guidelines laid out state-specific supervision, training, and/or certification requirements. In these guidelines, CMS stated, "Peer support services are an evidence-based mental health model of care, which consists of a qualified peer support provider who assists individuals with their recovery from mental illnesses and substance abuse disorders" (CMS, 2007). Medicaid-billable services delivered by peer providers may include care coordination, care management, individual and group counseling, whole-health behavior change, and peer-facilitated chronic disease self-management programs (Druss et al., 2010; Lorig, Sobel, Ritter, Laurent, & Hobbs, 2000). Peers are increasingly addressing the challenging problems related to high rates of smoking among adults with severe mental illnesses (Morris, 2009). Whole-health certified peer providers are becoming a vital part of integrated treatment teams and are serving in new settings. The contribution of peers through their unique understanding of service users' experiences and their ability to inspire hope, reduce stigma, and engage ambivalent service users is instrumental in promoting recovery, building resilience, improving outcomes, and reducing costs (Purington, 2016).

COMMUNITY HEALTH WORKERS

The American Public Health Association (APHA) defines a *community health worker* (CHW) as a "person who is a trusted member of and/or who has an unusually close understanding of the community served" and participates in the delivery of health-related services by working either directly with providers or with their partner organizations (APHA, 2016, p. 1). Similar to the peer workforce, the CHW workforce has community-based lived experiences with the health problems they are addressing. CHWs assist individuals and community organizations to build the knowledge, capacity, self-efficacy, and advocacy needed to impact the social determinants of health and help service structures address these challenges (APHA, 2016). Whether it is children with asthma or adult Medicaid recipients, CHWs have generated significantly improved health outcomes and cost savings for the health care system (Pittman, Sunderland, Broderick, & Barnett, 2015). However, similar to the struggles found with the adoption of peer providers, more specificity is needed regarding the essential job skills, scope of work, and practices so that CHWs can be designated for clinical care teams and funded through current and future billing mechanisms (Pittman et al., 2015).

PATIENT AND FAMILY NAVIGATORS

Newly defined roles such as *patient navigator* and *family navigator* are designed to span boundaries between patients and the health care financing and regulatory systems, as well as between patients and health care services, to overcome barriers to health insurance and health care. These important roles enable people, particularly the 25% of Americans who had been living without health insurance before passage of the ACA, to be recruited for health care insurance and to navigate the complex insurance system options. Patient and family navigator roles have also been creatively developed to help African-American women with positive breast cancer test results to seek and sustain care as a remedy to the racial disparities in breast cancer mortality and to help other populations (Jia, Yuan, Huang, Lu, Garner, & Meng, 2014).

TRAINING PROVIDERS FOR INTEGRATED HEALTH CARE

Workforce development does not take place in a vacuum. The most effective approach ensures an alignment of the values, knowledge, and skills of the workforce with the changing nature of the health care system. Many of the forces in play today will shape the needs of our future workforce, including the increasing number of ACOs, health homes, and patient-centered medical homes (see Chapter 5). Although the designs and models for each health care system vary, care coordination emerges as a critical core element in each. The current fragmented system is unlikely to achieve the Triple Aim without care coordination (Meyers et al., 2010).

These promising systems have, at their core, the need for a workforce prepared to function in networks and teams with care coordination. Through CMS, the ACA offers health care providers a range of ways to address the current fragmented system by promoting care coordination as a central service of a quality health care system (Brown et al., 2004). To achieve this goal, a clear definition of the principles, processes, and practices of care coordination are needed, including who will directly and indirectly play a role in care coordination and what knowledge and skills are needed. Not surprisingly, no single definition of care coordination has received widespread consensus.

Numerous studies have demonstrated that care coordination has a positive impact on health outcomes, overall costs, utilization of emergency care, and hospitalizations (Peikes, Chen, Schore, & Brown, 2009). Some of the key findings conclude that ongoing face-to-face interaction between service users and care coordinators to establish and maintain personal relationships is instrumental in achieving positive results. Targeted care coordination interventions are frequently most successful for high-risk, high-need individuals with chronic health conditions, behavioral health challenges, and chronic stress associated with poverty and social disconnection (Meyers et al., 2010). In the area of primary care, coordinated care that is comprehensive and initiated during the first contact with an individual is strongly associated with positive health outcomes and improved functioning of the health care system (Starfield, Shi, & Macinko, 2005).

There are two defining aspects of care coordination. The first relies on the transference and sharing of pertinent information from one provider to another, including communication about individual goals, medications, treatments, diagnoses, and precautions. The second aspect of care coordination concerns the establishment of accountability through the clear identification of team member roles and responsibilities. Care coordination is particularly important for individuals with complex physical and behavioral health needs who often require numerous services involving entities that rarely interact and that may face considerable challenges communicating and coordinating with each other.

To excel in care coordination, the workforce of the future needs to have competencies that allow for the development of strong relationships. Practitioners in direct care coordination or its supervision must have the knowledge and skills to assist people in accessing the full range of primary care and behavioral health services, as well as key supports in the social services system to address the social determinants of health, including the impacts of poverty, social isolation, discrimination, and racism on the overall wellbeing of individuals, families, and communities (see Chapter 3) (Clay, 2015).

A note of caution concerning the limits of coordinated care was suggested by a study of a highly coordinated system for adults struggling with substance use problems (Saitz et al., 2013). Individuals with severe substance use challenges were provided with an exhaustive array of coordinated and integrated health care supports. Researchers were surprised to discover that integrated health care coordination itself, without the presence of effective treatments delivered to the individual, demonstrated little benefit. The value of coordinated and integrated health care was directly related to the effectiveness and quality of the treatments for the specific substance use problem and the readiness of the individual to engage in treatment (Saitz et al., 2013). It appears that unless care coordination facilitates access to effective treatment interventions and fully engages the service user in his or her own care, the promises offered by a less fragmented system cannot be realized.

ORGANIZATIONAL READINESS

Establishment of best practice standards and competencies through formal classroom education, distance learning, and in-service training in the workplace alone is likely to be inadequate for ensuring quality practice in the absence of supportive organizational policies and procedures. Therefore, ongoing supervision designed to coach, mentor, and provide feedback on actual practice is an essential core competency of workforce development (Fixsen, Naoom, Blase, Friedman, & Wallace, 2005). Failure to recognize and develop comprehensive strategies to guide and reinforce the application of core competencies and best practices may result in a frustrated workforce with high levels of dissatisfaction and suboptimal performance (Fixsen et al., 2005).

A review of the research on competency development in a variety of industries, including human services, education, and medicine, concluded that "training by itself does not result in positive implementation outcomes (changes in practitioner behavior in the clinical setting) or intervention outcomes (benefits to consumers)" (Fixsen et al., 2005, p. 47). Learning new competencies for integrated health care needs supervisory feedback on performance in line with specific standards of best practices. We cannot rely on practitioners' self-assessment of skill and competency in delivering mental health and substance abuse treatment. It has often been found that practitioner self-assessment of competence bears little relationship to performance (Miller, Sorensen, Selzer, & Brigham, 2006).

To move past reliance on practitioner self-assessment, the existing system must address competency-focused supervision, which is characterized by clinical practice coaching that provides feedback on actual performance based on a set of best practice standards. Coaching is often provided during internships and other field learning opportunities. Unfortunately, ongoing supervision that is part of routine workforce development is often lacking, and when it does exist, it is usually unreimbursed (Miller et al., 2006). As professional training begins to adopt integrated health care competencies as part of its curriculum, field training approaches across all workforce levels will need to provide practice opportunities that include feedback mechanisms. This requires a significant shift in how medical and behavioral health practitioners are trained in the classroom and in the field. Ongoing supervision in the workplace must also be amended to include opportunities for supervisory feedback. In summary, the adoption of best practices in integrated health care organizations will be successful only when practitioners are prepared through coordinated training, coaching, and frequent performance reviews (Fixsen et al., 2005).

IMPLICATIONS FOR SOCIAL WORK

The changing health care system demands that providers and their professional associations and training institutions engage in honest self-examinations of their current alignments with the needed roles and competencies of integrated health care. Training must emphasize teamwork, coordination, and a whole-health perspective that recognizes the interdependence of mental health, substance use, and physical wellbeing. Social workers similarly need to engage in self-reflection to ensure that classroom curriculum, training, field placements, clinical practice, and the shaping of a professional identity align with the future of health care. The social work profession should articulate and demonstrate that the values and skills of social workers are indispensable to achieving the promise of integrated health care.

Although many of the core competencies described in this chapter are applicable to all medical and behavioral health practitioners, it is the perspective and value system of social work that stands out as a unique contribution to integrated health care. The long history of social work as a profession dedicated to advocating for social justice and equity means that the impacts of social determinants, resource insufficiency, racism, and discrimination in health are more likely to be recognized and addressed by this profession. The long-standing macro-systems perspective of social work, which emphasizes the importance of the individual's environmental context, mandates that care teams examine their institutional and social policies as critical factors in promoting health care access, quality, and outcomes and expand their role beyond that of a treatment team to one that advocates for systems changes.

CONCLUSIONS

The promise of integrated health care can be achieved only by a medical and behavioral health workforce (including peer and community health workers) that collectively possesses a set of values, knowledge, and skills designed to facilitate interprofessional teamwork and care coordination that is person-centered, system minded, and community focused. It requires the coordinated and comprehensive efforts of numerous stakeholders, including providers; federal, state, and local government agencies; universities; advocacy groups; accrediting, licensing, and regulating bodies; managed care organizations; researchers; and communities, each of which plays a critical role in the health care system and the preparation of and investment in the health care workforce.

The current way in which the medical and behavioral health workforce defines roles and competencies reinforces fragmentation through highly guarded professional spaces. As the health care system begins to break down the silos between behavioral and physical health systems of care, a national workforce development plan is critically needed. Despite some promising workforce initiatives promulgated by the ACA, we still need a national agenda and process to engage the key stakeholders in developing a comprehensive plan while the changes in the health care system are underway. This is essential to avoid serious misalignment between the needs of an integrated system of care and a workforce that is inadequately prepared to enable such a system to achieve its promise.

RESOURCES

Center for Integrated Health Solutions (CIHS), Substance Abuse and Mental Health Services Administration-Health Resources and Services Administration (SAMHSA-HRSA) http://www.integration.samhsa.gov/

Council on Social Work Education (CSWE) http://www.cswe.org/

The Innovation Center, Centers for Medicare & Medicaid Services (CMS) https://innovation.cms.gov

Institute for Healthcare Improvement (IHI) http://www.ihi.org

Integrated Primary & Behavioral Health, McSilver Institute for Poverty Policy and Research, New York University http://mcsilver.nyu.edu/integrated-primary-behavioral-health

National Alliance on Mental Illness (NAMI) http://www.nami.org/

National Association of Social Workers (NASW) http://www.socialworkers.org/

National Council for Behavioral Health (The National Council) http://www.thenationalcouncil.org/

National Implementation Research Network (NIRN) http://nirn.fpg.unc.edu/

REFERENCES

American Public Health Association. (2016). Community health workers. Retrieved from https://www.apha.org/apha-communities/member-sections/community-health-workers

Brown, R., Schore, J., Archibald, N., Chen, A., Peikes, D., Sautter, K., . . . Ensor, T. (2004). Coordinating care for Medicare beneficiaries: Early experiences of 15 demonstration programs, their patients, and providers. In L. Berenson (Ed.). *Report to Congress* (MPR Ref. No. 8756). Princeton, NJ: Mathematica Policy Research, Inc. Retrieved from https://innovation.cms.gov/files/reports/best-prac-congressional-report.pdf

Carter, R., Golant, S. K., & Cade, K. E. (2010). *Within our reach: Ending the mental health crisis.* New York, NY: Rodale.

Center for Integrated Health Solutions, Substance Abuse and Mental Health Services Administration-Health Resources and Services Administration. (2016a). About CIHS. Retrieved from http://www.integration.samhsa.gov/about-us/about-cihs

Center for Integrated Health Solutions, Substance Abuse and Mental Health Services Administration-Health Resources and Services Administration. (2016b). Peer providers. Retrieved from http://www.integration.samhsa.gov/workforce/team-members/peer-providers

Centers for Medicare & Medicaid Services. (2007). Letter on peer supports (SMDL No. 07-001). Retrieved from https://downloads.cms.gov/cmsgov/archived-downloads/SMDL/downloads/smd081507a.pdf

Clay, R. A. (2015). Fighting poverty. *Monitor on Psychology, 46*(7), 77–81.

Council on Social Work Education. (n.d.). Social Work and Integrated Behavioral Healthcare Project. Retrieved from http://www.cswe.org/CentersInitiatives/DataStatistics/58020.aspx

Diehl, S., Douglas, D., Hart, J. W., Carolla, B., Kimball, A., & Honberg, R. (2015). *State mental health legislation 2015: Trends, themes & effective practices.* Arlington, VA: National Alliance on Mental Illness. Retrieved from http://www.nami.org/About-NAMI/Publications-Reports/Public-Policy-Reports/State-Mental-Health-Legislation-2015/NAMI-StateMentalHealthLegislation2015.pdf

Druss, B. G., Zhao, L., von Esenwein, S. A., Bona, J. R., Fricks, L., Jenkins-Tucker, S., . . . Lorig, K. (2010). The Health and Recovery Peer (HARP) Program: A peer-led intervention to improve medical self-management for persons with serious mental illness. *Schizophrenia Research, 118,* 264–270. doi: 10.1016/j.schres.2010.01.026

Eiken, S., & Campbell, J. (2008). *Medicaid coverage of peer support for people with mental illness: Available research and state examples.* New York, NY: Thomson Reuters. Retrieved from http://nasuad.org/sites/nasuad/files/hcbs/files/150/7485/PeerSupport11-6.pdf

Fixsen, D. L., Naoom, S. F., Blase, K. A., Friedman, R. M., & Wallace, F. (2005). *Implementation research: A synthesis of the literature* (FMHI Pub. No. 231). Tampa, FL: University of South Florida, Louis de la Parte Florida Mental Health Institute, The National Implementation Research Network. Retrieved from http://ctndisseminationlibrary.org/PDF/nirnmonograph.pdf

Hoge, M. A., Morris, J. A., Laraia, M., Pomerantz, A., & Farley, T. (2014). *Core competencies for integrated behavioral health and primary care.* Washington, DC: Center for Integrated Health Solutions, Substance Abuse and Mental Health Services Adminsitration-Health Resources and Services Administration. Retrieved from http://www.integration.samhsa.gov/workforce/Integration_Competencies_Final.pdf

Humes, K. R., Jones, N. A., & Ramirez, R. R. (2011). *Overview of race and Hispanic origin: 2010* (Census Brief). New York, NY: U. S. Census Bureau, U.S. Department of Commerce.

Institute for Healthcare Improvement. (2016). The IHI Triple Aim. Retrieved from http://www.ihi.org/Engage/Initiatives/TripleAim/Pages/default.aspx

Institute of Medicine. (2012). *The mental health and substance use workforce for older adults: In whose hands?* (Report Brief). Washington, DC: National Academies Press. Retrieved from https://www.nationalacademies.org/hmd/~/media/Files/Report%20Files/2012/The-Mental-Health-and-Substance-Use-Workforce-for-Older-Adults/MHSU_olderadults_RB_FINAL.pdf

Jia L., Yuan B., Huang F., Lu Y., Garner P., & Meng Q. (2014). Strategies for expanding health insurance coverage in vulnerable populations (Review). *Cochrane Database of Systematic Reviews, 11,* Article No. CD008194. doi: 10.1002/14651858.CD008194.pub3

Lorig, K. R., Sobel, D. S., Ritter, P. L., Laurent, D., & Hobbs, M. (2000). Effect of a self-management program on patients with chronic disease. *Effective Clinical Practice, 4,* 256–262.

McSilver Institute for Poverty Policy and Research, New York University. (n.d.). Integrated primary and behavioral health. Retrieved from http://mcsilver.nyu.edu/integrated-primary-behavioral-health

Meyers, D., Peikes, D., Genevro, J., Peterson, G., Taylor, E. F., Lake, T., . . . Grumbach, K. (2010). *The roles of patient-centered medical homes and Accountable Care Organizations in coordinating patient care.* (AHRQ Pub. No. 11-M005-EF). Rockville, MD: Agency for Healthcare Research and Quality. Retrieved from https://pcmh.ahrq.gov/sites/default/files/attachments/Roles%20of%20PCMHs%20And%20ACOs%20in%20Coordinating%20Patient%20Care.pdf

Miller, W. R., Sorensen, J. L., Selzer, J. A., & Brigham, G. S. (2006). Disseminating evidence-based practices in substance abuse treatment: A review with suggestions. *Journal of Substance Abuse Treatment, 31,* 25–39. doi: 10.1016/j.jsat.2006.03.005

Morris, C. D. (2009). *The Peer-to-Peer Tobacco Dependence Recovery Program.* Washington, DC: Center for Integrated Health Solutions, Substance Abuse and Mental Health Services Administration-Health Resources and Servcies Administration. Retrieved from http://www.integration.samhsa.gov/Peer_to_Peer_Tobacco_Recovery_Program.pdf

Peikes, D., Chen, A., Schore, J., & Brown, R. (2009). Effects of care coordination on hospitalization, quality of care, and health care expenditures among Medicare beneficiaries: 15 Randomized trials. *Journal of the American Medical Association, 301*, 603–618. doi: 10.1001/jama.2009.126

Pittman, M., Sunderland, A., Broderick, A., & Barnett, K. (2015). *Bringing community health workers into the mainstream of U.S. health care.* Washington, DC: Institute of Medicine, The National Academy of Sciences. Retrieved from https://nam.edu/wp-content/uploads/2015/06/chwpaper3.pdf

Purington, K. (2016). *Using peers to support physical and mental health integration for adults with serious mental illness.* Washington, DC: National Academy for State Health Policy. Retrieved from http://nashp.org/wp-content/uploads/2016/01/Peer-Supports.pdf

Redhead, C. S., Lister S. A., Colello, K. J., Sarata, A. K., & Heisler, E. J. (2013). *Discretionary spending in the Patient Protection and Affordable Care Act (ACA).* Washington, DC: Congressional Research Service, Library of Congress. Retrieved from http://madisonproject.com/wp-content/uploads/2013/03/CRS-on-Obamacare-Discretionary-Spending-.pdf

Rural Health Information Hub. (2015, May 29). Federally Qualified Health Centers (FQHCs). Retrieved from https://www.ruralhealthinfo.org/topics/federally-qualified-health-centers

Saitz, R., Cheng, D. M., Winter, M., Kim, T. W., Meli, S. M., Allensworth-Davies, D., . . . Samet, J. H. (2013). Chronic care management for dependence on alcohol and other drugs: The AHEAD randomized trial. *Journal of the American Medical Association, 310*, 1156–1167. doi: 10.1001/jama.2013.277609

Starfield, B., Shi, L., & Macinko, J. (2005). Contribution of primary care to health systems and health. *The Milbank Quarterly, 83*, 457–502. doi: 10.1111/j.1468-0009.2005.00409.x

Substance Abuse and Mental Health Services Administration. (2012). *Mental health, United States, 2010* (HHS Pub. No. SMA 12-4681). Rockville, MD: Substance Abuse and Mental Health Services Administration. Retrieved from http://www.samhsa.gov/data/sites/default/files/MHUS2010/MHUS2010/MHUS-2010.pdf

Substance Abuse and Mental Health Services Administration (SAMHSA). (2013). *Report to Congress on the nation's substance abuse and mental health workforce issues.* Retrieved from https://store.samhsa.gov/shin/content/PEP13-RTC-BHWORK/PEP13-RTC-BHWORK.pdf

Substance Abuse and Mental Health Services Administration. (2016). SAMHSA's efforts in health care and health systems integration. Retrieved from http://www.samhsa.gov/health-care-health-systems-integration/samhsas-efforts

Uberoi, N., Finegold, K., & Gee, E. (2016). *Health insurance coverage and the Affordable Care Act, 2010-2016* (Issue Brief). Washington, DC: Office of the Assistant Secretary for Planning and Evaluation, U.S. Department of Health and Human Services. Retrieved from https://aspe.hhs.gov/sites/default/files/pdf/187551/ACA2010-2016.pdf

University of Massachusetts Medical School. (n.d.). Center for Integrated Primary Care. Retrieved from http://www.umassmed.edu/cipc/

University of Michigan School of Social Work. (2016). Web-based Certificate in Integrated Behavioral Health and Primary Care. Retrieved from http://ssw.umich.edu/offices/continuing-education/certificate-courses/integrated-behavioral-health-and-primary-care

PART III

INTEGRATED HEALTH CARE PRACTICES AND SETTINGS

CHAPTER 8

WORKING IN INTEGRATED HEALTH CARE SETTINGS

Neil S. Calman, Virna Little, and Elizabeth B. Matthews

During the past several decades, it has become evident that our health and behavioral health care systems are ill equipped to meet the increasingly complex health needs of the United States. Current estimates indicate that almost 20% of adult Americans are diagnosed with some form of mental illness within a 12-month period (Substance Abuse and Mental Health Services Administration, 2014). Of these individuals, up to 74% have a co-occurring chronic medical illness, and 50% have been diagnosed with two or more chronic conditions (Jones et al., 2014). These circumstances have far-reaching implications because research suggests that individuals with severe mental illnesses die an average of 25 years earlier than the general population—largely due to untreated but preventable medical conditions (Colton & Manderschied, 2006). These findings compel the development of a health care system that can effectively treat individuals with needs in multiple domains.

Motivated by the frequent co-occurrence of behavioral health and chronic medical conditions and the associated need for coordinated care, large-scale policy efforts have increasingly addressed the fragmentation of the nation's health and behavioral health care systems. Reform initiatives have called for incorporating models of integrated health care into routine practice, particularly since the enactment of the Patient Protection and Affordable Care Act (ACA) in 2010. This legislation supports the development of integrated health care across health care systems by increasing financial support for emerging models of integrated health care, such as patient-centered medical homes and accountable care organizations, and by encouraging a value-based payment system that rewards quality of care rather than the quantity of services provided. This chapter describes the various ways in which integrated health care can affect the structure of care settings and discusses the clinical tasks carried out by providers in these settings.

DEFINING INTEGRATED HEALTH CARE

The term *integrated health care* is most often used to describe any version of care in which two or more disciplines practice together. However, more than 175 definitions of integrated health care exist in the literature (Armitage, Suter, Oelke, & Adair, 2009), creating an arduous task for organizations and providers seeking to understand or implement integrated health care in their systems. At its simplest, integrated health care denotes primary and behavioral health care providers working together in a systemic way (Miller et al., 2016). In this context, the term *behavioral health* refers to the care and treatment of individuals for mental health, substance use, or psychosocial stressors in an integrated setting (Butler et al., 2008).

A report published by the Center for Integrated Health Solutions (Heath, Wise Romero, & Reynolds, 2013) created a useful framework for describing and categorizing levels of integrated health care. Building on previous examples (Blount, 2003; Doherty, McDaniel, & Baird, 1996), this model conceptualizes integrated health care along a continuum, ranging from services that are separate and minimally collaborative to those that have fully integrated practice spaces and clinical workflows (see Table 8.1). The framework was designed to provide a common language for components of integrated health care and to serve as a mechanism to reliably identify and compare the progressive stages of the integration process.

Tools such as this can help an organization assess its current status and develop and design strategies for achieving a more integrated system. Integration is often viewed solely as a clinical approach; however, as this framework illustrates, a truly integrated organization requires interdisciplinary collaboration across all organizational systems, not only clinical departments. Change must occur at the structural level, in terms of creating a physical environment that promotes integration, and at the clinical level, in terms of formulating the programs needed to ensure that all providers efficiently coordinate care.

EXPANDING ACCESS

Organizations are also motivated to adopt integrated models to expand access for service users and to create additional opportunities for them to engage with providers of various disciplines. However, many organizations have discovered that simply having services on site does not necessarily improve access to those services. Full provider schedules often prevent new service users from accessing appointments for weeks or months, but because of no-shows and cancellations, many opportunities for improving access to care are often missed. Several best practices are being adopted to mitigate this issue.

Same-day or next-day scheduling refers to a system in which individuals who seek or are referred to services are offered an appointment on either the same day or the following business day. This is considered to be the gold standard for improving access because it allows individuals to receive care when they need it most and reduces no-shows and cancellations, which become exponentially more likely with each additional day that an individual waits for an appointment. Alternatively, a clinic may adopt an open-access model

TABLE 8.1: Summary of Levels of Integration Framework

COORDINATED CARE — Key Element: Communication		CO-LOCATED CARE — Key Element: Physical Proximity		INTEGRATED CARE — Key Element: Practice Change	
Level 1	Level 2	Level 3	Level 4	Level 5	Level 6
Minimal Collaboration	Basic Collaboration at a Distance	Basic Onsite Collaboration	Close Onsite Collaboration with Some Integration	Close Onsite Collaboration Approaching Integration	Full Onsite Collaboration and Integration
Separate facilities	Separate facilities	Shared facilities, but not necessarily shared space	Shared space in shared facilities	Shared space in shared facilities, with some shared practice space	Shared space in shared facilities, with shared practice space
Separate systems	Separate systems	Separate systems	Some shared systems (e.g., medical records)	Some shared systems, along with active progression toward sharing one integrated system	One shared and integrated system
Communication and collaboration occur as needed	Communication and collaboration occur periodically to address specific issues	Communication and collaboration occur regularly to ensure continuity of care	Communication and collaboration occur regularly to develop coordinated plans for highest-risk service users	Communication and collaboration occur regularly as members of a care team	Communication and collaboration occur regularly as members of a care team and at the system, team, and individual levels
Separate treatment plans and clinical practices	Separate treatment plans and clinical practices but may be some sharing or overlapping	Separate treatment plans and clinical practices, with some shared elements	Possibly collaborative treatment plans and clinical practices for specific individuals or populations (e.g., those with more than one diagnosis)	Shared treatment plans and clinical practice guidelines	Single treatment plan and same clinical practice guidelines used for all service users
Service user's needs are treated separately, with few referrals	Service user's needs are treated separately, but information may be shared and some referrals may be made	Service user's needs are treated separately, but at the same site and with relatively frequent referrals	Service user's needs are treated separately, but at the same site and with some collaboration (e.g., warm handoffs)	Service user's needs are treated collectively by a care team for shared service users (e.g., those with more than one diagnosis)	Service user's needs are treated collectively by a care team for all service users
No systematic approach to coordination or collaboration	Some efforts to establish systematic information sharing	Integration efforts focus on physical co-location	Integration is supported through transdisciplinary problem solving	Integrated care is supported by most providers and leaders	Integrated care is embraced by all providers and leaders

Adapted from *A Standard Framework for Levels of Integrated Care* (p. 4), by B. Heath, P. Wise Romero, and K. A. Reynolds, 2013, Washington, DC: Center for Integrated Health Solutions, Substance Abuse and Mental Health Services Administration–Health Resources and Services Administration.

in which there are no scheduled appointments and individuals come in for care as needed or as they are able to attend. A completely open-access model for services such as psychiatric medication management or urgent primary care may work best when serving special populations such as homeless people, migrants, or street workers.

Most organizations develop blended models. Blended access utilizes open-access, walk-in opportunities, and scheduled appointments. This model allows individuals who struggle with precise appointment times to seek care when they need it or when they can access it; this is useful, for example, when there is limited ability to arrange transportation or child care. The ability to receive care "as able" can help keep service users engaged longer by avoiding frustrations associated with missing scheduled visits. Individuals who prefer appointments or need care at specific times (e.g., those who depend on scheduled transportation) also are accommodated in this model. Many organizations change individuals to more flexible open-access times if they miss a certain percentage of their scheduled appointments. The blended model is often preferable to providers because it allows them to avoid long stretches of missed or back-to-back appointments.

THE IMPACT MODEL OF INTEGRATION

The Improving Mood—Promoting Access to Collaborative Treatment (IMPACT) model, also known as the Collaborative Care model, is one of the most prevalent models of integrated health care in primary care settings. Although it was originally developed to identify and treat depression in seniors, collaborative care is now widely used for individuals of all ages. Based on a robust evidence base, an initial study found that twice as many people improved with collaborative care than with traditional care (Unützer et al., 2002).

IMPACT introduces two new members to the health care team: a depression care manager and a psychiatric consultant. In this model, individuals seeking primary care are routinely screened for depression using the Patient Health Questionnaire 9 (Spitzer, Kroenke, & Williams, 1999). Any individual experiencing depressive symptoms can then be referred to a depression care manager, who works with the individual to deliver brief interventions, such as problem-solving therapy and behavioral activation. Beyond these behavioral interventions, the depression care manager also coordinates regularly with a primary care provider and a psychiatric consultant if the individual is taking antidepressant medication. The depression care manager acts as an information hub, ensuring effective, timely, and accurate information exchange among the physician, the psychiatrist consultant, and the service user. Social workers are often the preferred candidates for this role. The IMPACT model has also been expanded to include other mental health diagnoses, such as anxiety, and incorporates the use of relevant tools such as the Generalized Anxiety Disorder 7 scale. Because of its expansive amount of supporting research and clearly defined roles, many primary care organizations choose IMPACT as their first official integration model.

As a result of IMPACT's success, many state and federal systems have recognized the effectiveness of Collaborative Care and have supported its development by expanding access grants to community health centers and increasing case rate funding for organizations that implement these models. More than 80 randomized trials have demonstrated the effectiveness of Collaborative Care, a model that, for the first time, is able to both identify and treat a mental health disorder within a primary care setting (Archer et al., 2012). The original IMPACT research project is widely considered to be the starting point of integrated health care in the United States and perhaps in the world.

STRUCTURAL INTEGRATION

Co-location is considered an early model of integration, which consists of moving multiple programs across disciplines into a single, shared location. However, the co-location model alone is limited in that it refers only to the physical location of services and research has consistently demonstrated that simply placing multiple disciplines together in one setting does little to improve outcomes (Krahn et al., 2006). Co-located providers often do not share records, nor do they take advantage of care coordination opportunities or adopt practices to meet the needs of an integrated setting. For example, a behavioral health provider co-located in primary care might provide traditional mental health services, such as long-term psychotherapy, rather than identifying best practices for behavioral health intervention in a primary care setting. Therefore, the co-location model can fail to bring about collaboration between primary and behavioral health providers, which is often considered to be the most crucial aspect of integrated health care to improve experiences and outcomes.

Although the co-location model is not effective on its own, a practice that has effectively co-located services can change its physical layout to facilitate collaboration. Research has shown that providers who practice in workspaces that are near each other are more likely to routinely communicate, share referrals, and easily accept handoffs (Gunn et al., 2015). To accommodate this new type of workspace, many clinics are being redesigned with distinct spaces for each team (sometimes referred to as *pods*) on a single practice floor. Compact practices require more resourceful solutions, such as swapping administrative primary care spaces and behavioral health offices to enable behavioral health providers to practice among the primary care team members. Some organizations have realized that not all primary care visits require an examination table, allowing behavioral health services to be delivered in an examination room that is not otherwise in use. *Multiuse rooms*, often referred to as *point-of-care rooms*, that meet the needs of all disciplines have become more common to optimize shared space among providers. When implementing integrated health care models, organizations should pay particular attention to the physical layout and proximity of disciplines to encourage collaboration and coordination among providers.

CLINICAL INTEGRATION

Integrated models of health care heavily rely on team-based approaches to deliver comprehensive services. Much like the overall concept of integration, professional collaboration exists on a spectrum. *Multidisciplinary care models* are practice settings in which multiple providers contribute to the care of an individual, although often with limited collaboration. In contrast, *interdisciplinary care models* involve direct cooperation among providers, such as case conferences or shared records.

At the other end of this spectrum is *transdisciplinary care*, which is the most advanced team-based model and is considered the gold standard of integrated health care settings. This model expands the care team to involve all providers, including primary care, behavioral health, dental, nursing, nutrition, health coaches, and community workers. Transdisciplinary care moves beyond multidisciplinary and interdisciplinary approaches by including specific education and training designed to prepare providers across all disciplines to support each other's services. Providers using this model are adept at establishing shared care plans with service users and appropriately drawing on the unique skill sets of each member of the care team. Another significant advantage of a transdisciplinary model is sharing of responsibilities across the service user's entire care team, which alleviates the burden on the individual provider.

Team-based care also requires shared liability, in which all providers are held accountable for all outcomes—even those outside their individual disciplines. One social worker practicing in New York described this experience: "I really understood what it was like to work on a team when for the first time in my career I was held accountable for all my patients getting a flu shot in our center—years ago I not only would not have asked but argued that it was not my responsibility and perhaps even that I was not qualified."

Although team-based care models are widely considered superior to traditional approaches, their implementation is hindered by the persistence of the fee-for-service (FFS)—or payment by the visit—reimbursement model. The care planning and coordination of services that are inherently prevalent in collaborative care are often viewed as unsustainable in an FFS environment because these tasks are typically not reimbursable.

PRACTICING IN AN INTEGRATED HEALTH CARE SETTING

THE WARM HANDOFF

To effectively collaborate, all programs, across all disciplines, must be easily accessible to every provider working within a system. For many years, the specialty mental health system was seen as inaccessible to most of the primary care community. Many community mental health providers did not coordinate with or refer to primary care providers; even those who did often received messages that the primary care providers were "too busy" to collaborate. As a result, primary care and mental health providers largely practiced in treatment silos for many years, with limited or ineffective referral processes.

It is well known that individuals who receive outside referrals from their providers often do not attend or keep those appointments. Some of these breaches can be attributed to social determinants (e.g., transportation or finances), the feeling that the referral is unnecessary, or a reluctance to engage with another provider in another setting.

Exacerbating this problem is the fact that individuals often feel a stigma about mental health services. Individuals who successfully follow through with an initial mental health referral often do not remain in care, and this information is seldom communicated to the referring primary care provider (Olfson & Marcus, 2010).

The luxury of being located in the same space with other health care professionals provides unique opportunities to enhance the effectiveness and success of behavioral health referrals. One of the best practices to emerge from the integrated health care models is the *warm handoff*. This is a mechanism through which physicians and other medical providers can engage behavioral health professionals in a primary care setting and vice versa; it can be initiated between any disciplines practicing in a co-located setting.

At the basic level, warm handoffs occur when a provider is invited to meet an individual during his or her visit with a provider from another discipline or when a provider escorts an individual to his or her visit with a provider from another discipline. Typically, this takes place during appointments as particular needs are identified. For example, a high score on a depression screening tool may prompt a physician or nurse to invite a behavioral health professional into the examination room to conduct an introduction and brief assessment.

A warm handoff has many benefits. It helps address pressing needs immediately and helps ensure that referrals are completed successfully by conducting them in real time. The resulting discussion occurs with two members of the care team present, facilitating information sharing, joint care planning, and service coordination as treatment continues.

Implementation of the warm handoff relies on the abilities of all providers across disciplines to refer an individual fluidly by introducing him or her to team members regardless of the reason for the current visit. To optimize this process, providers must work together and remain accessible to one another through shared work or through a structured system that can notify a provider when a warm handoff is needed (e.g., messages sent through a shared electronic health record system, pager, or cell phone).

The warm handoff is, however, accompanied by its own unique challenges. It complicates the management of preexisting scheduled appointments because warm handoffs occur unpredictably on an as-needed basis. This can be particularly difficult for behavioral health providers, many of whom are accustomed to conducting uninterrupted therapeutic sessions with prescheduled individuals. Reimbursement poses an additional obstacle because visits with multiple providers on the same day limit reimbursement options for the second provider in virtually all settings.

CLINICAL WORKFLOWS

The creation or expansion of an integrated health care system is largely shaped by the efficiency of its clinical workflows, which guide staff and delineate their roles in care processes. This is particularly important for situations in which providers across multiple disciplines are involved in a single appointment or play unique roles in treating the same illness or diagnosis. Workflows clarify who is responsible for what and help ensure that tasks follow established best practices and agency policies.

In a common integrated workflow concerning depression screening, medical assistants conduct the initial screening for depression and are subsequently guided to make evidence-based decisions, including a warm handoff to a behavioral health care provider, based on the severity of depressive symptoms. In addition to increasing the efficiency and effectiveness of care, establishing clear workflows can support integrated health care delivery by prompting providers to engage in transdisciplinary coordination at opportune, clinically relevant times.

EVIDENCE-BASED BRIEF INTERVENTIONS

Traditional behavioral health services often consist of regular, ongoing talk therapy. Although integrated health care settings do not preclude this form of care, behavioral health care providers in integrated settings are also frequently used to deliver targeted, brief behavioral interventions. In contrast to ongoing talk therapy, these interventions tend to be limited in time and focused on a specific area of behavior change. Sessions may last only 20 to 30 minutes and may be seamlessly incorporated into medical appointments as the result of warm handoffs.

The growth of integrated health and behavioral health settings has led to the emergence of several evidence-based practices that are commonly used to provide brief behavioral health treatment. The following sections review two of the most frequently used of these evidence-based practices: behavioral activation and problem-solving therapy (PST).

Behavioral activation. Behavioral activation is a brief, structured form of cognitive treatment that aims to increase rewarding and positive experiences, primarily by helping individuals identify and plan pleasurable activities (Martell, Dimidjian, & Herman-Dunn, 2013). Behavioral activation was initially developed as a treatment for depression, and it is based on the premise that depressive symptoms are both caused by and exacerbated by specific forms of avoidance behavior (Hopko, Lejuez, Ruggiero, & Eifert, 2003). For example, individuals experiencing depression may withdraw socially by not answering phone calls or avoiding friends and family. These behaviors increase feelings of loneliness and isolation, which worsen depressive symptoms by fulfilling doubts about self-worth or self-esteem that may underlie the illness (Veale, 2008). To combat this cycle, individuals are encouraged to plan weekly dinners with family or simply to take daily walks around the neighborhood to increase exposure to enjoyable social activity and reduce engagement in avoidance behaviors.

Lejuez, Hopko, Acierno, Daughters, and Pagogo (2011) developed a comprehensive treatment manual guiding clinicians through a behavioral activation intervention for individuals with depression. In their framework, treatment begins with psychoeducation to inform a service user of the rationale and elements of behavioral activation, followed by a discussion about the individual's values, preferences, and visions of how he or she would like to live their life. This information is then distilled into *activities*, or specific, manageable behaviors related to each individual's goals that can be accomplished on a daily basis. Examples include regular exercise, dietary changes, or deliberate plans to increase social activity.

Through frequent activity monitoring, service users and providers engage in collaborative discussions about planning and implementing positive behaviors and activities while identifying unhealthy patterns of behaviors that may contribute to symptoms. Individuals are encouraged to use family members and social supports as resources to continue working toward established behavioral goals. As sessions continue, service users and providers review progress, identify and dissolve barriers, and steadily advance toward more challenging activities. These discussions are often facilitated by the use of specific worksheets, such as activity monitoring logs or contracts that outline plans of action, and natural supports that have been mutually accepted and can help individuals accomplish their activity goals.

Behavioral activation has effectively reduced depressive symptoms in adults and often performed better than traditional cognitive therapy (Cuijpers, van Straten, & Warmerdam, 2007). Although most commonly used as a treatment for depression, research suggests that behavioral activation can also improve symptoms of anxiety, demonstrating the potential application of this intervention across a broader spectrum of behavioral health conditions (Hopko, Lejuez, & Hopko, 2004; Hopko, Lejuez, Ryba, Shorter, & Bell, 2016).

Problem-solving therapy. Much like behavioral activation, PST focuses on helping individuals develop and execute concrete plans to intervene on external factors affecting or leading to behavioral health symptoms. As its name implies, this cognitive intervention consists of developing pragmatic, problem-solving skills. A fundamental assumption of this model is that behavioral health symptoms are caused by ineffective or unhealthy coping mechanisms, which result in negative psychosocial consequences such as anxiety and depression (D'Zurilla & Goldfried, 1971). The principal task of PST is to help individuals correct ineffective problem-solving strategies in favor of rational problem-solving approaches. This is characterized by four stages:

1. Definition and articulation of a specific problem
2. Generation of alternative solutions
3. Engagement in decision making
4. Implementation and verification of ultimate solution (Nezu, 2004)

Throughout a PST intervention, clinicians support rational problem-solving efforts through a combination of didactic instruction and coaching, modeling and rehearsing problem-solving principles, and feedback and positive reinforcement (D'Zurilla & Nezu, 2010). The utility of PST has been demonstrated by its implementation in individual and group formats and by findings that suggest it effectively reduces symptoms of anxiety (Seekles, van Straten, Beekman, van Marwijk, & Cuijpers, 2011) and depression (Bell & D'Zurilla, 2009), including suicidal ideation (Fitzpatrick, Witte, & Schmidt, 2005).

Behavioral activation and PST are highly structured interventions that focus on concrete skill building. As such, providers from a wide range of disciplines can deliver these interventions (with adequate training). This approach is particularly well suited for integrated settings because care teams comprise a wide range of providers with varied professional training and backgrounds. Behavioral activation and PST are intended to be highly focused and time limited, making them well designed for the fast-paced environment of integrated health care settings.

Screening tools. To effectively identify those in need of behavioral health interventions, many organizations use standardized screening tools during a primary care triage or behavioral health intake process. Integrated primary care organizations use these instruments to help detect mental health disorders during routine primary care visits. The most recent guidelines from the U.S. Preventive Services Task Force recommend universal depression screening for all adults seeking primary care (Siu & U.S. Preventive Services Task Force, 2016), largely because individuals experiencing depressive symptoms are more likely to initially seek treatment from a primary care provider rather than a behavioral health care provider (Reilly et al., 2012). Therefore, primary care appointments offer an optimal gateway for connecting individuals in need of behavioral health treatment with qualified professionals. When this transition occurs in the context of an integrated primary care appointment, the stigma associated with mental illness can often be alleviated.

In addition to effectively identifying individuals with behavioral health symptoms, standardized screening tools allow all members of a transdisciplinary team to identify and discuss behavioral health diagnoses using the same language, thereby providing a consistent way to track behavioral health outcomes. One example of a screening tool used by both primary care and behavioral health care providers is the Patient Health Questionnaire 9. Containing only nine items—including an item screening for suicidality—this instrument can be administered quickly by a wide range of professionals, and it has been shown over time to be an effective tool in integrated settings for identifying and treating individuals with depression (Kroenke, Spitzer, & Williams, 2003).

IMPLICATIONS FOR SOCIAL WORK

The Colorado Consensus Conference established the following eight core competencies that are critical for behavioral health care providers practicing in integrated primary care settings:

1. Identify and assess behavioral health needs as part of a primary care team.
2. Engage and activate service users in their care.
3. Work as a primary care team member to create and implement care plans that address behavioral health factors.
4. Observe and improve care team function and relationships.
5. Communicate effectively with other providers, staff, and service users.
6. Provide efficient and effective care delivery that meets the needs of the population of the primary care setting.
7. Provide culturally responsive, whole-person, and family-oriented care.
8. Understand, value, and adapt to the diverse professional cultures of an integrated health care team (Miller et al., 2016).

Although many of these functions are consistent with the core values of social work practice, many social workers have not been trained to practice on a team, develop shared care plans, or actively address physical health concerns. This calls for a revised educational curriculum that can adequately prepare emerging social workers to practice in the unique context of integrated health care. The successful behavioral health care provider in a primary care setting is flexible, able to accommodate the fast pace of primary care, and prepared to share accountability and responsibility for the full range of service users' medical and behavioral health symptoms. Although this may seem like a marked departure from traditional social work practice, adopting a culturally sensitive, person-in-environment perspective is already fundamental to social work training and the discipline at large. For this reason, social workers are particularly equipped to create care plans that seamlessly identify and relate the unique biological, psychological, and social needs of each individual service user.

CONCLUSIONS

Although the term *integrated health care* has come to have many meanings, recent frameworks have attempted to identify common terminologies and mechanisms in order to categorize levels of integration. At its core, integrated health care focuses on transdisciplinary, team-based services in which providers across disciplines work together with an individual to achieve common, mutually accepted goals. Integrated health care seeks to break down traditional distinctions between physical and behavioral health services in favor of a whole-person approach in which all aspects of an individual's health are addressed by a cohesive team of professionals.

Organizations transitioning to an integrated model of care must be prepared to make changes at all levels of their care system, including physical environment, program structure, and clinical workflows. Social workers in integrated settings can no longer think of themselves as exclusively mental health or substance abuse counselors and must instead reconceptualize their role as a critical member of a health care team, with the goal of helping individuals achieve a comprehensive state of wellness.

There are several challenges for organizations transitioning to integrated models of care—most notably the current payment system, which is predominantly FFS. Many of the care coordination activities that are essential to the success of integrated health care, such as case conferences, are not considered reimbursable by major insurers. Limitations on the number of providers that can be seen on 1 day create additional obstacles to delivering team-based care. As payment mechanisms slowly shift to reward quality instead of quantity of care, it is expected that some of these challenges will be alleviated, allowing integrated health care to become increasingly more routine.

RESOURCES

Advancing Integrated Mental Health Solutions (The AIMS Center), University of Washington https:// aims.uw.edu/

Excellence in Motivational Interviewing (MINT) www.motivationalinterviewing.org

Federally Qualified Health Center (FQHC) Link http://www.fqhc.org/

Integrated Care Resource Center (ICRC), Centers for Medicare & Medicaid Services (CMS) http://www.integratedcareresourcecenter.com/Default.aspx

Patient-Centered Primary Care Collaborative (PCPCC) https://www.pcpcc.org/

REFERENCES

Archer, J., Bower, P., Gilbody, S., Lovell, K., Richards, D., Gask, L., . . . Coventry, P. (2012). Collaborative care for depression and anxiety problems. *Cochrane Database of Systematic Reviews*(10). doi: 10.1002/14651858.CD006525.pub2

Armitage, G. D., Suter, E., Oelke, N. D., & Adair, C. E. (2009). Health systems integration: State of the evidence. *International Journal of Integrated Care, 9*(2), e82. doi: 10.5334/ijic.316/

Bell, A. C., & D'Zurilla, T. J. (2009). Problem-solving therapy for depression: A meta-analysis. *Clinical Psychology Review, 29*, 348–353. doi: 10.1016/j.cpr.2009.02.003

Blount, A. (2003). Integrated primary care: Organizing the evidence. *Families, Systems & Health, 21*, 121–133. doi: 10.1037/1091-7527.21.2.121

Butler, M., Kane, R. L., McAlpine, D., Kathol, R. G., Fu, S. S., Hagedorn, H., & Wilt, T. J. (2008). *Integration of mental health/substance abuse and primary care.* (AHRQ Pub. No. 09-E003, Evidence Report/Technology Assessment No. 173). Rockville, MD: Agency for Healthcare Research and Quality. Retrieved from http://www.ahrq.gov/sites/default/files/wysiwyg/research/findings/evidence-based-reports/mhsapc-evidence-report.pdf

Colton, C. W., & Manderscheid, R. W. (2006). Congruencies in increased mortality rates, years of potential life lost, and causes of death among public mental health clients in eight states. *Preventing Chronic Disease, 3*(2), A42. Available from https://www.cdc.gov/pcd/issues/2006/apr/05_0180.htm

Cuijpers, P., van Straten, A., & Warmerdam, L. (2007). Behavioral activation treatments of depression: A meta-analysis. *Clinical Psychology Review, 27*, 318–326. doi: 10.1016/j.cpr.2006.11.001

Doherty, W. J., McDaniel, S. H., & Baird, M. A. (1996). Five levels of primary care/behavioral healthcare collaboration. *Behavioral Healthcare Tomorrow, 5*, 25–28. Retrieved from http://www1.genesishealth.com/pdf/mh_reynolds_resource_dohertybaird_051110.pdf

D'Zurilla, T. J., & Goldfried, M. R. (1971). Problem solving and behavior modification. *Journal of Abnormal Psychology, 78*, 107–126. doi: 10.1037/h0031360

D'Zurilla, T. J., & Nezu, A. M. (2010). Problem-solving therapy. In K. S. Dobson (Ed.), *Handbook of cognitive-behavioral therapies* (3rd ed., pp. 197–225). New York, NY: Guilford Press.

Fitzpatrick, K. K., Witte, T. K., & Schmidt, N. B. (2005). Randomized controlled trial of a brief problem-orientation intervention for suicidal ideation. *Behavior Therapy, 36*, 323–333. doi: 10.1016/S0005-7894(05)80114-5

Gunn, R., Davis, M. M., Hall, J., Heintzman, J., Muench, J., Smeds, B., . . . Cohen, D. J. (2015). Designing clinical space for the delivery of integrated behavioral health and primary care. *Journal of the American Board of Family Medicine 28*(S1), S52–S62. doi: 10.3122/jabfm.2015.S1.150053

Heath, B., Wise Romero, P., & Reynolds, K. A. (2013). *A standard framework for levels of integrated healthcare.* Washington, DC: Center for Integrated Health Solutions, Substance Abuse and Mental Health Services Administration–Health Resources and Services Administration. Retrieved from http://www.integration.samhsa.gov/integrated-care-models/A_Standard_Framework_for_Levels_of_Integrated_Healthcare.pdf

Hopko, D. R., Lejuez, C. W., & Hopko, S. D. (2004). Behavioral activation as an intervention for coexistent depressive and anxiety symptoms. *Clinical Case Studies, 3*, 37–48. doi: 10.1177/1534650103258969

Hopko, D. R., Lejuez, C. W., Ruggiero, K. J., & Eifert, G. H. (2003). Contemporary behavioral activation treatments for depression: Procedures, principles, and progress. *Clinical Psychology Review, 23*, 699–717. doi: 10.1016/S0272-7358(03)00070-9

Hopko, D. R., Lejuez, C. W., Ryba, M. M., Shorter, R. L., & Bell, J. L. (2016). Support for the efficacy of behavioral activation in treating anxiety in breast cancer patients. *Clinical Psychologist, 20*, 17–26. doi: 10.1111/cp.12083

Jones, D. R., Macias, C., Barreira, P. J., Fisher, W. H., Hargreaves, W. A., & Harding, C. M. (2004). Prevalence, severity, and co-occurrence of chronic physical health problems of persons with serious mental illness. *Psychiatric Services, 55*, 1250–1257. doi: 10.1176/appi.ps.55.11.1250

Krahn, D. D., Bartels, S. J., Coakley, E., Oslin, D. W., Chen, H., McIntyre, J., . . . Levkoff, S. E. (2006). PRISM-E: Comparison of integrated care and enhanced specialty referral models in depression outcomes. *Psychiatric Services, 57*, 946–953. 10.1176/ps.2006.57.7.946

Kroenke, K., Spitzer, R. L., & Williams, J. B. (2003). The Patient Health Questionnaire-2: Validity of a two-item depression screener. *Medical Care, 41*, 1284–1292. doi: 10.1097/01.MLR.0000093487.78664.3C

Lejuez, C. W., Hopko, D. R., Acierno, R., Daughters, S. B., & Pagoto, S. L. (2011). Ten year revision of the brief behavioral activation treatment for depression: Revised treatment manual. *Behavior Modification, 35*, 111–161. doi: 10.1177/0145445510390929

Martell, C. R., Dimidjian, S., & Herman-Dunn, R. (2013). *Behavioral activation for depression: A clinician's guide.* New York, NY: The Guilford Press.

Miller, B. F., Gilchrist, E. C., Ross, K. M., Wong, S. L., Blount, A., & Peek, C. J. (2016). *Core competencies for behavioral health providers working in primary care.* Aurora, CO: Eugene S. Farley, Jr., Health Policy Center, University of Colorado. Retrieved from http://farleyhealthpolicycenter.org/wp-content/uploads/2016/02/Core-Competencies-for-Behavioral-Health-Providers-Working-in-Primary-Care.pdf

Nezu, A. M. (2004). Problem solving and behavior therapy revisited. *Behavior Therapy, 35*, 1–33. doi: 10.1016/S0005-7894(04)80002-9

Olfson, M., & Marcus, S. C. (2010). National trends in outpatient psychotherapy. *The American Journal of Psychiatry, 167*, 1456–1463. doi: 10.1176/appi.ajp.2010.10040570

Reilly, S., Planner, C., Hann, M., Reeves, D., Nazareth, I., & Lester, H. (2012). The role of primary care in service provision for people with severe mental illness in the United Kingdom. *PLoS One, 7*, e36468. doi: 10.1371/journal.pone.0036468

Seekles, W., van Straten, A., Beekman, A., van Marwijk, H., & Cuijpers, P. (2011). Effectiveness of guided self-help for depression and anxiety disorders in primary care: A pragmatic randomized controlled trial. *Psychiatry Research, 187*, 113–120. doi: 10.1016/j.psychres.2010.11.015

Siu, A. L., & U.S. Preventive Services Task Force. (2016). Screening for depression in adults: U.S. Preventive Services Task Force recommendation statement. *Journal of the American Medical Association, 315*, 380–387. doi: 10.1001/jama.2015.18392

Spitzer, R. L., Kroenke, K., & Williams, J.B.W. (1999). Validation and utility of a self–report version of PRIME-MD: The PHQ primary care study. *Journal of the American Medical Association, 282*, 1737–1744. doi: 10.1001/jama.282.18.1737

Substance Abuse and Mental Health Services Administration (SAMSA). (2014). *Results from the 2013 national survey on drug use and health: Mental health findings* (HHS Publication No. [SMA] 14-4887). Rockville, MD: Substance Abuse and Mental Health Services Administration. Retrieved from http://www.samhsa.gov/data/sites/default/files/NSDUHmhfr2013/NSDUHmhfr2013.pdf

University of Washington Psychiatry and Behavioral Sciences Division of Integrated Care and Public Health. (2016). Advancing Integrated Mental Health Solutions. Retrieved from https://aims.uw.edu.

Unützer, J., Katon, W., Callahan, C. M., Williams, J. W., Hunkeler, E., Harpole, L., . . . Langston, C. (2002). Collaborative care management of late-life depression in the primary care setting: A randomized controlled trial. *Journal of the American Medical Association, 288*, 2836–2845. doi: 10.1001/jama.288.22.2836

Veale, D. (2008). Behavioural activation for depression. *Advances in Psychiatric Treatment, 14*, 29–36. doi: 10.1192/apt.bp.107.004051

CHAPTER 9

SCREENING AND BRIEF INTERVENTIONS

Evan Senreich and Shulamith Lala Ashenberg Straussner

An integrated health care approach aims to seamlessly provide a coordinated system of physical health, mental health, and substance misuse prevention and treatment. The model emphasizes the fundamental connection between mind and body in all aspects of health care (Stanhope, Videka, Thorning, & McKay, 2015). This chapter considers how social workers can provide screenings, brief interventions, and referrals to treatment according to an integrated health care model. Specific procedures and tools are elucidated for use in primary care settings and in the many other types of institutions and agencies in which social workers are employed.

The following case example highlights major deficits in the current U.S. health care system, which has historically not adhered to an integrated health care framework. It also demonstrates the need for social workers to become an intrinsic part of an integrated health care model through effective screening, intervention, and referral of individuals in all fields of practice.

CASE VIGNETTE

Joan is a 54-year-old divorced woman who was diagnosed six months ago with breast cancer. She had a turbulent relationship with her husband that ended eight years ago. Her two grown children live in different parts of the country with their partners and children. Joan experienced serious bouts of depression over the course of her marriage, which worsened after she divorced and her children moved away. Her use of alcohol increased to the point that she met the *Diagnostic and Statistical Manual of Mental Disorders*, fifth edition (DSM-5) criteria for alcohol use disorder of moderate severity.

Joan was brought up to believe that one does not share personal problems with others. She has been able to maintain her job working in a large department store, but most of her close friends have distanced themselves from her. After she was diagnosed with breast cancer, she underwent a mastectomy and subsequent radiation therapy at a large hospital center. During this process, Joan completed more than one screening form at the hospital that asked about depression and anxiety and her use of alcohol. She indicated that she was experiencing some depression but minimized her alcohol use. Based on her answers, a hospital social worker came to see her before a radiation therapy session and asked about her depression. The social worker recommended that she see a psychotherapist, and Joan told her that she would consider doing this. Joan subsequently called her managed care company and obtained the name of a clinical social worker in her neighborhood. The social worker was a goal-oriented cognitive-behavioral therapist who became frustrated with Joan's resistance to completing weekly homework assignments and her refusal to attend Alcoholics Anonymous meetings. Joan found the sessions to be upsetting, and she stopped going after several visits.

The therapist subsequently sent Joan a termination letter recommending that she attend a substance abuse treatment program, but Joan ignored this recommendation. She kept her follow-up appointments with her oncologist and her primary care physician, but no one at their offices asked her about her depression or alcohol use.

Joan felt mutilated after her cancer surgery, stopped dating men, and isolated herself. On the weekends, she stayed alone in her apartment and drank heavily. One night, she ran out of alcohol and went to a local bar to drink. She became heavily intoxicated and was hit by a car crossing the street while walking home, sustaining serious injuries.

In the scenario just described, health care professionals, including social workers, were performing their functions in an overwhelmed, fragmented system in which there is little meaningful communication between physical health, mental health, and substance abuse treatment providers. This case example demonstrates how Western conceptualizations of wellness falsely separate physical and emotional health. Although there is no guarantee that the end of this story would have been different in an integrated health care system, it is important to pose some hypothetical questions to consider what changes in the U.S. health care system are necessary and what the role of social workers should be in that system:

- What if the hospital social worker had been able to follow-up with Joan over time regarding her treatment for depression and recommend to Joan's primary care physician and oncologist that they monitor Joan's depression on an ongoing basis?
- What if the hospital social worker had been trained in a more effective screening method to elicit from Joan more accurate information about her alcohol misuse?
- What if the clinical social worker in the community had used a person-centered, motivational interviewing, or harm-reduction approach in working with Joan?
- What if the clinical social worker had tried to personally speak to Joan in a concerned way to expedite referral to another therapist or program?
- What if the clinical social worker had been able to notify Joan's primary care physician regarding the need for further treatment to address her depression and alcohol misuse?
- What if Joan's primary care physician's office had social workers on staff serving the function of care coordinator for all patients and regularly interacting with each patient to ensure that all physical health, mental health, and substance use wellness needs were being addressed on an ongoing basis?

It appears that social workers trained in providing effective screenings, brief interventions, and referrals to treatment at the different physical and behavioral health care venues with which Joan interfaced could have made a substantial difference in the quality of treatment Joan received.

SCREENING, BRIEF INTERVENTION, AND REFERRAL: DEFINITIONS

Before discussing how social workers in an integrated health care system can provide the functions of screening, brief intervention, and referral to treatment for physical health, mental health, and substance use issues, it is important to define these three functions. Screening, brief intervention, and referral to treatment, often referred to as the SBIRT protocol, is an increasingly used evidence-based practice founded on the principles of motivational interviewing (MI). It was created to screen individuals for substance misuse and to provide brief interventions for those for whom alcohol or other drug use has become problematic. Although SBIRT was designed specifically for problems related to substance misuse and has been endorsed as an evidence-based approach by the U.S. government (Substance Abuse and Mental Health Services Administration [SAMHSA], 2016), the concepts of screening, brief intervention, and referral to treatment can also be applied to mental and physical health issues in an integrated health care model.

SCREENING

Mosby's Dictionary of Medicine, Nursing, and Health Professions (Mosby, 2013) defines screening as "a preliminary procedure, such as a test or examination, to detect the most characteristic sign or signs of a disorder that may require further investigation" (p. 1607). In an integrated health care model, social workers screen for a wide range of mental health, physical health, and substance use problems. SAMHSA and the U.S. Health Resources and Services Administration (HRSA) have stated the following:

> Despite the high prevalence of mental health and substance use problems, too many Americans go without treatment—in part because their disorders go undiagnosed. Regular screenings in primary care and other healthcare settings enable earlier identification of mental health and substance use disorders, which translates into earlier care. Screenings should be provided to people of all ages, even the young and the elderly (Center for Integrated Health Solutions, n.d., p. 1).

Screening usually involves the use of validated, standardized instruments completed by the service user alone or in the presence of the clinician. However, screening can also involve in-depth interviewing by a health professional without the use of a screening instrument. If a standardized written or online instrument is being used, it is essential that an interview with a clinician directly follows the service user's completion of the screening tool.

A brief intervention can be defined as "brief counseling that raises awareness of risks and motivates clients toward acknowledgement of [a] problem" (Pacific Southwest Addiction Technology Transfer Center [PS-ATTC], 2011, p. 6). A SAMHSA (2013a) publication stated that "brief interventions are 1 to 5 sessions in length, [lasting] from a few minutes to an hour" (p. 7), and that an MI approach should be used. Brief interventions typically have one of two functions:

1. For problems that do not need lengthy, in-depth treatment, the purpose of brief interventions is to motivate an individual to take action to ameliorate the problem. For example, for someone who is misusing alcohol but does not meet the DSM-5 criteria for moderate or severe alcohol use disorder, a brief intervention may be all that is needed for the individual to reduce use (Gauthier et al., 2011). Other examples are motivating individuals to exercise, meditate, eat healthier, or take medication regularly.
2. For problems that need ongoing treatment, the purpose of brief interventions is to motivate individuals to accept referrals to appropriate providers and to do so in a way that is consonant with their views of the problem and the steps that need to be taken to alleviate it.

The modality of MI is associated with brief interventions. MI is a person-centered psychotherapy that is specifically designed to resolve individuals' ambivalence about making necessary changes in their lives (Miller & Rollnick, 2013). Developed in the 1980s by Miller and Rollnick as an approach to substance abuse treatment, it is now used for almost any issue for which individuals have ambivalence about change, and it is focused on individuals' creating their own specific action plans to bring about change.

In the first edition (1991) of Miller and Rollnick's textbook, *Motivational Interviewing,* five principles were presented:

1. Expressing empathy (about individuals' ambivalence to change)
2. Developing discrepancy (between individuals' substance misuse and life goals)
3. Avoiding argumentation
4. Rolling with resistance
5. Supporting individuals' self-efficacy

In the third (2013) edition of the textbook, emphasis was placed on the use of four core interviewing skills (with the acronym of OARS):

1. Open-ended questions (O)
2. Affirmations (A)
3. Reflections (R), which are statements demonstrating understanding of the deep meaning of what the service user is saying
4. Summarizing (S)

MI is a gentle, encouraging, nonconfrontational modality that helps individuals create and carry out plans for change regarding troublesome issues in their lives.

REFERRALS

Referrals are "procedures to help patients access specialized care" (PS-ATTC, 2011, p. 6). In an integrated health care system, the goal of the brief intervention is often referral to an appropriate specialty area to meet the service user's needs. To facilitate success, recent literature has emphasized the need for a *warm handoff referral*, also referred to as active referral to treatment (ART) (Boston University School of Public Health, 2015). This may include introducing an individual to a mental health or substance abuse care provider in person (Horevitz, Organista, & Arean, 2015; Richter et al., 2012) (see Chapter 8). Because this is not often possible, calling the specialist's office together with the service user and arranging for follow-up with the service user to ensure that the referral successfully took place is far more effective than simply providing names and telephone numbers.

ART also involves continual reaching out to an individual until the referral has successfully taken place (Boston University School of Public Health, 2015). In the case example, neither of the social workers engaged in a warm handoff referral process with Joan. The hospital social worker merely advised her to see a psychotherapist, and the clinical social worker mailed her a letter recommending substance abuse treatment.

FUNCTIONS FOR SOCIAL WORKERS IN AN INTEGRATED HEALTH CARE APPROACH

Social work education—with its emphasis on systems theory, ecological assessment, and a strengths-based, person-centered approach—is well suited to train providers for the unifying tasks necessary in an integrated health care model. Social workers frequently perform the function of a case manager, organizing individuals' services in many health and social service settings. This function can be expanded in an integrated health care approach to include a care-coordinating role in primary health care settings and a role as provider of integrated health care screenings and brief interventions in all nonmedical settings.

Social workers can ensure that each service user's physical health, mental health, and substance abuse treatment needs are being addressed in a holistic way in all fields of practice. For example, social workers employed as clinicians in mental health agencies need to screen for substance misuse and medical issues, whereas social workers in substance abuse programs need to screen for mental health and physical problems. Social workers in schools, senior citizen centers, shelters, child welfare programs, criminal justice programs, and other settings need to integrate SBIRT concepts for physical health, mental health, and substance misuse into their routine work.

In addition to providing SBIRT services in an integrated health care model, social workers need to follow through with service users to ensure that they do not become lost in the cracks of the fragmented health care system, as described previously in the case of Joan. Although it would have been ideal for Joan to have received the services of a care coordinator in her primary care physician's office, both social workers with whom she interacted could have taken on more responsibility to ensure that her mental health and substance misuse issues were being addressed to the greatest possible degree.

The following sections describe procedures for performing SBIRT services specifically addressing mental health problems, substance use problems, and physical health problems.

ADDRESSING MENTAL HEALTH PROBLEMS

Integration of effective, comprehensive screening for mental health problems into a primary care setting with a large patient population and a limited number of social workers can be daunting. The likelihood of an individual's mental health needs being met often depends on whether a primary care physician emphasizes the individual's emotional wellbeing. If an integrated health care approach is to be instituted as a national model of health care, the social work profession will need to advocate for a greater number of social workers in primary health care settings.

The following strategies are recommended for providing SBIRT services in a primary care setting, although most of the procedures discussed apply to social workers in all settings. The principal difference is that in most fields of practice, a physician is not present on site.

SCREENING

The use of validated written or online screening instruments for mental health problems can help in a primary care setting as long as clinicians understand that they represent *adjuncts* to effective assessment and diagnosis, not the assessment itself. These tools can alert clinicians to potential mental health problems. The use of these screens is not recommended without an in-person interview directly following the screening.

Many primary care settings have an individual complete a depression scale as part of the intake package. There are several such scales, including the Burns Depression Checklist (Burns, 1999), and the Beck Depression Inventory (BDI) (Beck, Steer, & Garbin, 1988). Because depression is a common mental health issue that can have serious and possibly lethal consequences if not treated correctly, use of these scales is a positive development. However, the use of a depression scale alone, or even with an additional anxiety measure such as the Generalized Anxiety Disorder 7 (GAD-7) scale (Spitzer, Kroenke, Williams, & Lowe, 2006) or the Beck Anxiety Inventory (Beck, Epstein, Brown, & Steer, 1988), is not sufficient. It is more effective to use an instrument that screens for a variety of psychiatric conditions. The Substance Abuse and Mental Health Services Administration–Health Resources and Services Administration's (SAMHSA-HRSA) Center for Integrated Health Solutions (n.d.) provides several mental health screens on its website, and the interdisciplinary team in a primary care facility should carefully choose the ones they think will be most helpful in alerting staff to service users' mental health problems.

In many primary care facilities, a nurse or physician's assistant sees an individual before the physician does. However, each service user should also be screened for mental health and substance use problems before being seen by a doctor. The screening can be conducted by a social worker. Before social workers ask individuals about their mental health conditions and use of substances, they should request permission to do so. If an individual does not wish to discuss any of these issues, the social worker must respect that choice.

Ideally, the social worker should see individuals alone, ask them why they are seeing the physician, and then ask how they have been feeling emotionally in the past several months. This survey should include questions about recent stressors and service users' reactions to their physical problems. The social worker should inquire about the individual's family life and social support system. Asking an individual about a typical day in their life usually reveals much information. If an individual expresses emotional distress, a suicide assessment should be performed. If service users are forthcoming about their mental health issues, it may not be necessary to review the results of formal screening instruments with them. It is more advisable for the social worker to follow what service users are saying, conveying an understanding of their issues in a person-centered way.

There are two situations in which the social worker should review the results of the screening instruments with the service user. First, if there is considerable discrepancy between the screening results and what the individual verbally reports, the social worker should inquire about the incongruence. Second, the results of the screening instruments should be shared if the service user asks for them. If the screening results are shared, social workers need to ask service users what they think about the results and discuss their reactions. All patients assessed for alcohol and drug problems should receive their screening results.

Although validated screening instruments are being used, the levels of severity of the mental health problems that are revealed by the scores do not necessarily reflect the subjective experience of the affected individual. For example, individuals who score in mild ranges of depression or anxiety may be feeling very depressed or anxious. Conversely, a person whose score denotes depression may not be consciously aware of it or label it as such. Different scales for the same mental health symptom can produce different results in the same person, even if both scales have been validated. An individual may also score differently on different days because symptoms can be greatly affected by what is occurring in the person's life on any given day.

In many health care settings, if the results of service users' written mental health screening scales do not demonstrate a problem, no one will verbally screen them for emotional issues, and significant mental health issues may be missed. Ideally, social workers should interview all individuals as part of a mental health assessment and not rely solely on screening instruments.

Individuals of all ages should be screened for mental health issues. When working with children and adolescents, the screening process most likely would also involve the individual's caregivers. Social workers need to use their judgment regarding when to see children and adolescents alone and when to have sessions with caregivers or other family members. Numerous mental health screening instruments are available for children and adolescents, and most include a section to be filled out by their caregivers. Specialized screening instruments are also available for the assessment of older adults. An example is the Geriatric Depression Scale (GDS) (Sheikh et al., 1991). Because depression in this age group sometimes manifests as dementia, it is essential that a thorough mental health assessment be performed for all such individuals.

BRIEF INTERVENTION AND REFERRAL

After it has been established that there is a mental health issue, the social worker in a primary care setting should perform a brief intervention. Use of a person-centered framework is advisable because it is essential for service users themselves to ultimately choose how they plan to ameliorate their mental health issues, if at all. Whether it is the use of psychotropic medication, individual or group psychotherapy, family or couple's therapy, exercise, meditation, yoga, or some other modality, the service user's perceptions and wishes must be respected. Before the interview is completed, a plan should be written out and given to the individual. Follow-up phone calls and visits should be arranged to monitor the service user's progress.

After the interview, the social worker needs to communicate with the physician concerning the results of the mental health screening and the treatment plan. The physician needs to include this treatment plan in a discussion with the service user and reinforce the referral.

A warm handoff referral is important. If the primary care setting has a behavioral health department, physically walking the individual to that department is ideal. However, because this is rarely the case, the social worker and the service user should call the mental health provider together and arrange for an appointment. Social workers must call the service user several days later to find out whether the appointment was actually fulfilled.

The warm handoff referral does not only apply to mental health programs. If an individual decides that he or she would like to join a gym or engage in meditation or yoga, a selection of resources should be provided. The social worker and the service user can contact these resources together, and the social worker should follow-up with the individual shortly afterward.

If service users who manifest psychiatric issues opt for no mental health intervention, the social worker can contract with the individuals to follow-up with them if they agree. Social workers can also ask them whether they wish to have their family members contacted about the problem.

CASE VIGNETTE

The following vignette illustrates the use of an integrated health care approach for a patient experiencing anxiety and depression in a primary health care setting.

Mario is a 63-year-old man who recently underwent cardiac bypass surgery. The operation went well, and three months later he visited his physician at a primary care clinic. As he checked in for his appointment, he was given medical, mental health, and substance misuse questionnaires to complete. They included the brief PHQ-4 depression and anxiety scale (Kroenke, Spitzer, Williams, & Lowe, 2009), and the CAGE-AID, a commonly used, brief substance misuse screening tool. Mario was then interviewed by a physician's assistant, who reviewed his medical issues. A social worker then entered the office and interviewed him. Before meeting Mario, the social worker reviewed the results of the screening instruments, which indicated he was experiencing mild depression and moderate anxiety and did not indicate substance misuse problems.

The social worker began the screening part of the interview by asking Mario for permission to discuss emotional issues with him. After he agreed, the social worker asked Mario how he had been feeling emotionally over the past several weeks. Mario indicated that he had been feeling extremely anxious and a little depressed. They discussed how he worried excessively about death even though the surgery was successful and he had already returned to work. Mario stated that, even when he was not worrying, he often felt his body was shaking inside. Sometimes he felt disconnected from the world. His wife had been complaining about his worrying and his distant mood, even calling his relatives and telling them that they must calm him down and "put some sense in his head." When asked about his use of alcohol and drugs, Mario stated that he used to drink occasionally but had not had a drop of alcohol since the surgery. The social worker did not review the results of the screening instruments with him, and he did not ask for this information. Mario did not wish to have his wife contacted.

As part of the brief intervention, the social worker validated Mario's experience, saying that many people who undergo cardiac surgery have depression and anxiety afterward and that he was not experiencing anything unusual. The social worker then informed him about various treatment options, including the possibility of medications for his depression and anxiety. Mario expressed concern that psychotropic medications could affect his heart, but he was willing to speak to the physician about them. He also stated that a referral to a psychotherapist would be a good idea because he would welcome having someone to speak to about his anxiety. Mario discussed how going to work was very beneficial for him because it distracted him from his worries and he enjoyed socializing with his colleagues. Given his social nature, the social worker informed Mario about Mended Hearts, a free monthly support group for people who have undergone cardiac surgery. Together, they looked online for a meeting that would fit his schedule, and he agreed to attend.

As part of a warm handoff referral, the social worker and Mario together performed a search online and found a private psychotherapist whose profile Mario liked. Mario left a message on the therapist's voicemail for an appointment. The social worker asked Mario if she could call him in a week to find out how he was feeling and about his reactions to seeing the psychotherapist and attending the support group. He felt grateful for this offer. After the interview, the social worker spoke to the physician about Mario's anxiety and depression and his desire to discuss psychotropic medications with the physician despite fears about taking them. The social worker also told the physician about the referrals to the private psychotherapist and support group. The physician followed-up with these issues during the next meeting with Mario.

ADDRESSING SUBSTANCE MISUSE PROBLEMS

To effectively screen and provide brief interventions for substance-using individuals, the evidence-based protocol known as SBIRT is already in place. It was originally designed for use by physicians (SAMHSA, 2016), but more recently SAMHSA has strongly encouraged its use by other health professionals such as nurses, social workers, psychologists, counselors, and dentists. It is appropriate for use by social workers in most fields of practice and with adolescents and adults of all ages. SBIRT is based on MI, and social workers need some training in this modality to use it effectively. Based on guidelines provided by SAMHSA (2013b), the use of SBIRT to address substance use problems is described in the following sections.

SCREENING

SBIRT's screening protocol is universal. This means that social workers should screen all individuals in health and social service settings regarding substance misuse issues, not just those whom clinicians already suspect are abusing alcohol or drugs. Although SBIRT should be performed in the context of a person-centered interview by the clinician, it is a good idea to have the service user complete a short substance misuse assessment screening form in the waiting room along with the mental health questionnaires. The CAGE-AID questionnaire is a four-question substance misuse prescreen instrument that can be used for this purpose. The Alcohol Use Disorders Identification Test-C (AUDIT-C) (Bush, Kivlahan, McDonell, Fihn, & Bradley, 1998), can also be used in the waiting room as a pre-screening tool for alcohol misuse. These instruments may help indicate that an individual has substance use problems that need to be explored further.

Regardless of the setting, after the social worker has asked the individual for permission to discuss mental health and substance misuse issues, the clinician should first screen for mental health difficulties. Using the SBIRT protocol, the social worker should then perform an in-person alcohol and drug use prescreening. This begins with two questions: "Do you sometimes drink beer, wine, or other alcoholic beverages?" (SAMHSA, 2013b, Session 2, p. 11) and "How many times in the past year have you used an illegal drug or prescription medication for nonmedical reasons?" (SAMHSA, 2013b, Session 2, p. 24). If the answers to these questions are "no" and "never," respectively, the SBIRT screening is finished.

If the service user states that he or she drinks alcohol, the social worker should perform the following prescreening procedures to determine whether a formal alcohol screening tool is necessary:

1. The clinician first asks, "During how many days do you drink alcohol in the course of an average week?" and "How much do you drink on those days?" For

adult men younger than 65 years of age, 14 or fewer drinks per week is considered safe drinking. For all adult women and for men age 65 or older, maximum of seven drinks per week is considered safe. For teenagers, any drinking is considered hazardous. If individuals drink at levels greater than these amounts, a formal alcohol screening needs to be performed.

2. If the individual does not drink at the aforementioned levels, the social worker asks men younger than 65 years of age how many days in the past year they have consumed five or more drinks in one day. If the individual states that he has done this *at least once in the prior year*, a formal screening needs to be performed. Similarly, the social worker asks men age 65 or older and all women how many days in the past year they have consumed four or more drinks in one day. If they have done this *at least once in the prior year*, a formal alcohol screening needs to be performed. Any alcohol consumption by teenagers warrants a formal alcohol screening.

3. In performing the prescreening procedures, the social worker needs to understand and convey to the service user that "one drink" is equivalent to 12 ounces of beer, 5 ounces of wine, or 1.5 ounces of 80-proof spirits (i.e., one jigger or shot) (SAMHSA, 2013b, Session 2, p. 17).

If the results of the prescreening indicate that a formal alcohol screening needs to be performed, there are numerous tools from which to choose. For adults, the AUDIT is commonly used, particularly the 10-item version. The World Health Organization's (WHO) Alcohol, Smoking, and Substance Involvement and Screening Test (ASSIST) (WHO ASSIST Working Group, 2002), is another commonly used tool. For adolescents, the CRAFFT questionnaire (using six key items: car, relax, alone, forget, friends, trouble) may be used (Knight, Sherritt, Shrier, Harris, & Chang, 2002). The 10-item Short Michigan Alcohol Screening Test Geriatric Version (SMAST-G) was created for screening individuals age 65 or older (Vermont Department of Health, 2016).

If individuals affirm their use of illegal drugs or prescription medications for nonmedical reasons, the social worker should ask which drugs are being used and how frequently. Any use of drugs necessitates application of a formal screening instrument. A commonly used screening tool is the 10-item Drug Abuse Screening Test (DAST). The ASSIST (for adults) and CRAFFT (for teenagers) questionnaires can be used for assessing both drug and alcohol use.

The social worker should make using these scales as collaborative a process as possible. The social worker should show the instrument to the service user and explain its function, perhaps also demonstrating the scoring procedure. SBIRT applications are available on smartphones and computers, and the social worker can complete the screening tools together with the service user on a screen. Sharing the score with the individual and explaining what the score signifies become part of the brief intervention. When performing any of these prescreening or screening procedures, it is important to maintain a warm, nonjudgmental attitude, using the principles of a person-centered approach.

The SBIRT brief intervention is also referred to as the brief negotiated interview (BNI) (SAMHSA, 2013b, Session 6, p. 8). This process is divided into four steps:

1. Building rapport
2. Providing feedback
3. Building readiness to change
4. Negotiating a plan for change

If the alcohol and drug screenings do not indicate risky substance misuse, there is no need for a brief intervention unless individuals manifest biopsychosocial problems due to their substance misuse despite their scores.

In the building rapport phase, the clinician asks service users in a matter-of-fact way how the use of alcohol or drugs fits into their life. In line with MI principles, the social worker first asks what the individual likes about using the substance and then what he or she does not like about it. The order of these two questions needs to be followed so that service users end up talking about the difficulties caused by their substance use. The social worker summarizes what individuals have stated in an empathic way, first reflecting what they like and then what they do not like about using alcohol or drugs.

In the providing feedback phase, the social worker discusses the results of the formal screening instruments. It can help for the clinician to have visual aid cards with diagrams showing the different levels of alcohol and drug use corresponding to the scores on the screening tools: low-risk or healthy use, at-risk use, harmful use, and dependent use.

It is important to ask service users how they feel about their scores and risk categories. After obtaining permission from service users to do so, the social worker can provide feedback about the level of substance use and the harms that this can create. The social worker must then ask what the individual thinks and feels about the feedback.

In the building readiness to change phase, the social worker obtains a sense of what aspects of substance-using behaviors, if any, the service user wants to eradicate or modify. This can begin with a question such as, "Can we talk for a few minutes about any desire you may have to make a change in your marijuana use?" In this phase, social workers need to ascertain what changes individuals want to make while being careful not to push their own agendas.

A technique called *the ruler* is often used. It is derived from solution-focused therapy (Shafer & Jordan, 2014). The social worker questions service users regarding their desire to change their substance-using behaviors, on a scale from 0 to 10 (some use a scale from 1 to 10). Clinicians can use different kinds of rulers. Using the *importance ruler*, the social worker asks a question such as, "How important is it for you to cut down on your alcohol use on a scale from 0 to 10, in which 0 is not important at all and 10 is very important?" Using the *readiness ruler*, a worker can ask, "How ready are you to make a change in your cocaine use?" There is also a *confidence ruler*, which measures individuals' perceived ability to make the change that they have proposed, and a *commitment ruler*, which measures individuals' belief that they can remain committed to their change plan.

Whatever numbers on the ruler service users choose in their responses, the social worker always asks why they chose that number rather than a lower number. For example, if an individual states that he or she is at a five in regard to readiness to reduce alcohol consumption, the social worker would ask, "Why did you choose a five and not a two?" This induces the service user to discuss reasons for wanting to make the change. The social worker never asks why individuals did not choose a *higher* number because this would encourage them to discuss reasons for *not* making a change. If an individual chooses a low number (i.e., less than three), the social worker can ask, "What would need to happen in your life for it to be important to you to change your alcohol use?" Responses to the ruler questions should result in a discussion about the aspects of substance abuse the service user wishes to change. The social worker must respect the service user's point of view of what needs to be changed, even if the change seems less than adequate to the social worker.

In the negotiating a plan for change phase, the social worker encourages service users to formulate a plan for reducing or stopping their substance misuse. It is important that the service user, not the social worker, creates this plan. The clinician can solidify the plan by asking practical questions about how the service user will carry it out and how motivation for this change can be maintained. The social worker should elicit as many details as possible in the change plan. After the plan is completed, the social worker or the service user should write down the plan on paper, and it should be given to the service user. A date should be arranged when the service user will return to or contact the social worker to discuss whether and how the plan was followed. If on that date the plan has not been followed, a new plan should be created if the service user desires to do so.

In SBIRT, the social worker must express respect for service users who do not desire to change their substance misuse. This creates an environment in which individuals feel understood and leaves the door open to discussing their alcohol and drug misuse in the future. It is a good idea for social workers to ask service users who do not wish to change their substance misuse for permission to discuss the issue in the future.

A warm handoff referral is crucial, with the social worker ideally accompanying the service user to a substance abuse treatment program. If this is not possible, calling the program with the service user present is essential, and the social worker must follow-up to find out whether the service user began treatment. In the brief intervention, the explicit goal of the plan may be for the service user to begin substance abuse treatment. For example, when using the readiness ruler, the social worker can ask, "On a scale of 0 to 10, how ready are you to begin an outpatient substance abuse program three times a week?"

CASE VIGNETTE

The following scenario regarding the use of SBIRT takes place at a high school rather than a primary care facility. However, the procedures are almost identical in other settings.

Alex is a 16-year-old student in a public high school. His grades have been dropping steadily over the past 18 months, and he has been failing courses. A teacher requested that Alex see a social worker because he seems fatigued and preoccupied in class and sometimes falls asleep. When Alex meets the social worker, Amanda, he appears guarded but shares that there has been conflict in his home between him and his stepfather and that he has recently been arguing with his mother as well. He has two younger half-siblings whom he gets along with, but he believes that his parents favor them. Alex states that he has friends in school and likes socializing with them. However, he is vague about his tiredness in class and not completing homework assignments.

The social worker and Alex discuss his mood, and he agrees that he feels depressed about his family situation and being a year behind in school. As the social worker continues to be empathic and to focus on Alex's perceptions of his life situation, he appears more relaxed and less guarded. The social worker asks Alex whether she can ask him a few questions about his alcohol and drug use. She tells him that his answers will be confidential and will not negatively affect his standing in school in any way. Before she asks the prescreening questions, Alex states that he sometimes smokes marijuana but does not like alcohol or use other drugs.

The social worker asks Alex whether she can ask him a few questions about his marijuana use and he agrees. She asks him the six questions from the CRAFFT instrument. She then asks Alex to tell her about how marijuana fits into his life. Alex says that it relaxes him with all of the tension that is occurring in his household. More importantly, he finds it fun to smoke marijuana with his friends. As Alex reveals what he likes about marijuana, she reflects, "So marijuana helps you relax from all of the tension you are experiencing at home and helps you have fun with your friends." Alex agrees. She then asks Alex what he does not like about smoking marijuana, and he states that when he smokes in the morning, he cannot concentrate in his classes. He also has trouble completing homework when smoking after school. He further reveals that much of the fighting in his household lately revolves around his marijuana use and declining grades. Amanda reflects on what he told her and then asks him, "On a scale of 0 to 10, how important it is to you that you graduate high school?" Alex gives this a 10. She asks Alex why a 10 and not a 7. He states that he is aware that he will never have sufficient income without a high school diploma and discusses his career plans, which require college.

Amanda reviews Alex's score on the CRAFFT, showing him on a chart that his score of 4 indicates a very high probability of hazardous drug use. Alex states that he is aware that his marijuana use is affecting his ability to function in school, but he does not want to stop using it. Amanda then asks Alex, on a scale of 0 to 10, how important it is for him to not stop using marijuana but to reduce his use in a way that he can succeed in his classes. Alex gives this a 7. Amanda asks why a 7 and not a 4. Alex then reiterates the importance of passing his classes. She asks Alex to devise a plan to reduce his marijuana use so that it does not heavily interfere with his school functioning. He immediately states that he must not smoke marijuana in the morning before going to school. Beyond this, he is not certain what to do. The social worker asks him, on a scale of 0 to 10, how confident he feels that he could commit to not using marijuana before school each day in the next week. He states an 8. Alex writes this goal on a card. They discuss what triggers might occur for him to smoke marijuana in the morning, and he devises strategies to counter these triggers. Alex writes these strategies on the card as well. The social worker asks Alex to create a title for the card that will help him meet his goal, and he writes: "Graduating From High School." They agree to meet in one week to discuss his problems at home, his depression, and his goal of not smoking marijuana before school.

ADDRESSING PHYSICAL HEALTH PROBLEMS

There has been far more emphasis in the literature on the inclusion of mental health and substance misuse screenings for individuals in primary care settings than on the inclusion of physical health screenings in mental health, substance misuse, and social service settings. Moreover, it is not easy to find appropriate physical health screening instruments online for social workers to use in nonprimary care settings. This is unfortunate because studies have clearly demonstrated that individuals with mental health and substance use problems have substantially shorter life expectancies due to physical illnesses (Colton & Manderscheid, 2006; Hayes et al., 2011; Miller, Paschall, & Svendsen, 2006). For example, in a study in Maryland, the life expectancy of individuals with severe mental illnesses was 51.8 years (Daumit et al., 2010). The primary goal of the physical health screening and brief intervention process in nonmedical settings is to ensure that individuals are referred to and monitored by physicians and allied health professionals for their medical issues.

SCREENING

The most important aspect of screening for physical health problems is asking service users when they last had an appointment with a physician and what the reason was for the visit. Despite the prevalence of serious health issues and underuse of primary health care services among the populations with whom social workers interface, many social workers do not routinely ask these simple questions. The questions should be included on all intake and assessment forms.

These questions should be followed by asking service users about physical symptoms that they are experiencing and concerns they may have about their health. The service users' responses need to be explored in depth. One comprehensive screening tool that was developed to assess the physical health issues of individuals in mental health facilities is the Physical Health Check (PHC) (Rethink Mental Illness, 2014). This tool can be used in other types of agencies and institutions. A discussion of the results of a physical health screening can point to the need for service users to seek consultation from a physician.

Clinicians need to ask all individuals about their history of tobacco use and any desire they have to quit. It is also important to ask about any sleep difficulties and how these problems are affecting their lives. Social workers need to ask service users when they last visited a dental facility and discuss the service users' dental health. Because it may be overlooked in other health screenings, dental health needs to be explored as a separate question.

Social workers also should discuss issues of diet and exercise with each service user. The PHC screen includes questions about these issues. Social workers should encourage service users to use available resources to learn how to improve their eating habits and find ways to carry out simple exercise regimens.

After screening is complete, a simple plan should be created to address physical health concerns. As with brief interventions for mental health and substance misuse problems, a collaborative, person-centered approach such as MI should be used. The social worker should begin by asking service users their opinions of the screening discussion that just occurred and what aspects of their physical health they wish to address. If service users omit physical health areas that the social worker thinks may be problematic, the social worker should ask the service users' thoughts and feelings about addressing those issues. However, the service users' opinions must ultimately be respected. It is often helpful for the social worker and the service user to write down the service user's plan for dealing with physical health issues. A copy of this plan should be given to the service user and can be used as part of the review process in the next session. The concepts of warm handoff referrals and follow-up plans are of paramount importance.

CASE VIGNETTE

The following vignette illustrates how a screening and brief intervention for physical health problems can be performed by a social worker in a non-medical setting.

Suzanne is a 55-year old woman who recently began treatment at an outpatient substance abuse program. Although she smoked marijuana recreationally for most of her adult life, she never felt she had a drug problem until she began a relationship five years earlier with a man named Joe who was crack cocaine dependent and encouraged her to smoke crack with him. Shortly before beginning treatment, she left her partner and moved in with her 78-year-old mother.

Anthony was assigned to be her social worker. The agency had recently added more in-depth questions about physical health as part of the intake process, including the PHC (Rethink Mental Illness, 2014). During their first session, in addition to the substance misuse and mental health assessments, Anthony reviewed Suzanne's responses to the PHC and discussed the fact that she had not seen a physician in more than five years. She expressed great concern about this, adding that she had not seen a gynecologist and had not received any screening for breast or cervical cancer for many years. Suzanne mentioned having bouts of diarrhea over the last year, and although she had seen some blood in her stool, she had never had a colonoscopy. She stated that her diet had been very unhealthy during the past five years and that she had lost at least 30 pounds since she started using crack. However, her recent move to her mother's apartment had resulted in an improvement in her diet because her mother ensured that she was eating better.

Suzanne stated that she wanted to exercise but was feeling overwhelmed by coming to the substance abuse program four days each week and felt tired much of the time since she stopped smoking crack. She also discussed smoking about 10 cigarettes daily for the past 30 years and stated that she could not imagine reducing her tobacco use at this time. She also discussed how her teeth were "falling apart" and how this greatly disturbed her. She had had an emergency extraction of an infected tooth the previous year but no preventative or restorative dental work since she met Joe. Her sleep pattern has been a problem, and she frequently wakes up in the middle of the night and cannot fall back asleep.

Suzanne agreed to make an appointment with a primary care physician regarding her intestinal problems. She stated that she was feeling very anxious about this and needed to address this issue first before she could think about other physical issues and her dental problems. However, her lack of exercise also bothered her, and she wanted to change that. For the time being, Suzanne came up with a plan to walk home from the substance abuse clinic, a distance of about one mile on the four days that she attended the program. Anthony asked Suzanne to write down her plan for the next two weeks, which included seeing a physician to begin addressing her intestinal problems and walking home from the program four days each week. They discussed which primary care physician she could see, and she stated that she would make an appointment with her mother's physician. Together, they looked online for the physician's phone number, and Suzanne called for an appointment from the office.

CONCLUSIONS

Screening, brief intervention, and referral to treatment for mental health, substance misuse, and physical health problems are major components of an integrated health care model. The purpose of these processes is not to add to the administrative and paperwork burden of social workers and health care providers but to approach mental health, substance misuse, and physical health problems in a holistic way, with fewer serious issues falling through the chasms of a fragmented health care system.

Training of all social workers in the proper use of screening and assessment processes and the use of valid instruments is essential. For this to be achieved, a parallel process of addressing the holistic wellness needs of social workers must also be encouraged. In a person-centered approach, both service users and service providers need to meet in an environment where they feel cherished and respected. In a practical sense, this means that sufficient funding must be provided to support a well-trained and adequate social work and health care workforce. If this is accomplished, dissemination of an integrated health care model has the potential to save billions of dollars on health care costs and improve the lives of a vast portion of the U.S. population.

RESOURCES

Behavioral Health-Assessment and Scoring Instruments, Nationwide Children's http://www.nationwide-childrens.org/mental-health-assessment-and-scoring-instruments

Center for Integrated Health Solutions (CIHS), Substance Abuse and Mental Health Services–Health Resources and Services Administration (SAMHSA-HRSA) http://www.integration.samhsa.gov/

Child and Youth Mental Health Tools & Resources, General Practice Services Committee (GPSC) http://www.gpscbc.ca/what-we-do/professional-development/psp/modules/child-and-youth-mental-health/tools-resources

Children's Mental Health Screening, Minnesota Department of Human Services http://www.dhs.state.mn.us/main/idcplg?IdcService=GET_DYNAMIC_CONVERSION&RevisionSelectionMethod=LatestReleased&dDocName=dhs16_149102

Clinical Tools, Teen Mental Health.org http://teenmentalhealth.org/care/health-professionals/clinical-tools

Mental Health Screening Tools, Mental Health America (MHA) http://www.mentalhealthamerica.net/mental-health-screening-tools

Screening, Brief Intervention and Referral to Treatment, New York State Office of Alcoholism and Substance Abuse Services (OASAS) https://www.oasas.ny.gov/adMed/sbirt/index.cfm

Screening, Brief Intervention, and Referral to Treatment (SBIRT), Substance Abuse and Mental Health Services Administration (SAMHSA) http://www.samhsa.gov/sbirt

Screening, Brief Intervention & Referral to Treatment (SBIRT), Vermont Department of Health http://sbirt.vermont.gov/

Screening, Diagnostic Assessment and Interview Tools, Iowa Coalition on Mental Health & Aging http://www.public-health.uiowa.edu/icmha/outreach/screening.html

Screening Tools, Behavioral Health Evolution http://www.bhevolution.org/public/screening_tools.page

REFERENCES

Beck, A. T., Steer, R. A., & Garbin, M. G. (1988). Psychometric properties of the Beck Depression Inventory: Twenty-five years of evaluation. *Clinical Psychology Review, 8,* 77–100.

Beck, A. T., Epstein, N., Brown, G. & Steer, R. A. (1988). An inventory for measuring clinical anxiety: Psychometric properties. *Journal of Consulting and Clinical Psychology, 56,* 893–897.

Boston University School of Public Health. (2015). Active referral to treatment. Retrieved from http://www.bu.edu/bniart/sbirt-in-health-care/sbirt-active-referral-treatment-art/

Burns, D. D. (1999). *Feeling good: The new mood therapy.* New York, NY: Avon Books.

Bush, K, Kivlahan, D.R., McDonell, M. B., Fihn, S. D., & Bradley, K. A. (1998). The AUDIT alcohol consumption questions (AUDIT-C): an effective brief screening test for problem drinking. Ambulatory Care Quality Improvement Project (ACQUIP). Alcohol Use Disorders Identification Test. *Archives of Internal Medicine, 158,* 1789–1795.

Center for Integrated Health Solutions, Substance Abuse and Mental Health Services Administration-Health Resources & Services. (n.d.). Screening tools. Retrieved from http://www.integration.samhsa.gov/clinical-practice/screening-tools

Colton, C. W., & Manderscheid, R. W. (2006). Congruencies in increased mortality rates, years of potential life lost, and causes of death among public mental health clients in eight states. *Preventing Chronic Disease, 3,* A42.

Daumit, G. L., Anthony, C. B., Ford, D. E., Fahey, M., Skinner, E. A., Lehman, A. F., . . . Steinwachs, D. M. (2010). Pattern of mortality in a sample of Maryland residents with severe mental illness. *Psychiatry Research, 176,* 242–245. doi: 10.1016/j.psychres.2009.01.006

Gauthier, G., Palacios-Boix, J., Charney, D. A., Negrete, J. C., Pentney, H., & Gill, K. J. (2011). Comparison of brief and standard interventions for drug and alcohol dependence: Considerations for primary care service delivery. *Canadian Journal of Community Mental Health, 30*(1), 93–104. doi: 10.7870/cjcmh-2011-0007

Hayes, R. D., Chang, C. K., Fernandes, A., Broadbent, M., Lee, W., Hotopf, M., & Stewart, R.(2011). Associations between substance use disorder sub-groups, life expectancy and all-cause mortality in a large British specialist mental healthcare service. *Drug and Alcohol Dependence, 118,* 56–61. doi: 10.1016/j.drugalcdep.2011.02.021

Horevitz, E., Organista, K. C., & Arean, P. A. (2015). Depression treatment uptake in integrated primary care: How a "warm handoff" and other factors affect decision making by Latinos. *Psychiatric Services, 66,* 824–830. doi: 10.1176/appi.ps.201400085

Knight JR; Sherritt L; Shrier LA//Harris SK//Chang G. (2002). Validity of the CRAFFT substance abuse screening test among adolescent clinic patients. *Archives of Pediatrics & Adolescent, 156,* 607–614.

Kroenke, K., Spitzer, R. L., Williams, J. B. W. & Lowe, B. (2009). An Ultra-Brief Screening Scale for Anxiety and Depression: The PHQ–4. Psychosomatics 50, Issue 6, 613–621. DOI: http://dx.doi.org/10.1016/S0033-3182(09)70864-3

Miller, B. J., Paschall, C. B., & Svendsen, D. P. (2006). Mortality and medical comorbidity among patients with serious mental illness. *Psychiatric Services, 57,* 1482–1487. doi: 10.1176/ps.2006.57.10.1482

Miller, W. R., & Rollnick, S. (1991). *Motivational interviewing: Preparing people to change addictive behavior* (1st ed.). New York, NY: Guilford Press.

Miller, W. R., & Rollnick, S. (2013). *Motivational interviewing: Helping people change* (3rd ed.). New York, NY: Guilford Press.

Mosby, Inc. (2013). *Mosby's dictionary of medicine, nursing & health professions* (9th ed.). St. Louis, Mo: Elsevier/Mosby.

Pacific Southwest Addiction Technology Transfer Center. (2011). *Screening, brief intervention, and referral to treatment (SBIRT) training: Participant guide.* Los Angeles, CA: Pacific Southwest Addiction Technology Transfer Center, Integrated Substance Abuse Programs, University of California, Los Angeles. Retrieved from http://attcnetwork.org/regcenters/productDocs/11/Participant%20Guide%202012-01-20.pdf

Rethink Mental Illness. (2014). *Physical Health Check tool.* Retrieved from https://www.rethink.org/media/1137219/Physical%20Health%20Check%202014.pdf

Richter, K. P., Faseru, B., Mussulman, L. M., Ellerbeck, E. F., Shireman, T. I., Hunt, J. J., ... Cook, D. J. (2012). Using "warm handoffs" to link hospitalized smokers with tobacco treatment after discharge: Study protocol of a randomized controlled trial. *Trials, 13,* 127. doi: 10.1186/1745-6215-13-127.

Shafer, K. C., & Jordan, S. A. S. (2014). Working with mandated clients with substance use disorders: A solution focused approach. In S. L. A. Straussner (Ed.), *Clinical work with substance abusing clients* (pp. 202–224). New York, NY: Guilford Press.

Sheikh, J. I., Yesavage, J. A., Brooks, J. O., Friedman, L. F., Gratzinger, P., Hill, R. D., ... Crook, T. (1991). Proposed factor structure of the Geriatric Depression Scale. *International Psychogeriatrics, 3,* 23–28. doi: 10.1017/S1041610291000480

Spitzer, R. L., Kroenke, K., Williams, J. B. W., & Lowe, B. (2006). A brief measure for assessing generalized anxiety disorder. *Archives of Internal Medicine, 166,* 1092–1097. doi: 10.1001/archinte.166.10.1092

Stanhope, V., Videka, L., Thorning, H., & McKay, M. (2015). Moving toward integrated health: An opportunity for social work. *Social Work in Health Care, 54,* 383–407. doi: 10.1080/00981389.2015.1025122

Substance Abuse and Mental Health Services Administration. (2013a). *Screening, brief intervention, and referral to treatment (SBIRT) medical professional training program: Request for applications* (RFA No. TI-13-002). Rockville, MD: Substance Abuse and Mental Health Services Administration.

Substance Abuse and Mental Health Services Administration. (2013b). *Teaching SBIRT: SAMHSA core curriculum.* Rockville, MD: Substance Abuse and Mental Health Services Administration.

Substance Abuse and Mental Health Services Administration. (2016). Screening, brief intervention, and referral to treatment (SBIRT). Retrieved from http://www.samhsa.gov/sbirt

Vermont Department of Health. (2016). SMAST-G—Short Michigan Alcohol Screening Test–Geriatric Version. Retrieved from http://sbirt.vermont.gov/screening-forms/older-adult-alcohol-screening-instrument

WHO ASSIST Working Group (2002). The Alcohol, Smoking and Substance Involvement Screening Test (ASSIST): Development, reliability and feasibility. *Addiction, 97* (9): 1183-1194.

CHAPTER 10

PERSON-CENTERED CARE

Victoria Stanhope and Mimi Choy-Brown

Person-centered care (PCC) is one of the driving principles behind health care reform in the United States and throughout the world (World Health Organization, 2015). The phrase *person-centered care* appears frequently in the legislative language of the Patient Protection and Affordable Care Act (ACA) and was specifically referenced by President Barack Obama in his last State of the Union address in 2016. The term is immediately appealing, and the tendency is for most providers to say they take a person-centered approach to care—who would say they do not? However, when one delves deeper, it becomes clear that PCC requires a paradigmatic shift in how we have traditionally approached health care. The approach is value-based, requiring both providers and systems to take account of people's subjective experiences of health and health care. A commitment to caring for the whole person is needed, along with the skills necessary to take a multidimensional approach beyond simply focusing on a set of symptoms. In integrated health care, PCC is a key benchmark of quality. To realize it in practice, we must have a comprehensive understanding of what this perspective entails rather than simply rendering it as an appealing but vague goal.

The Institute of Medicine (2001) has defined PCC as "care that is respectful of and responsive to individual patient preferences, needs, and values and ensuring values guide all clinical decisions" (p. 6). This is the most widely used definition across settings and has informed further clarification of PCC philosophy and practice. The philosophy of PCC asserts that care is "of the person (of the totality of the person's health, both ill and positive), by the person (with clinicians adopting humanistic and ethical attitudes and extending themselves as full human beings), for the person (assisting the fulfillment of the person's life goals), and with the person (in respectful collaboration with the person who consults)" (Adams & Grieder, 2014, p. 6). Concepts closely related to PCC are the service user's experience, service user's engagement, shared decision making, and decision support. Overall, PCC anchors the services we provide in the experiences of service users and empowers them to make decisions that reflect their own identities and values. Although PCC is aligned with social work values, the medical model within which most social workers operate has often neglected the perspective of the individual and placed individuals in a passive role with respect to their health care.

This chapter provides an overview of how PCC has evolved in different fields of practice and focuses on one aspect of this approach, person-centered care planning (PCCP). PCCP first emerged in the field of developmental disabilities but has become increasingly influential in the area of mental health. Having one unified service plan is key to the coordinated care approach; therefore, strategies to ensure that the service plan and planning process are person-centered can drive the integration of a whole-person orientation across service settings. PCCP targets the plan and the planning process, is well specified, and allows providers to meet the needs of the people they are serving as well as the needs of their organizations in terms of reimbursement requirements.

Dissemination of PCC approaches is supported by a growing evidence base. Shared decision-making and decision supports, two important aspects of integrated health approaches that are closely related to the person-centered approach, are also discussed in this chapter.

EVOLUTION OF PERSON-CENTERED CARE

PCC evolved in different fields of practice, and different terminologies have been used. In medicine, we often see the term *patient-centered care*, which is conceptually the same as PCC but uses the medical term *patient*. Instead of *care planning*, the medical field often refers to this phase as *treatment planning*, reflecting the more narrow medical approach rather than the broader activities involved in a holistic care approach, which can include natural supports and activities in the community. This chapter refers mainly to PCC, which captures the approach across settings and resonates more with social work and recovery-oriented methods.

MEDICINE

The first references to patient-centered care emerged in the 1950s, and the term was formally introduced in the 1970s (Balint, Hunt, Joyce, Marinker, & Woodcock, 1970). However, it was not until the Institute of Medicine's 2001 report, *Crossing the Quality Chasm: A New Health System for the 21st Century,* which proposed patient-centeredness as one of six aims in improving the health care system, that the medical field fully embraced the notion that the service user's experience is central to quality care. Advocates for PCC had strong arguments on ethical, empirical, and economic grounds, stating that PCC is not merely nice to have but necessary (Balik, Conway, Zipperer, & Watson, 2011). Service user movements asserted the right of people to have control over their health care, which can be captured by the following maxims:

1. The needs of the patient come first.
2. Nothing about the patient without the patient.
3. Every patient is the only patient (Berwick, 2009).

There is now a robust literature supporting the premise that people have better outcomes if they have more input into their care, including positive experiences with quality of care and good relationships with their providers (Davidson et al., 2012). This is particularly true for people with chronic illnesses, who have demonstrated greater ability to manage their conditions, better mental health outcomes, and shorter length of hospital stays when they are more actively involved in their care (Balik et al., 2001). Moreover, the financial benefits to the system become apparent when we consider how service disengagement, which is often the result of service users' feeling that providers do not listen or take their needs into account, leads to costly no-shows for clinics and increases in high-cost emergency care.

Mead and Bower (2000) offered an alternative to the biomedical model that largely determines clinical methods according to standardized diagnostic criteria focused on pathology. First, they used a key lens of social work, the *biopsychosocial perspective*, which argues that social and psychological factors must inform diagnosis and assessment (see Chapter 2). Employing this more holistic approach, providers are prompted to engage with the whole lives of their service users. Second, providers must view the *patient as a person*, which means seeing the illness through the service user's eyes. Third, providers should share power and responsibility, shifting the paradigm from the passive patient to a mutual collaboration in which both clinician and service user take responsibility for the course of treatment. Fourth, providers must pay attention to the therapeutic alliance based on Rogers' theory that empathy, congruence, and unconditional positive regard are key to effecting change in service users (Rogers, 1967).

There has been a particular focus on PCC among nurses and social workers working with the elderly. In nursing homes and assisted living facilities, the aim of person-centeredness is to mitigate the impact of institutionalization by giving people as much control as possible over their life and health care and adapting to their needs and preferences. McCormack (2003) developed a framework of PCC for nurses that is underpinned by the concept of *authentic consciousness*, a Kantian notion based on "a consideration of the person's life as a whole to help sustain meaning in life" (p. 204). This act of integrating individuals' life experience to ensure that their decisions reflect their values and beliefs is central to person-centered decision-making. Other aspects of PCC are informed flexibility (i.e., new information integrated into decision-making), sympathetic presence (i.e., interpersonal skills demonstrating the value of the individual's perspective), mutuality (i.e., equal importance of both parties in decision-making), transparency (i.e., explicitly stating underlying motivations and expectations), and negotiation (i.e., accepting that there is no final arbiter for decisions). This approach resonates strongly with the social work core value of the dignity and worth of an individual. With humanistic approaches to care becoming more prominent across all health care professions, social workers will have increased credibility and opportunities to share their expertise.

INTELLECTUAL AND DEVELOPMENTAL DISABILITIES

One of the earliest articulations of PCCP emerged in the 1990s as an intervention for people with intellectual and developmental disabilities. By that time, care for people with developmental disabilities had moved beyond an exclusive focus on custodial care. Providers thought that interventions could remedy individual functional deficits but still missed a focus on the individual preferences of those receiving care. At the same time, the normalization movement was taking hold, which advocated for the rights of people with developmental disabilities to participate fully in the community, spurred on by a series of Supreme Court cases prompting deinstitutionalization and the development of individual program plans. However, Smull and Lakin (2002) described how these plans quickly "began to be written to the rule—not to help the person achieve a lifestyle . . . It became important for plans to meet criteria, not for them to be useful" (p. 363). It became clear that mandating a practice is not sufficient and that for value-oriented practices such as PCCP, providers must believe in the practice and possess the requisite skills for implementing the practice. Later care models started to develop more comprehensive guidance about PCCP, reinforcing the core belief that people with intellectual and developmental disabilities have the right to determine the course of their lives (Taylor & Taylor, 2013).

MENTAL HEALTH

The increasing prominence of PCCP in the mental health field resulted from the recovery movement. In the 1960s, people who had experienced an oppressive and paternalistic system of care started to challenge the notion that their lives should be defined by their diagnoses and that they should be consigned to lives without hope or fulfillment. These activists have referred to themselves in various ways: some as service users, some as psychiatric survivors of the mental health system, and some as ex-patients—meaning that they are no longer defined by the service system. Rooted in the protest and civil rights movements, their voices challenged prevailing mental health practices to embrace the idea that people with mental illnesses can recover in a deeply existential sense—that their lives can regain meaning and purpose. As asserted by Deegan (1996), people can be the drivers of their own unique recovery paths: "Those of us who have been diagnosed are not objects to be acted on. We are fully human subjects who can act and, in acting, change our situation. We are human beings, and we can speak for ourselves" (p. 92). Mental health recovery has also been informed by the psychiatric rehabilitation movement, which has focused on how people can live full and satisfying lives in the community, focusing on their education, work, and social pursuits.

Gradually, the recovery message was heard by mainstream policy makers who were grappling with the same quality chasm that was afflicting the medical system. In 2003, the President's New Freedom Commission Report recommended wholesale reform of the mental health system oriented toward the goal of recovery (New Freedom Commission on Mental Health, 2003). This was followed by the Substance Abuse and Mental Health Services Administration's consensus statement, which proposed the 10 fundamental components of recovery, one of which is person-centeredness (U.S. Department of Health and Human Services, 2004).

Reorienting a system to recovery requires wholesale reform of programs, services, financing, and clinical practices. Many states (supported by federal transformation grants) implemented changes throughout their system (Davidson et al., 2007). PCCP in many ways lies at the heart of this transformation by embedding the recovery approach into the care planning process. Over the past decade, PCCP has developed into a well-specified practice that has been disseminated throughout the country (Tondora, Miller, Slade, & Davidson, 2014). As mental health care shifts toward a more integrated health care approach, PCC and PCCP have become even more salient.

INTEGRATED HEALTH CARE

In the era of health care reform, with its focus on integration, PCC has become a central strategy. Renewed appreciation for the power of healing relationships among providers, individuals, and their families and an understanding that the needs of people with complex difficulties cannot be met without their cooperation are now uniformly accepted. There is a consensus that PCC is a key quality dimension, and experts think that it will "bend the cost curve" through higher rates of engagement (Engelberg Center for Health Care Reform, 2016). Much of this thinking originates from the Chronic Care Model (see Chapter 2), which demonstrates that quality is intrinsically related to how involved people feel about their care, the way they communicate with their provider, and most importantly, the extent to which they feel empowered to make decisions that are right for them. Decisions about health care are often complicated and deeply personal. PCCP creates an authentic process for both the service user and the provider.

Three key aspects of the Chronic Care Model that rest on PCC are *activation*, which ensures that individuals are fully engaged in their care process; *self-management*, which refers to all of the steps a person takes to pursue wellness; and *decision support*, which is focused on helping people to negotiate difficult decisions by being fully informed (Wagner, Austin, & Von Korff, 1996). As an organizing principle, person-centeredness extends beyond the individual and his or her relationship with the provider to address how healthy lives can be promoted at the population level.

Throughout the ACA, there are frequent references to *patient-centeredness, patient engagement,* and *patient satisfaction* with regard to how care should be organized, delivered, and evaluated. The law directs the U.S. Department of Health and Human Services to develop a unified framework to guide service user involvement in all aspects of health care decision-making across various programs and models. Built into the defining features of the patient-centered medical homes and health homes is their ability to deliver PCC. The standards for health homes delineated in the ACA by the Centers for Medicare and Medicaid Services (CMS) specifically state that "services must be quality driven, cost effective, culturally appropriate, person- and family-centered, and evidence-based." PCC has become an important benchmark for integrated health models determining whether a group can receive a designation (e.g., health home) and their level of funding.

The National Quality Forum is working with CMS to develop individual measures that will capture the quality of care from the service user's perspective, including experience, satisfaction, and activation in his or her own care. Epstein, Fiscella, Lesser, and Stange (2010) identified six aspects of PCC that can be measured: fostering healing relationships, exchanging information, responding to emotions, managing uncertainty, making decisions, and enabling self-management. One example of an integrated health care model evaluated with these more subjective measures can be seen in the quality metrics that determine payment from the Medicaid Shared Savings Program for accountable care organizations; within the 33 quality metrics, 7 are related to the service user's experience and 1 specifically focuses on shared decision-making.

The challenges of how to understand and implement PCC point to the need for more conceptual and intervention research in this area. In response, the ACA established the Patient-Centered Outcomes Research Institute (PCORI), which was specifically created to provide answers to the questions service users have about their health care (see Chapter 17). PCORI focuses on person-centered outcomes, comparative effectiveness research, and the communication and dissemination of knowledge about effective treatments (Clancy & Collins, 2010). PCORI adheres to the person-centered tenet—nothing about me, without me—by funding only research with service user engagement at all levels. The ACA has taken the idea of PCC to heart with specific provisions embedding this principle in all aspects of service delivery and research. However, despite the mandates, many providers have struggled to understand what PCC means in daily practice, indicating the need for well-specified practices that capture the spirit and the specifics of PCC.

PERSON-CENTERED CARE PLANNING

PCCP, also referred to as recovery planning or treatment planning, is a well-specified behavioral health intervention that translates PCC principles into practical tools and practices that can be used by behavioral health providers. The service plan is used across evidence-based practices to map the work that the provider, the person in recovery, and potentially his or her family and friends will complete toward the individual's goals. PCCP targets this service plan document and the process of service planning in behavioral health service settings. The following discussion provides an overview of essential PCCP principles and sample practices. More sample practices and tools can be found in the texts by Adams and Grieder (2014) and by Tondora et al. (2014).

PCCP principles mirror and grow from the evolution of the person-centered approach throughout health care settings and emphasize holism, empowerment, and equity in the service user–provider exchange. PCCP emerges from the values of mental health recovery that envision a behavioral health service system that is more humane, hopeful, and inclusive. From these principles, PCCP integrates practical service planning tools and practices with other recovery-oriented, evidence-based practices (e.g., shared decision-making, motivational interviewing, Wellness Recovery Action Planning) to drive the transition to use of recovery-oriented approaches. The service planning process must include shared decision-making with active participation; empowerment of all parties; and attention to trust, exchange, and humanity in the therapeutic relationship.

The therapeutic relationship between a person in recovery and his or her providers has been essential to the success of the PCCP process and behavioral health services in general (Stanhope, Barrenger, Salzer, & Marcus, 2013). Historically, people have had experiences of providers building helpful, trusting relationships, especially with social workers who explicitly value the service user–provider relationship. However, PCCP pushes providers to further emphasize the humanistic interchange between people by challenging traditional clinical boundaries. Such boundaries can reinforce the paternalistic nature of the service user–provider exchange and undermine the recovering person's engagement, activation, and collaboration (Tondora et al., 2014). In contrast, an interchange that mutually acknowledges the humanity of all parties creates the context for collaborative identification of goals, assessment of the service users' strengths and values, and shared understanding of where they are and where they want to go.

Before the service plan is written, the first step in PCCP is a strengths-based assessment of the person in recovery based on the provider's understanding of the relevant information. As Adams and Grieder (2014) stated, "Any plan is only as good as the assessment" (p. 39). Ideally, the service plan can map the collaborative work or journey ahead, and it must be built on a firm foundation of understanding and respecting the person in recovery as the expert on his or her own experiences (see Figure 10.1).

In contrast to traditional, problem- and diagnosis-focused service plans, the person-centered assessment grows from Saleebey's (1996) strengths-based interview and begins with the elicitation of an individual's strengths, values, skills, talents, hopes, dreams, and what is meaningful in his or her life. From there, the assessment moves into what is getting in the way of achieving the recovery goals (Tondora et al., 2014). This potentially unstructured conversation, focused on asset-based questions, can inform an integrated summary or a richer narrative hypothesis of what is going on for this individual and how to move forward toward his or her goals (Adams & Grieder, 2014).

From this narrative understanding and in the context of a collaborative alliance, the service plan document is developed. This document outlines the goals, objectives, services, and activities to be completed by the provider, the person in recovery, and natural supports such as family and friends (if endorsed). These activities should be connected directly to

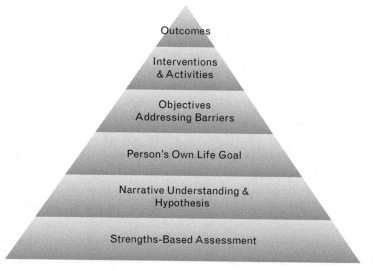

FIGURE 10.1: Model of the person-centered plan. Adapted from *Treatment Planning for Person-Centered Care: Shared Decision Making for Whole Health* (2nd ed., p. 60), by N. Adams and D. Grieder, 2014, Cambridge, MA: Academic Press. Copyright 2014 by Elsevier, Inc.

ameliorate identified barriers to achieving the proposed goal. The emphasis on naturally occurring activities (e.g., a bowling league as opposed to a socialization therapeutic group) and supporters (e.g., family) reflects a key PCCP principle of promoting community inclusion. By focusing the plan on community integration, the results are socially valued roles for people in recovery rather than a parallel existence in behavioral health services. The language used in the plan is important for engaging the person in recovery and must be understandable; jargon should be limited, and all necessary terms should be explained. The language should reflect recovery-oriented values (e.g., "a person with schizophrenia" rather than "a schizophrenic"). Language is particularly important for writing the individual's life goal.

The development and identification of a meaningful life goal reflects a significant departure from the traditional service planning process. Goals in traditional service plans have often been dictated by uniform agency domains and tended to focus on symptom reduction. The life goals must be important to the individual, must be stated in his or her own words, and must include life beyond services (e.g., hopes, dreams, visions of life) as the focus of the plan. This orientation promotes humanistic considerations and shifts the focus from problems that only services can help resolve to a holistic approach that considers valued social roles, inclusion in the community, and the person's life in context. Framing the work in this way guides service planning to maintain the expertise of the individual in identifying his or her own life goals, reinforces the central PCCP principles, and motivates people to engage in the activities necessary to work toward their goals (Tondora et al., 2014). After setting the goal, the plan outlines the strengths of the individual and the family that can aid in achieving the goal and the barriers that will challenge their efforts. These strengths and barriers are directly reflected in the objectives and interventions highlighted in the service user's plan.

In subsequent components of the plan, the services provided and the roles of the person in recovery and his or her supporters are detailed. Rigorous documentation standards required by funding bodies (e.g., CMS) are reflected in these sections to ensure that the services are (a) appropriate to a person's needs, (b) effective, (c) efficient in the use of resources, and (d) likely to help the person. The service plan organizes all of the information about what and where services will be delivered (Adams & Grieder, 2014) and ensures that the four documentation criteria, known as *medical necessity*, are detailed. Objectives, which are identified within each goal, typically relate to identified barriers that inhibit goal attainment and conform to behavioral criteria: They are specific, measurable, attainable, realistic, and time-framed (SMART). For example, if an individual wants to get a job and lacks the required skills, the objective could address skill development (i.e., barrier) in service of the goal (i.e., job attainment). The interventions required to meet that objective reflect the specific activities and services that will be completed as well as when and by whom (i.e., identification and coordination of skills training).

In PCCP, objectives and interventions go beyond service participation and include opportunities for the service user and his or her natural supports to build on strengths and contribute to meeting goals. Connections between the interventions and the individual's identified life goals should be explicit; this promotes a transparent and holistic approach in which all activities are linked to meaningful improvements in the individual's daily life. In this way, the PCC plan functions as a transformative tool that engages and activates the person in recovery (Adams & Grieder, 2014) by enlisting strengths, hopes, and dreams for a meaningful life beyond services.

In the following case example, Ms. R, an older adult woman, has been referred by a community provider to a setting that combines behavioral and physical health services. The brief assessment and excerpt from a sample person-centered plan offer an illustration of the PCCP concepts in an integrated health care setting.

CASE VIGNETTE

Ms. R is a 50-year-old, white woman who has never been married and has two adult sons. She lives alone and has recently reconnected with her sons, with whom she had lost contact, despite significant challenges caused by her poor physical and mental health and ongoing substance use. She laughs easily with her neighbors. She likes to cook and go to the movies, and she has a new interest in gardening.

Ms. R is facing a diagnosis of breast cancer with a good chance of recovery with treatment. She is struggling to cope with this news along with feelings of hopelessness and sadness. She recently increased her use of alcohol and prescription drugs, including Klonopin (a tranquilizer used to control seizures and panic disorder), which has strained her relationships and her ability to follow-up on health care. The housing provider referred her to an integrated health care setting for additional support to help her coordinate, cope with, and manage her medical and behavioral health needs.

Ms. R was first hospitalized for psychiatric reasons at age 16 and has since struggled with hospitalizations due to major depression and incarcerations due to offenses related to her substance use. She lost custody of her two children to her cousin due to her criminal justice involvement. She has maintained ties with her cousin, who raised the children.

EXCERPT FROM MS. R'S SERVICE PLAN

Goal #1. I want to be healthy so I can spend time with my sons.

Strengths. Ms. R loves her children and is motivated to address her health needs. She has persevered when faced with obstacles to accessing medical care and has successfully advocated for her care. She is an affable person who easily builds relationships with providers, neighbors, and family, and she has the capacity to follow through on treatment. Ms. R has the support of her sons, who are willing to attend appointments with her. She is action oriented and motivated to address her current substance use and has a history of extended abstinence.

Barriers or assessed needs. Ms. R's increased mental health symptoms (i.e., depression and anxiety) have been disruptive, and she has recently begun using more alcohol and benzodiazepines (e.g., up to 8 mg of Klonopin), and this has been straining her relationships and interfering with her ability to attend her appointments. She expresses that she is experiencing intense anxiety about the cancer treatment and its possible side effects.

Objectives. In 3 months, Ms. R will reduce her use of alcohol and Klonopin as evidenced by her self-report and communication with family members.

INTERVENTIONS AND ACTION STEPS

PROFESSIONAL SERVICES AND SUPPORTS

1. Amy (primary clinician) will meet weekly with Ms. R for the next 3 months to assist her in identifying and managing her co-occurring mental health symptoms and alcohol and substance use that interfere with her relationships and use of health care services.

2. Anastasia (psychiatrist) will meet monthly with Ms. R for the next 3 months to monitor her medication regimen and to discuss the risks and benefits of various anxiety management options. She will also coordinate with the oncologist and primary care physician to ensure continuity of care.

3. Rachel (behavioral health home [BHH] care coordinator) will meet weekly with Ms. R for the next 3 months to provide a range of BHH services. Rachel will conduct a primary health assessment and offer person-centered medicine to Ms. R in a way that respects her history. She will follow-up on all needed health evaluations (e.g., blood work, x-rays services) and interventions (e.g., chemotherapy). If needed, she will work with Ms. R to identify and use community health supports and services (e.g., home health aide, cancer peer support group). She will provide a warm handoff referral to these providers to ensure continuity of care, support Ms. R with information about the new providers, and facilitate introductions.

4. John (benefits specialist) will coordinate with Ms. R and Rachel monthly to help manage and resolve any insurance or billing issues that arise as Ms. R accesses multiple physicians and specialists to address her health care needs. He will track and collect all required documentation to assist in supporting Ms. R in her contact with billing and insurance representatives.

5. Alex (primary care physician) will meet with Ms. R twice in the next 3 months and as needed to assess her general physical condition. He will also coordinate with Ms. R, Rachel, and Anastasia to ensure that Ms. R's anxiety and cancer treatments are managed appropriately.

6. Jane (oncologist) will meet with Ms. R twice in the next 2 months and as needed to discuss the treatment options and potential side effects. She will also coordinate with Ms. R, Rachel, Anastasia, and Alex to ensure that the anxiety related to the treatment options and side effects are managed appropriately.

7. Jeanelle (peer specialist) will help Ms. R interact with her doctors and address any questions or needs that arise in order to weigh intervention options and side effects. She will also assist Ms. R with recording information from appointments and necessary follow-ups and will attend appointments with Ms. R when her family is unable to be with her to provide encouragement and support for her anxiety.

SELF-DIRECTED AND NATURAL SUPPORT ACTIONS

1. Payton (Ms. R's son) will accompany Ms. R to at least one half of her appointments in the next 3 months to provide comfort and support, given her anxiety around accessing health care services on her own. Ms. R will give Payton at least 1 week of notice before an appointment so that he can make arrangements to be there.
2. Ms. R will go to a community garden or the botanic garden with Payton to relax, explore, and get involved in gardening there.
3. Ms. R will, in the next month, cook one meal with her family to enjoy together.
4. Ms. R will talk to her friend Mr. V, with whom she drinks alcohol and uses Klonopin, about her plan to stop using and ask for his support.
5. Ms. R will also talk to two other friends about her plan to stop using benzodiazepines and ask for their emotional support.

EVIDENCE BASE FOR PERSON-CENTERED CARE PLANNING

There is a growing evidence base to support the effectiveness of PCCP for improving treatment processes and clinical outcomes. Research has demonstrated improvement in the ability to articulate preferences when PCCP is used with people who have developmental disabilities, as well as positive outcomes with regard to expanding social networks and increasing community integration (Claes, Van Hove, Vandevelde, van Loon, & Schalock, 2010). A systematic review of personalized care planning for people with chronic illnesses encompassed 19 studies, finding that the intervention improved self-management capabilities in terms of self-efficacy and self-care activities, reduced depression, and had a moderately positive effect on physical health outcomes (Coulter et al., 2015).

In community mental health settings, there have been two randomized controlled trials. The first study examined PCCP among low-income adults of Hispanic or African origin in a peer-run community integration program and showed that PCCP was effective in increasing participants' active involvement in the care planning process and increasing inclusion in the planning process for housing, employment, and education (Tondora et al., 2014). In the second study, ten community health clinics were randomized to receive either training in PCCP and collaborative documentation, or treatment as usual. The clinics in the experimental condition showed a significant increase in medication adherence over time compared with those in the control condition. There was also a significant decrease in no-shows among the clinics in the experimental condition (Stanhope, Ingoglia, Schmelter, & Marcus, 2013). As PCCP continues to be adopted, there will be more opportunities to explore the effectiveness of the practice in real-world settings.

IMPLEMENTATION OF PERSON-CENTERED CARE PLANNING

Although states are shifting their health service systems to align with PCCP, many barriers can impede the translation of evidence-based practices into community behavioral health and integrated health care settings. The implementation and dissemination literature has identified a variety of potential barriers in the outer system, the organization, the individuals involved, the implementation process, and the intervention itself (Damschroder et al., 2009). Although knowledge of PCCP implementation remains in a nascent stage, scholarship in recovery-oriented practice has found that some external funding requirements are contrary to the implementation of such practice in behavioral health settings (Khoury & Rodriguez del Barrio, 2015), and barriers have been identified in leadership, organizational culture, and staff turnover during implementation efforts (Aarons, Sommerfeld, & Willging, 2011; Whitley, Gingerich, Lutz, & Mueser, 2009). Moreover, many challenges have been encountered regarding PCCP implementation among individual providers.

Although PCCP practices are well specified, they do require that providers believe in the spirit of recovery-oriented practice. From decades of experience implementing PCCP in behavioral health systems nationally and internationally, Tondora, Miller, and Davidson (2012) identified the top concerns of providers working in the field. Some of these concerns are consistent with barriers that face the implementation of evidence-based practices, including salience of the intervention (e.g., How is this different from what I was doing before?), funding barriers (e.g., Will our funders pay for this?), and organizational readiness to integrate a new practice (e.g., organizational infrastructure to change the electronic health records). Providers also voice concerns about the spirit and values of mental health recovery (e.g., people are too sick to recover) that necessitate training and ongoing consultation to support and sustain changes in practice (Tondora et al., 2012).

DECISION-MAKING

Decision-making lies at the heart of PCC and PCCP. How individuals make decisions about their health care, including overall decisions regarding what type of treatment or support they receive and daily decisions regarding the general management of their wellness, can have far more impact on their health than the actions of their providers. In accordance with the social work value of self-determination, all providers have an ethical imperative to deliver care that gives people real and meaningful choices about their health (Deegan & Drake, 2006). This has been notably absent in traditional mental health care, in which stigma and paternalistic attitudes have often deprived people of the power to make choices about their mental health. The health care system is moving away from the attitude that "the doctor knows best" and toward a paradigm of shared decision-making.

This modality becomes particularly important in the context of caring for people with chronic illnesses who are faced with ongoing decisions concerning their health and long-term relationships with providers. The frequent decision points about health behaviors (e.g., whether to take medications) and the increased opportunities to revisit decisions are different from the decision-making process when one is faced with an acute health crisis (Charles, Gafni, & Whelan, 1997). Key to these decisions are the individual's preferences and life circumstances, placing the onus on providers to understand these health care decisions in the context of the whole person.

SHARED DECISION-MAKING

Shared decision-making is "an approach in which the clinician and the patient go through all phases of decision making together, in which they share the preference for treatment and reach an agreement on treatment choice" (Joosten et al., 2008, p. 220). This type of decision-making is essentially collaborative, which distinguishes it from the traditional medical model (in which the provider decides) and the informed medical model (in which the provider gives information only). The expertise of both parties is necessary for the sharing of information; providers contribute knowledge about possible treatments and outcomes, and service users contribute their own wellness experiences, including what has worked for them and is consistent with their values and preferences. Building from this shared knowledge, the provider and the individual can move toward consensus, both with active roles in deciding among possible options. However, all of these activities of shared decision-making are predicated on a strong therapeutic alliance. Without a trusting context, service users may be reluctant to enter into a process with so much at stake and potential for decisional conflict (Stanhope et al., 2013). Some have referred to this as *relational decision making*, stressing the role of the relationship to empower individuals to share fully about their hopes for their lives and enable providers to frame decisions in that context. The implementation of shared decision-making demands some groundwork to ensure that both the provider and the person receiving care have the required skills and willingness to enter into an authentic process.

Despite the complexities, there is evidence to support the notion that shared decision-making is the more effective way to deliver care in physical and behavioral health settings. In terms of improving the treatment process, shared decision-making has been shown to improve service user satisfaction, sense of choice, autonomy, and knowledge and to decrease decisional conflict (Davidson et al., 2012; Malm, Ivarsson, Allebeck, & Falloon, 2003; Stein et al., 2013). Shared decision-making has also been associated with positive outcomes, including improved adherence to depression medication and social functioning and decreased rates of hospital readmission and use of emergency services (Angell, Matthews, Stanhope, & Rowe, 2015). However, questions remain about the inherent presumption of rationality underlying shared decision-making. Social psychologists have demonstrated that individuals often make decisions automatically without being aware of a process of weighing options. Particularly in high-stake situations, people are influenced by a potentially complex web of factors that is not reducible to logic, including perceptions about who they are and who they can become. In response to the challenges involved in this sense-making process, particularly during short physician visits, decision aids have been developed to facilitate decision-making processes.

DECISION AIDS

Decision aids are increasingly being used in medicine, particularly when a decision is preference sensitive, meaning that not enough evidence exists to support one course over another (O'Connor, Légaré, & Stacey, 2003). Decision aids primarily lay out options and likely outcomes to help people make decisions, but they can also help service users clarify their own values, weigh benefits and harms given what is important to them, and communicate with providers. They can take many forms, including workbooks, videos, and computer applications. Although most decision aids have been used in medical settings, they are appearing in behavioral health settings.

One example of a mental health decision aid combines web technology and peer support to help people work collaboratively with their psychiatrists to make treatment decisions. The decision aid, Common Ground, was developed by the leading recovery advocate, Patricia Deegan (Deegan, Rapp, Holter, & Riefer, 2008). Before an appointment, a person has the opportunity to use the software program remotely or at the clinic. The program prompts individuals to complete a survey that asks how they are doing in their recovery, what is their "personal medicine" (i.e., activities that help them stay well), and what is their "power statement" (i.e., declaration of goals for using psychiatric medicine). From this, a one-page report is produced for the individual and the psychiatrist that can be used to inform the visit. The program can also generate a personal medicine card that provides the individual with suggestions and resources for additional help. Peer staff members are present at the computer terminals for consultation and additional decision support. The whole process is designed to enhance the decision-making process by extending the time and the tools someone has beyond a 15- to 20-minute psychiatric appointment.

In a qualitative study, participants reported that Common Ground helped them to "amplify their voice" and more efficiently focus on their primary concerns during visits (Deegan, 2010). Overall, decision aids have had a demonstrated impact on increasing knowledge, decreasing decisional conflict, creating more realistic expectations, and making people more active in the process (O'Connor et al., 2003).

IMPLICATIONS FOR SOCIAL WORK

The PCC approach and its underlying philosophy are congruent with social work ethics. PCC and social work share the fundamental value of the dignity and worth of people and the belief that all people have the right to determine their own lives, charting their own paths toward meaning and purpose. Social work and PCC also share the understanding of the primacy of the therapeutic relationship in healing processes. Mounting

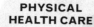

PHYSICAL HEALTH CARE

BEHAVIORAL HEALTH CARE

– Patient as Person
– Biopsychosocial Perspective
– Healing Relationships
– Decision Support
– Self-Management
– Mutuality & Collaboration
– Self-Determination
– Use of Self

SOCIAL WORK

FIGURE 10.2: Person-centered care.

evidence supports the notion that healing is found in established relationships of mutual trust and collaboration.

PCCP provides important tools and strategies to build on relational skills and guide social workers in applying and enacting these values in integrated health care settings. PCCP also enlists and integrates other commonly taught practices and perspectives in social work education. The foundation of PCCP, as elucidated in its logic model, is the strengths-based assessment that includes an individual's capacities, interests, hopes, visions, and values in addition to potential barriers or adversities (Saleebey, 1996). Both aspects reinforce the notion that social workers approach their work with a holistic perspective that values the experiences of the individual and seeks to broaden possibilities for choice and control. Consideration of the whole person beyond their clinical psychiatric symptoms—including values, hopes, and environmental considerations—is shared and consistent with ecological systems theory, an influential perspective in social work education and scholarship (Bronfenbrenner, 1979). Consequently, much conceptual overlap exists between social work and person-centered approaches to service provision (see Figure 10.2).

In practice, PCCP tools can provide critical guidance for integrating these approaches in various settings. Given the conceptual overlap with social work approaches, social workers are poised to lead the integration of PCC in these settings with strong skills in the disciplined use of self, therapeutic alliances, strengths-based biopsychosocial assessments, and a firm grounding in the underlying philosophy and values. As PCC is increasingly adopted, social workers employed in health service settings are challenged to reflect on their own practices and guard against the widespread barrier of believing that they already provide PCC.

CONCLUSIONS

The prominence of PCC in all aspects of integrated health care represents considerable progress in understanding how important relationships are to the processes and outcomes of service delivery. The challenge is to make PCC a reality rather than an aspiration, which means giving the workforce concrete tools that place the service user in the driver's seat. One such practice is PCCP, which brings recovery principles to a core activity of all services and provides a unifying process for integrated health care. Although PCCP is an aspect of direct care, its successful implementation rests on the alignment of policies, funding streams, resources, and organizational factors. Another key component for the successful dissemination of PCC practices is having the measures to capture the extent to which they have penetrated practice. As more funding is tied to PCC, the onus will be placed on agencies to demonstrate that they are meeting the criteria for PCC. As with any value-based approach, quantifying the more abstract dimensions of care is a challenge for both researchers and policy makers. This challenge must be met if we are to transform the health care system into one that places individuals firmly at the center of their care and empowers them to make decisions that are meaningful and further their life goals.

RESOURCES

Common Ground, Pat Deegan PhD & Associates (PDA) https://www.patdeegan.com/commonground

Person-Centered Outcomes Research Institute (PCORI) http://www.pcori.org

Person Centered Planning: Practice and Resources, New York State Office of Mental Health (OMH) https://www.omh.ny.gov/omhweb/pros/Person_Centered_Workbook/

Recovery and Recovery Support, Substance Abuse and Mental Health Services Administration (SAMHSA) http://www.samhsa.gov/recovery

Why Shared Decision Making? Informed Medical Decisions Foundation http://www.informedmedicaldecisions.org/shareddecisionmaking.aspx

Yale Program for Recovery and Community Health, Yale School of Medicine http://medicine.yale.edu/psychiatry/prch/

REFERENCES

Aarons, G. A., Sommerfeld, D. H., & Willging, C. E. (2011). The soft underbelly of system change: The role of leadership and organizational climate in turnover during statewide behavioral health reform. *Psychological Services, 8*, 269–281. doi: 10.1037/a0026196

Adams, N., & Grieder, D. (2014). *Treatment planning for person-centered care: Shared decision making for whole health* (2nd ed.). Waltham, MA: Academic Press.

Angell, B., Matthews, E., Stanhope, V., & Rowe, M. (2015). Shared decision making. In P. W. Corrigan (Ed.), *Person-centered care for mental illness: The evolution of adherence and self-determination.* Washington, DC: American Psychological Association.

Balik, B., Conway, J., Zipperer, L., & Watson, J. (2011). *Achieving an exceptional patient and family experience of inpatient hospital care* (IHI Innovation Series white paper). Cambridge, MA: Institute for Healthcare. Available from http://www.ihi.org/resources/pages/ihiwhitepapers/achievingexceptionalpatientfamilyexperienceinpatienthospitalcarewhitepaper.aspx

Balint, M., Hunt, J., Joyce, D., Marinker, M., & Woodcock, J. (1970). *Treatment or diagnosis: A study of repeat prescriptions in general practice.* Philadelphia, PA: J. B. Lippincott.

Berwick, D. M. (2009). What "patient-centered" should mean: Confessions of an extremist. *Health Affairs, 28*, w555–w565. doi: 10.1377/hlthaff.28.4.w555

Bronfenbrenner, U. (1979). *The ecology of human development: Experiments by nature and design.* Cambridge, MA: Harvard University.

Charles, C., Gafni, A., & Whelan, T. (1997). Shared decision-making in the medical encounter: What does it mean? (Or it takes at least two to tango). *Social Science & Medicine, 44*, 681–692. doi: 10.1016/S0277-9536(96)00221-3

Claes, C., Van Hove, G., Vandevelde, S., van Loon, J., & Schalock, R. L. (2010). Person-centered planning: Analysis of research and effectiveness. *Intellectual and Developmental Disabilities, 48*, 432–453. doi: 10.1352/1934-9556-48.6.432

Clancy, C., & Collins, F. S. (2010). Patient-Centered Outcomes Research Institute: The intersection of science and health care. *Science Translational Medicine, 2*, 37cm18. doi: 10.1126/scitranslmed.3001235

Coulter, A., Entwistle, V. A., Eccles, A., Ryan, S., Shepperd, S., & Perera, R. (2015). Personalised care planning for adults with chronic or long-term health conditions. *Cochrane Database of Systematic Reviews, 3*, CD010523. doi: 10.1002/14651858.CD010523.pub2

Damschroder, L. J., Aron, D. C., Keith, R. E., Kirsh, S. R., Alexander, J. A., & Lowery, J. C. (2009). Fostering implementation of health services research findings into practice: A consolidated framework for advancing implementation science. *Implementation Science, 4*, 50. doi: 10.1186/1748-5908-4-50

Davidson, L., Roe, D., Stern, E., Zisman-Ilani, Y., O'Connell, M., & Corrigan, P. W. (2012). If I choose it, am I more likely to use it? *The International Journal of Person Centered Medicine, 2*, 577–592. doi: 10.5750/ijpcm.v2i3.201

Davidson, L., Tondora, J., O'Connell, M. J., Kirk, T., Jr., Rockholz, P., & Evans, A. C. (2007). Creating a recovery-oriented system of behavioral health care: Moving from concept to reality. *Psychiatric Rehabilitation Journal, 31*, 23–31. doi: 10.2975/31.1.2007.23.31

Deegan, P. E. (1996). Recovery as a journey of the heart. *Psychiatric Rehabilitation Journal, 19*, 91–97. doi: 10.1037/h0101301

Deegan, P. E., & Drake, R. E. (2006). Shared decision making and medication management in the recovery process. *Psychiatric Services, 57*, 1636–1639. doi: 10.1176/ps.2006.57.11.1636

Deegan, P. E., Rapp, C., Holter, M., & Riefer, M. (2008). Best practices: A program to support shared decision making in an outpatient psychiatric medication clinic. *Psychiatric Services, 59*, 603–605. doi: 10.1176/appi.ps.59.6.603

Deegan, P. E. (2010). A web application to support recovery and shared decision making in psychiatric medication clinics. *Psychiatric Rehabilitation Journal, 34*, 23–28. doi: 10.2975/34.1.2010.23.28

Engelberg Center for Health Care Reform. (2016). *Bending the curve: Person-centered health care reform: A framework for improving care and slowing health care cost growth.* Washington, DC: Engelberg Center for Health Care Reform, The Brookings Institution. Retrieved from https://www.brookings.edu/wp-content/uploads/2016/06/person_centered_health_care_reform-1.pdf

Epstein, R. M., Fiscella, K., Lesser, C. S., & Stange, K. C. (2010). Why the nation needs a policy push on patient-centered health care. *Health Affairs, 29*, 1489–1495. doi: 10.1377/hlthaff.2009.0888

Institute of Medicine. (2001). *Crossing the quality chasm: A new health system for the 21st century.* Washington, DC: National Academy Press. doi: 10.17226/10027

Joosten, E. A. G., DeFuentes-Merillas, L., de Weert, G. H., Sensky, T., van der Staak, C. P. F., & de Jong, C. A. J. (2008). Systematic review of the effects of shared decision-making on patient satisfaction, treatment adherence and health status. *Psychotherapy and Psychosomatics, 77*, 219. doi: 10.1159/000126073

Khoury, E., & Rodriguez del Barrio, L. (2015). Recovery-oriented mental health practice: A social work perspective. *British Journal of Social Work, 45*(Suppl. 1), 27–44. doi: 10.1093/bjsw/bcv092

Malm, U., Ivarsson, B., Allebeck, P., & Falloon, I. R. H. (2003). Integrated care in schizophrenia: A 2-year randomized controlled study of two community-based treatment programs. *Acta Psychiatrica Scandinavica, 107*, 415–423. doi: 10.1034/j.1600-0447.2003.00085.x

McCormack, B. (2003). A conceptual framework for person-centred practice with older people. *International Journal of Nursing Practice, 9*, 202–209. doi: 10.1046/j.1440-172X.2003.00423.x

Mead, N., & Bower, P. (2000). Patient-centredness: A conceptual framework and review of the empirical literature. *Social Science & Medicine, 51*, 1087–1110. doi: 10.1016/S0277-9536(00)00098-8

New Freedom Commission on Mental Health. (2003). *Achieving the promise: Transforming mental health care in America: Final report* (DHHS Pub. No. SMA-03-3832). Rockville, MD: New Freedom Commission on Mental Health, U.S. Department of Health and Human Services.

O'Connor, A. M., Légaré, F., & Stacey, D. (2003). Risk communication in practice: The contribution of decision aids. *British Medical Journal, 327*, 736–740. doi: 10.1136/bmj.327.7417.736

O'Connor, A. M., Stacey, D., Entwistle, V., Llewellyn-Thomas, H., Rovner, D., Holmes-Rovner, M., . . . Jones, J. (2003). Decision aids for people facing health treatment or screening decisions (Review). *Cochrane Database of Systematic Reviews, 1*, CD001431. doi: 0.1002/14651858.CD001431

Rogers, C. R. (1967). *On becoming a person: A therapist's view of psychotherapy.* London, England: Constable.

Saleebey, D. (1996). The strengths perspective in social work practice: Extensions and cautions. *Social Work, 41*, 296–305. doi: 10.1093/sw/41.3.296

Smull, M., & Lakin, K. C. (2002). Public policy and person-centered planning. In S. Holburn & P. M. Vietze (Eds.), *Person-centered planning: Research, practice and future directions* (pp. 379–398). Baltimore, MD: Paul H. Brookes.

Stanhope, V., Barrenger, S. L., Salzer, M. S., & Marcus, S. C. (2013). Examining the relationship between choice, therapeutic alliance and outcomes in mental health services. *Journal of Personalized Medicine, 3*, 191–202. doi: 10.3390/jpm3030191

Stanhope, V., Ingoglia, C., Schmelter, B., & Marcus, S. C. (2013). Impact of person-centered planning and collaborative documentation on treatment adherence. *Psychiatric Services, 64*, 76–79. doi: 10.1176/appi.ps.201100489

Stein, B. D., Kogan, J. N., Mihalyo, M. J., Schuster, J., Deegan, P. E., Sorbero, M. J., & Drake, R. E. (2013). Use of a computerized medication shared decision making tool in community mental health settings: Impact on psychotropic medication adherence. *Community Mental Health Journal, 49*, 185–192. doi: 10.1007/s10597-012-9528-8

Taylor, J. E., & Taylor, J. A. (2013). Person-centered planning: Evidence-based practice, challenges, and potential for the 21st century. *Journal of Social Work in Disability & Rehabilitation, 12*, 213–235. doi: 10.1080/1536710X.2013.810102

Tondora, J., Miller, R., Slade, M., & Davidson, L. (2014). *Partnering for recovery in mental health: A practical guide to person-centered planning.* Hoboken, NJ: John Wiley & Sons.

Tondora, J., Miller, R., & Davidson L. (2012). The top ten concerns about person-centered care planning in mental health systems. *International Journal of Person Centered Medicine, 2*, 410–420. doi: 10.5750/ijpcm.v2i3.132

U.S. Department of Health and Human Services. (2004). National consensus statement on mental health recovery. Rockville, MD: Substance Abuse and Mental Health Services Administration.

Wagner, E. H., Austin, B. T., & Von Korff, M. (1996). Organizing care for patients with chronic illness. *The Milbank Quarterly, 74*, 511–544. doi: 10.2307/3350391

Whitley, R., Gingerich, S., Lutz, W. J., & Mueser, K. T. (2009). Implementing the illness management and recovery program in community mental health settings: Facilitators and barriers. *Psychiatric Services, 60*, 202–209. doi: 10.1176/ps.2009.60.2.202

World Health Organization. (2015). *WHO global strategy on integrated people-centred health services 2016– 2026: Placing people and communities at the centre of health services* (Executive Summary). Geneva, Switzerland: World Health Organization. Retrieved from http://apps.who.int/iris/bitstream/10665/ 180984/1/WHO_HIS_SDS_2015.20_eng.pdf

CHAPTER 11

EVIDENCE-BASED SOCIAL WORK PRACTICE IN INTEGRATED HEALTH CARE

Shelly A. Wiechelt and Shulamith Lala Ashenberg Straussner

Humans are complex beings with integrated physical, psychological, and social aspects. Individuals sometimes experience problems and challenges in one or more of these areas. Until recently, mental and physical problems were divided into separate fields (i.e., health, mental health, and substance use), and care for these problems was provided by separate and distinct treatment providers with little or no care coordination. Inattention to the integrated nature of these problems and lack of care coordination contributed to poor outcomes.

Mental health and substance use problems carried more stigma than physical health problems, and third-party payors provided less coverage for care. This situation is changing gradually since the Mental Health and Addiction Equity Act of 2008 and the Patient Protection and Affordable Care Act (ACA) of 2010 facilitated the reduction of stigma for behavioral health problems and fueled an already emerging impetus to provide integrated health care in the United States.

Integrated health care involves teams of primary care providers and behavioral health clinicians working together with individuals and their families to address physical health and behavioral health problems in primary care settings using evidence-based practice (EBP) approaches (Safety Net Medical Home Initiative, 2013). Behavioral health is fundamentally about mental and emotional wellbeing and the promotion of psychological wellness (Substance Abuse and Mental Health Services Administration [SAMHSA], 2014b). Behavioral health problems include substance misuse, substance use disorders, mental disorders, psychological or emotional distress, and life stressors and crises. There are several models of integrated health care in primary care settings, ranging from co-located care settings to collaborative care models with various degrees of integration (see Chapter 8). Care team members include the service user, primary care provider, behavioral health care provider (who provides care management and behavioral interventions), and, ideally, a psychiatric prescriber, front desk staff, medical assistants, and peer support specialists.

Social workers are well suited to provide integrated health care in general and specifically within the behavioral health care provider role. The notion of person-centered holistic care from a biopsychosocial perspective is consistent with social work's values, ethics, and person-centered, strengths-based practice perspective (Saleebey, 2002). The care management aspect of the behavioral health care provider role involves care coordination, supportive counseling, tracking of individual care, and facilitation of referrals. These tasks are consistent with social work case management, and clinical social workers are well suited for the behavioral intervention aspect of the behavioral health care provider role as well. They are trained to draw on existing theory and research regarding human problems in social contexts, work with service users to identify goals and strategies for healing, and evaluate progress and outcomes.

Integrated health care is underpinned by evidence-based practices and interventions (Stanhope, Videka, Thorning, & Mckay, 2015), concepts that are relatively new but are being rapidly accepted in the field of social work. This chapter provides information on EBP for social workers in integrated health care settings. It begins with a general discussion of EBP in social work and then describes several evidence-based approaches and interventions that are useful for social work practice in primary care settings. A case example is presented to further corroborate the utility of EBP in integrated health care.

EVIDENCE-BASED PRACTICE

Evidence-based practice (EBP) is rooted in the field of medicine, where it began to be used formally in 1992 (Straus, Richardson, Glasziou, & Haynes, 2011). The original emphasis of evidence-based medicine (EBM) was to teach medical residents to critically appraise existing scientific evidence to address a given medical problem. Over time, EBM evolved beyond a focus on scientific evidence alone to include clinical expertise, service user values, and individual circumstances when selecting an intervention. This shifted the process from EBM to EBP (Mullen, Bledsoe, & Bellamy, 2008; Straus et al., 2011). Currently, most health care and helping professions (including social work) strive to engage in EBP. Correctly applied, EBP is congruent with social work values, ethics, and practice perspectives (Drisko & Grady, 2015). It is important to understand the distinction between EBP, which is a clinical or practice-focused decision-making process, and *an* EBP, which refers to a specific practice or intervention that has been studied empirically using rigorous research methods (e.g., randomized controlled clinical trials, meta-analyses) and has been shown to be effective for a given group of service users (Drisko & Grady, 2012; Royse, Thyer, & Padgett, 2016).

EBP for social workers is a process in which social workers apply their clinical expertise to consider the service user's clinical state, needs, circumstances, values, and expectations. They also draw on current research evidence, including scientific studies, databases of EBPs, clinical outcomes, measures to be incorporated into the psychosocial assessment, and the psychosocial assessment itself (Drisko & Grady, 2012; Royse et al., 2016;

Rubin, 2008). EBP includes a critical collaboration of the social worker with the service user to identify the best course of action. The decision-making model of EBP in social work involves the following steps:

1. Identify service user issues, problems, and characteristics.
2. Formulate a well-designed, answerable question aimed at identifying appropriate interventions.
3. Gather, assess, and appraise evidence for interventions.
4. Integrate evidence with the social worker's practice experience and the service user's characteristics, values, and situation.
5. Monitor progress and evaluate effectiveness. (Gibbs, 2003)

Because this model closely parallels the model used in medicine (Straus et al., 2011), it may be readily applied in collaboration with medical teams in integrated health care settings.

Of the various EBPs used, a few are widely applicable and frequently used to help individuals dealing with medical, substance use, and psychiatric issues:

- Motivational interviewing (MI)
- Cognitive-behavioral therapy (CBT)
- Trauma-informed care (TIC)
- Wellness Self-Management (WSM) and Wellness Self-Management Plus (WSM+)
- Mindfulness

MOTIVATIONAL INTERVIEWING

Motivational interviewing (MI) is fundamentally a way of "being with and for people" (Miller & Rollnick, 2002). It is a person-centered counseling style that is used to address individuals' ambivalence about change, thereby facilitating such a change (Miller & Rollnick, 2013). Although MI is a primary treatment, it is also used as a tool to enhance readiness or responsiveness to another treatment (Prochaska, DiClemente, & Norcross, 1992), and it can be integrated into other treatments, such as assertive community treatment (Manthey, Blajeski, & Monroe-DeVita, 2012). Numerous research studies, including more than 200 clinical trials, systematic reviews, and meta-analyses, indicate that MI is effective for facilitating change in individuals across a broad range of settings and problems (Burke, Arkowitz, & Dunn, 2002; Miller & Rollnick, 2013). It is noteworthy that MI was originally developed to address addictive behavior and that much research demonstrates that MI is effective for mental health, substance use, and physical problems. This substantial body of research supports the utility of MI in integrated health care settings.

According to Miller and Rollnick (2013), MI is underpinned by a philosophical spirit that involves partnership, acceptance, compassion, evocation, and autonomy. The clinician and service user engage in a conversation together in which they explore the service user's story, strengths, ideas, goals for change, and ambivalence about change. The clinician holds and communicates an attitude of unconditional positive regard and gives priority to the service user's needs. The service user's rights to self-determination and freedom of choice are respected. Mind and heart brought forth in the context of the therapeutic relationship are important in the spirit of MI.

MI is organized around four processes:

1. *Engaging,* which is the process whereby the clinician and the service user establish a positive connection and working relationship for therapy
2. *Focusing,* which is about working together with the service user to identify change targets
3. *Evoking,* which is directed at drawing out the service user's intrinsic motivation and capacity for change
4. *Planning,* which occurs when readiness for change is in view, fosters commitment for the change, and specifies a clear plan of change

Individuals typically want to change and do not want to change, and they engage in talk that supports change (i.e., change talk) or supports the status quo (i.e., sustain talk). The familiar phrase, "roll with resistance," is no longer emphasized in descriptions of the MI approach (Miller & Rollnick, 2013). Rather, the approach to working with ambivalence emphasizes recognizing, evoking, and supporting change talk while reflecting or responding in such a way as to maintain and evoke more change talk. Sustain talk is not pathological resistance; it is simply the other side of ambivalence. The point of MI is to acknowledge the normalcy of ambivalence and work to cultivate change talk, which essentially leads to individuals' talking themselves into change.

Clinicians who argue against the service user's sustain talk are unwittingly supporting the status quo. For example, if a social worker tries to facilitate change in the behavior of an individual who misuses alcohol by presenting arguments against the individual's sustain talk about how alcohol use is beneficial, the social worker is likely to create a situation in which the individual feels misunderstood and antagonistic and becomes fixed in the "no change" stance. The worker would be more likely to move the service user toward change by reflecting the service user's own desire to change and inquiring about how alcohol use may be detrimental. The idea is to move the service user through ambivalence toward change by means of his or her own thought process and talk.

The core skills used to facilitate change in MI are commonly used therapeutic techniques known by the acronym OARS (Matulich, 2013):

- *Open questions,* which consists of asking open-ended questions designed to elicit the service user's thoughts, ideas, and feelings rather than asking questions that elicit short answers. The aim is to engage the service user in the conversation and generate exploration of ambivalence about needed changes.
- *Affirming,* which consists of recognizing and affirming the service user's strengths, efforts, and ideas (e.g., "I know it took a lot of courage for you to talk about this"). It is important to encourage the service user to be self-affirming.
- *Reflective listening,* which consists of reflecting on what the service user says in response to the open-ended questions; it should be provided in a conversational,

affirming, confidence-building style. This is similar to active listening skills in social work.

- *Summarizing*, which consists of using reflection to bring together multiple ideas or points that the service user has made regarding a specific issue, linking current comments to earlier comments, and transitioning to ending a session or shifting a conversation.

Informing and advising is a fifth core skill needed to conduct MI (Miller & Rollnick, 2013; Rollnick, Miller, & Butler, 2008). Information and advice are provided to service users at their request and with full recognition that it is up to them how to use the information. The clinician helps service users to explore, consider, and evaluate the information while allowing them to come to their own conclusions.

The spirit and practice of MI fit well with social work ethics, values, and practices, and MI is a useful tool for social workers practicing in integrated health care systems (Wahab, 2005). At the same time, there are some aspects of MI that may pose challenges for social workers attempting to implement it in integrated health care settings. For example, the traditional intake and assessment process that involves a series of questions is contraindicated in MI; it is seen as a disengaging rather than engaging strategy. Integrated health care settings may involve shorter periods of contact and treatment than traditional psychotherapy settings, thereby limiting the time available to build therapeutic relationships and explore opportunities to facilitate change.

COGNITIVE-BEHAVIORAL THERAPY

Cognitive-behavioral therapy (CBT) is one of the most widely researched treatment approaches used for various emotional and behavioral problems that affect the individual's daily life (SAMHSA, n.d.). Many CBT approaches have proved to be effective with problems such as substance use, smoking, obsessive-compulsive disorders, phobias, anxiety, depression, distress associated with acute psychosis, trauma-related disorders, sorrow associated with end-stage cancer, type 2 diabetes, epilepsy, and chronic pain (SAMHSA, n.d.).

According to the cognitive-behavioral model, individuals' moods and behaviors are contingent on their thoughts and beliefs. Psychological problems arise when thoughts and beliefs are dysfunctional. CBT attempts to reduce self-defeating behavior by modifying cognitive distortions and maladaptive beliefs and by teaching techniques of thought control (Beck, 2011; Liese, 2014). A core element of CBT is teaching individuals how to cope with life stressors more productively. This is achieved by helping the individual to identify and anticipate high-risk situations that may trigger their unhelpful behavior and then to apply an array of self-control skills, such as emotional regulation, anger management, practical problem solving, and substance refusal. The focus is not on reducing stressors that are out of service users' control (e.g., a physical illness or a substance-using family member) but on improving their own functioning given the reality of the situation (Beck, 2011). Among the numerous CBT approaches with strong evidence for effectiveness are contingency management therapy, acceptance and commitment therapy, the

Seeking Safety program (Najavits, 2002), and CBT for late-life depression (CBT-LLD) (SAMHSA, n.d.).

TRAUMA-INFORMED CARE

Trauma-informed care (TIC) is an approach to practice and service delivery that is congruent with EBP and social work in that it is strengths-based, person-centered, and recovery-oriented. There is clear evidence that traumatic experiences are interwoven into individuals' physical, mental health, and substance use problems and that failure to consider the role of trauma in these problems results in poorer outcomes (Wiechelt, 2014). The landmark Adverse Childhood Experiences (ACEs) study showed a positive association between the number of ACEs and negative health outcomes across a broad spectrum of disorders and risky health behaviors, including smoking, alcohol and drug use, depression, obesity, diabetes, heart disease, stroke, and cancer (Felitti et al., 1998).

Psychologically, *trauma* refers to an experience that is emotionally painful, distressful, or shocking and that is usually accompanied by long-term negative mental and/or physical (including neurological) consequences (Straussner & Calnan, 2014). Traumatic stressors may take different forms (e.g., life-threatening incident, serious injury, sexual violation), and individuals may experience them directly, witness them occurring to others, or learn about them occurring to a family member or close friend (American Psychiatric Association, 2013). Trauma may be a single event, a series of events, or a chronic condition. It can affect individuals, families, communities, and cultures, and it can be transmitted across generations (SAMHSA, 2014b). Individuals who experience traumatic events may develop reactions that meet diagnostic criteria for trauma-induced or stressor-related disorders, such as posttraumatic stress disorder (PTSD) and other mental disorders such as anxiety, mood, substance use, dissociative, eating, somatization, and personality disorders. Individuals may also experience medical problems and physical symptoms.

Some individuals may not meet diagnostic criteria for any trauma-related mental disorder but nonetheless experience significant challenges in their lives as a result of trauma. Hence, it is important for clinicians and systems to be sensitive to the possibility that each of their service users may be profoundly affected by trauma. It is important to recognize when trauma is involved in the behavioral or physical health problems of individuals coming to treatment and to design service delivery systems that are trauma-informed so that the individual is not re-traumatized.

TIC is both an intervention and an organizational approach to delivering care. According to SAMHSA (2015), a program, organization, or system that is trauma-informed is one that

1. *Realizes* the widespread impact of trauma and understands potential paths for recovery
2. *Recognizes* the signs and symptoms of trauma in service users, families, staff, and others involved with the system
3. *Responds* by fully integrating knowledge about trauma into policies, procedures, and practices
4. *Seeks* to actively resist repeating the traumatization

There are several models for adopting TIC in a variety of settings. The key components of TIC are as follows:

- Safety—establishing a physically and emotionally safe environment, protecting individuals from abuse and potential retraumatization due to insensitive processes, validating and expressing service users' needs, and teaching service users skills for self-soothing and calming down
- Choice—supporting choice autonomy and control and allowing individuals to choose when, where, how, and from whom they will receive treatment and services
- Collaboration—engaging service users in treatment planning, evaluating progress and any decisions that affect them, and equalizing power between staff and service users and between staff and administrators
- Trustworthiness—holding appropriate interpersonal boundaries; being clear, consistent, and dependable; promoting transparency of organizational processes and decisions; and facilitating trust among all who are involved with the organization
- Empowerment—helping individuals identify and apply strengths, providing skill building to increase opportunities, and recognizing and fostering resilience
- Diversity—incorporating diversity-based resources into treatment planning; recognizing historical trauma; and considering and respecting differences in gender, race, ethnicity, religion, culture, class, ability, sexual orientation, language, and socioeconomic status (Elliot, Bjelajac, Fallot, Markoff, & Reed, 2005; SAMHSA, 2014a, 2014b, 2016)

To implement TIC, all facets of the organization and program operations must be designed to be sensitive to trauma issues and triggers by incorporating the key components listed. All staff members need to be trauma aware, including receptionists, custodians, clinicians, and administrators. Being trauma aware involves understanding the general effects of trauma, how trauma symptoms may manifest, how trauma may affect an individual in social contexts, and how intake, assessment, and intervention processes may affect an individual who has experienced trauma. Trauma screening should be done universally. The trauma-informed system may employ individuals who have expertise in trauma-specific interventions or may operate using a trauma-informed approach and then refer individuals for trauma-specific treatment. The entire organization must integrate trauma-informed approaches in all domains, including governance, policies, procedures, leadership, workforce development (e.g., hiring practices, supervision, training), interventions, engagement of service users, collaboration with other providers, care coordination, quality assurance, financing, and evaluation (Institute for Health and Recovery, 2012).

Social workers who practice in integrated health care settings should work with the multidisciplinary team and office administration to deliver TIC. Several resources are available to facilitate the planning process (e.g., Institute for Health and Recovery, 2012). Care should be taken to reduce the likelihood that any process in the office or organization could retraumatize or "trigger" individuals who have experienced trauma. Common processes in medical environments that may be triggering for trauma survivors and require particular care and responsiveness by staff include disrobing, being touched, and experiencing invasive procedures. Sights, sounds, and smells (e.g., medical equipment, sirens, rubbing alcohol) may also be triggers (Huang, Sharp, & Gunther, 2013). A particular concern in multidisciplinary settings is redundant assessment processes in which individuals must keep retelling their traumatic stories. It is prudent to develop intake, screening, and assessment procedures that gather necessary data only once.

Given the overwhelming evidence that trauma is often at the nexus of mental health problems, substance use disorders, and physical health problems, social workers in integrated health care settings should make TIC a priority in their practice. Social workers should obtain training on selecting and conducting trauma screenings, administering assessment measures, and providing trauma-specific and evidence-based interventions.

WELLNESS SELF-MANAGEMENT

The Wellness Self-Management (WSM) program is a recovery-oriented curriculum designed to help adults manage severe mental illnesses (Salerno, Margolies, & Cleek, 2008). It is based on Illness Management and Recovery (IMR), which is a well-established EBP designed to help adults manage severe mental illnesses and achieve specific goals (Mueser & Gingerich, 2003). WSM is a group-based program that is delivered with the use of a workbook. The workbook is organized into three major chapters:

1. Addressing Recovery
2. Mental Health Wellness
3. Relapse Prevention

It contains 57 lessons in 19 topic areas, such as "Understanding What Helps and What Hinders Recovery," "Finding and Using Coping Skills That Work," and "Understanding the Connection Between Physical and Mental Health." Each lesson is formatted to begin with topical information, followed by a personalized worksheet and an "actions" step to practice and continue learning between sessions. Salerno et al. reported in 2011 that the WSM program was well received by clinicians and service users and that 75% of service users made significant progress on their goals through the program.

The WSM+ program, which is an adaptation of the original WSM program, was developed to provide individuals who have substance use and mental health problems with knowledge and skills to enhance their recovery (Salerno et al., 2010). Similar to its predecessor, it contains three major chapters:

1. Recovery
2. Mental Health Wellness, Substance Use Harm Reduction, and Relapse Prevention
3. Living a Healthy Lifestyle and Recovery

Like WSM, it has 57 lessons divided into 18 topic areas, including "Understanding Stress and Relapse," "Making Mental Health and Substance Abuse Services Work for You," and "Using Physical Healthcare to Stay Healthy." The lesson format is the same as that of WSM.

The WSM and WSM+ programs are manualized workbooks that are designed to be delivered in group settings. The recovery focus of these programs—and particularly the integration of health, mental health, and substance use issues in WSM+—make them valuable tools and resources for social workers in integrated health care settings.

MINDFULNESS

Mindfulness is about being present with yourself, free of judgment, and in the moment—aware of who you are through a systematic process of self-observation, self-inquiry, and mindful action (Kabat-Zinn, 1994). Mindfulness is typically associated with meditation practice, but they are not necessarily the same. Mindfulness is a central component of Buddhist and yoga practices, but it is also a state of being that can be attained outside of any religious or spiritual practice.

Mindfulness is a component of manualized evidence-based interventions such as dialectical behavior therapy (Linehan, 1993), and it is the main focus or active component ingredient in others, such as mindfulness-based stress reduction (MBSR) (Kabat-Zinn, 1990) and mindfulness-based cognitive therapy (MBCT) (Segal, Williams, & Teasdale, 2002). A plethora of mindfulness-based interventions (MBIs) has emerged in recent years across a range of problems and populations with various levels of research support. Dimidjian and Segal (2015) cautioned against overly optimistic interpretations of the effectiveness of MBIs across various problems. Some existing research may have been affected by lack of control groups or low intervention fidelity, among other limitations. Randomized controlled clinical trials offer a higher level of support regarding the efficacy of the intervention, but efficacy may be limited in terms of generalizability across a range of problems and specificity about mindfulness as the key active ingredient in the intervention.

MBSR and MBCT are the most widely researched MBIs and have the best evidence for effectiveness. MBSR was developed by Kabat-Zinn, Lipworth, and Burney (1985) for working with individuals who were experiencing chronic pain (Kabat-Zinn, 1990). The intervention is now widely applied to reducing psychological distress due to medical conditions, physical pain, or life events. It is designed to reduce stress, anxiety symptoms, depression symptoms, and negative affect as well as improve self-esteem, mental health, and general functioning.

Segal, Williams, and Teasdale (2002) built on the framework of MBSR and integrated CBT to create MBCT. MBCT was designed to reduce residual depressive symptoms, prevent depression relapses, reduce other comorbid psychiatric symptoms, facilitate tapering and discontinuation of antidepressant medications, and improve physical and psychological quality of life.

MBSR and MBCT are group-based, manualized interventions that are delivered in weekly sessions. MBSR consists of 10 sessions over eight weeks. MBCT includes an initial one-on-one orientation session, eight weekly sessions, and up to four follow-up group sessions. Mindfulness meditation is central to both interventions, and it is recommended that individuals who lead these interventions maintain their own meditation practice.

Systematic reviews and meta-analyses indicate that MBIs are generally effective for physical health, mental health, and substance use problems (Chiesa & Serretti, 2014; Gotink et al., 2015; Wyatt, Harper, & Weatherhead, 2014). Much of the research involves randomized controlled trials of MBSR and MBCT and shows that these interventions are effective at reducing stress, anxiety, and depression while increasing quality of life for individuals with chronic health problems (Gotink et al., 2015). They have reduced pain levels among individuals with chronic pain and lowered blood pressure levels among those with hypertension. Although the findings are less robust, MBSR and MBCT are also associated with reductions in substance use problems (Chiesa & Serretti, 2014). Overall, it appears that individuals do better in treatment if their comfort with MBIs is assessed and discussed with them before treatment (Wyatt et al., 2014). They also should be oriented to the MBI processes and the potential physiological and psychological effects that they may experience before receiving the treatment.

CASE VIGNETTE

Edna is a 35-year-old single, white woman who presented to the health center with a chief complaint of stomach pain and frequent vomiting. During the medical assessment, Edna indicated that she consumed four or five alcoholic drinks on a daily basis; the physician also noted that Edna appeared to be depressed. The physician determined that the medical diagnosis was stomach ulcers and was concerned about Edna's alcohol use and the possibility of clinical depression. A social worker was consulted about the case to further assess and address the intersecting physical health, substance use, and mental health problems that Edna was experiencing.

The social worker engaged in EBP by partnering with Edna to identify her strengths and challenges. She found out that Edna had a bachelor of arts degree in psychology and was employed as an insurance agent. Edna had received warnings at work about her frequent absenteeism and tardiness, which she related to her depression. She was recently divorced from her husband of five years and acknowledged that her husband disliked her alcohol use and that it contributed to their divorce. At the time of the social worker's assessment, Edna lived alone but had frequent contact with her parents and elder sister, who lived nearby.

The social worker administered assessment measures on alcohol use problems and on depression—the Addiction Severity Index-Lite (McLellan, Luborsky, Woody, & O'Brien, 1980) and the Beck's Depression Inventory (Beck, Ward, Mendelson, Mock, & Erbaugh, 1961). The clinical interview and scores on the assessment measures indicated that Edna met criteria for an alcohol use disorder of moderate severity and was experiencing persistent depressive disorder, previously known as dysthymia. In discussing the results of the assessment measures, Edna was able to recognize that her ulcer, alcohol use, and depression were interrelated and that she needed help to address those issues.

Concerned about potential issues of trauma, which are common among individuals who have substance use and mental health problems, the social worker administered a research-based trauma screen, the PTSD Checklist for DSM-5 (Weathers et al., 2013).

Although Edna did not meet the criteria for a diagnosis of PTSD, she did reveal having been sexually abused as a child by her uncle and experiencing some trauma-related symptoms that were still present at the time of assessment. The social worker and the physician conferred about Edna's depression, and the physician prescribed antidepressant medication.

During the following weeks, using an MI approach, the social worker helped Edna to explore her ambivalence about changing her drinking behavior. After a few sessions, Edna expressed a desire to enter treatment for her substance use and trauma-related issues. Edna agreed with the physician's recommendation that she first check into an inpatient unit to detoxify from her alcohol use. Together with the social worker, she decided that, on discharge, she would enroll at a nearby outpatient treatment center that offered an intensive program for women using the Seeking Safety program, an evidence-based, cognitive-behavioral treatment that incorporates interpersonal and case management domains to address problems with substance use and trauma (Najavits, 2002).

The social worker helped Edna secure the support of her family and facilitated her admission to the outpatient treatment program after detoxification. Edna continued to see the physician in the health clinic to receive treatment for her ulcers. She also met with the social worker during her visits to receive support and to evaluate her symptoms of depression and the progress in her recovery from her alcohol use disorder.

CONCLUSIONS

Integrated health care is an innovative way to deliver high-quality health care that addresses the whole person. Use of multidisciplinary teams of health and behavioral health professionals brings specialized skills to bear on complex intersecting physical health, substance use, and mental health problems, thereby improving outcomes. Integrated health care is underpinned by EBP approaches and evidence-based interventions.

Social workers who use EBP are well suited for working in integrated health care settings. They can work with individuals to identify their treatment needs and recovery pathways for intersecting physical health, substance use, and mental health problems. They can implement evidence-based interventions such as MI, TIC, CBT, and mindfulness; engage families in the treatment process; and deliver case management services. Integrated health care appears to be the new direction for health care delivery in the United States, and evidence-based social work is a key component for its success.

RESOURCES

Evidence-Based Behavioral Practice (EBBP), Northwestern University http://www.ebbp.org/

Evidence Based Practice for Public Health, University of Massachusetts Medical School http://library.umassmed.edu/ebpph/

Evidence-Based Practice in Social Work, University of South Carolina (USC) School of Social Work https://sowkebp.wordpress.com/definitions/

National Registry of Evidence-based Programs and Practices (NREPP), Substance Abuse and Mental Health Services Administration (SAMHSA) http://www.samhsa.gov/nrepp

Organized, Evidence-Based Care: Behavioral Health Integration, Safety Net Medical Home Initiative http://www.integration.samhsa.gov/news/Implementation-Guide-Behavioral-Health-Integration.pdf

Star Model Research, Health Science Center, University of Texas (UT)—San Antonio School of Nursing http://nursing.uthscsa.edu/onrs/starmodel/

REFERENCES

American Psychiatric Association. (2013). *Diagnostic and statistical manual of mental disorders* (5th ed.). Arlington, VA: American Psychiatric Association. doi: 10.1176/appi.books.9780890425596

Beck, A. T., Ward, C. H., Mendelson, M., Mock, J., & Erbaugh, J. (1961). An inventory for measuring depression. *Archives of General Psychiatry, 4,* 561–571. doi: 10.1001/archpsyc.1961.01710120031004

Beck, J. S. (2011). *Cognitive behavior therapy: Basics and beyond* (2nd ed.). New York, NY: Guilford Press.

Burke, B. L., Arkowitz, H., & Dunn, C. (2002). The efficacy of motivational interviewing and its adaptations: What we know so far. In W. R. Miller & S. Rollnick (Eds.), *Motivational interviewing: Preparing people for change* (2nd ed., pp. 217–250). New York: Guilford Press.

Chiesa, A., & Serretti, A. (2014). Are mindfulness-based interventions effective for substance use disorders? A systematic review of the evidence. *Substance Use & Misuse, 49,* 492–512. doi: 10.3109/10826084.2013.770027

Dimidjian, S., & Segal, Z. V. (2015). Prospects for a clinical science of mindfulness-based intervention. *American Psychologist, 70,* 593–620. doi: 10.1037/a0039589

Drisko, J. W., & Grady, M. D. (2012). *Evidence-based practice in clinical social work.* New York, NY: Springer.

Drisko, J. W., & Grady, M. D. (2015). Evidence-based practice in social work: A contemporary perspective. *Clinical Social Work Journal, 43,* 274–282. doi: 10.1007/s10615-015-0548-z

Elliot, D. E., Bjelajac, P., Fallot, R. D., Markoff, L. S., & Reed, B. G. (2005). Trauma-informed or trauma-denied: Principles and implementation of trauma-informed services for women. *Journal of Community Psychology, 33,* 461–477. doi: 10.1002/jcop.20063

Felitti, V. J., Anda, R. F., Nordenberg, D., Williamson, D. F., Spitz, A. M., Edwards, V., . . . Marks, J. S. (1998). Relationship of childhood abuse and household dysfunction to many of the leading causes of death in adults: The Adverse Childhood Experiences (ACE) Study. *American Journal of Preventive Medicine, 14,* 245–258. doi: 10.1016/S0749-3797(98)00017-8

Gibbs, L. (2003). *Evidence-based practice for the helping professions: A practical guide with integrated media.* Pacific Grove, CA: Brooks/Cole.

Gotink, R. A., Chu, P., Busschbach, J.J.V., Benson, H., Fricchione, G. L., & Hunink, M.G.M. (2015). Standardised mindfulness-based interventions in healthcare: An overview of systematic reviews and meta-analyses of RCTs. *PLOS One, 10*(4), e0124344. doi: 10.1371/journal.pone.0124344

Huang, L. N., Sharp, C. S., & Gunther, T. (2013). It's just good medicine: Trauma-informed primary care [Powerpoint slides]. Retrieved from http://www.integration.samhsa.gov/about-us/CIHS_TIC_Webinar_PDF.pdf

Institute for Health and Recovery. (2012). *Developing trauma-informed organizations: A tool kit* (2nd ed.). Cambridge, MA: Institute for Health and Recovery.

Kabat-Zinn, J. (1990). *Full catastrophe living: Using the wisdom of your body and mind to face stress, pain, and illness.* New York, NY: Delacorte Press.

Kabat-Zinn, J. (1994). *Wherever you go, there you are: Mindfulness meditation in everyday life.* New York, NY: Hyperion.

Kabat-Zinn, J., Lipworth, L., & Burney, R. (1985). The clinical use of mindfulness meditation for the self-regulation of chronic pain. *Journal of Behavioral Medicine, 8,* 163-190. doi: 10.1007/BF00845519

Liese, B. S. (2014). Cognitive-behavioral therapy for people with addictions. In S.L.A. Straussner (Ed.), *Clinical work with substance-abusing clients* (3rd ed., pp. 225–250). New York, NY: Guilford Press.

Linehan, M. M. (1993). *Cognitive-behavioral treatment of borderline personality disorder.* New York, NY: Guilford Press.

Manthey, T. J., Blajeski, S., & Monroe-DeVita, M. (2012). Motivational interviewing and assertive community treatment: A case for training ACT teams. *International Journal of Psychosocial Rehabilitation, 16,* 5–16. Retrieved from http://www.psychosocial.com/index.htm

Matulich, B. (2013, May 30). *Introduction to motivational interviewing* [Video file]. Retrieved from https://www.youtube.com/watch?v=s3MCJZ7OGRk#t=867

McLellan, A. T., Luborsky, L., Woody, G. E., & O'Brien, C. P. (1980). An improved diagnostic evaluation instrument for substance abuse patients: The Addiction Severity Index. *Journal of Nervous and Mental Disease, 168,* 26–33. Retrieved from http://journals.lww.com/jonmd/pages/default.aspx

Miller, W. R., & Rollnick, S. (2002). *Motivational interviewing: Preparing people for change* (2nd ed.). New York, NY: Guilford Press.

Miller, W. R., & Rollnick, S. (2013). *Motivational interviewing: Helping people change* (3rd ed.). New York, NY: Guilford Press.

Mueser, K., & Gingerich, S. (2003). *Illness management and recovery Evidence-Based Practices (EBP) Kit.* Washington, DC: Substance Abuse and Mental Health Services Administration. Retrieved from http://store.samhsa.gov/product/Illness-Management-and-Recovery-Evidence-Based-Practices-EBP-KIT/SMA09-4463

Mullen, E. J., Bledsoe, S. E., & Bellamy, J. L. (2008). Implementing evidence-based social work practice. *Research on Social Work Practice, 18,* 325–338. doi: 10.1177/1049731506297827

Najavits, L. M. (2002). *Seeking safety: A treatment manual for PTSD and substance abuse.* New York, NY: Guilford Press.

Prochaska, J. O., DiClemente, C. C., & Norcross, J. C. (1992). In search of how people change. Applications to addictive behaviors. *American Psychologist, 47,* 1102–1114.

Rollnick, S., Miller, W. R., & Butler, C. C. (2008). *Motivational interviewing in healthcare: Helping patients change behavior.* New York, NY: Guilford Press.

Royse, D., Thyer, B. A., & Padgett, D. K. (2016). *Program evaluation: An introduction to evidence-based approach* (6th ed.). Boston: Cengage Learning.

Rubin, A. (2008). *Practitioner's guide to using research for evidence-based practice.* Hoboken, NJ: John Wiley & Sons.

Safety Net Medical Home Initiative. (2013). *Organized, evidence-based care: Planning care for individual patients and whole populations* (Implementation Guide). Retrieved from http://www.safetynetmedicalhome.org/sites/default/files/Implementation-Guide-Evidence-Based-Care.pdf

Saleebey, D. (2002). *The strengths perspective in social work practice.* Boston, MA: Allyn and Bacon.

Salerno, A., Margolies, P., & Cleek, A. (2008). *Wellness self-management personal workbook* (2nd ed.). New York, NY: New York State Office of Mental Health & Urban Institute for Behavioral Health. Retrieved from http://vet2vetusa.org/LinkClick.aspx?fileticket=aY9UPl%2BL6uY%3D&tabid=67

Salerno, A., Margolies, P., Cleek, A., Pollock, M., Gopalan, G., & Jackson, C. (2011). Wellness self-management: An adaptation of the Illness Management and Recovery practice in New York State. *Psychiatric Services, 62,* 456–458. doi: 10.1176/appi.ps.62.5.456

Salerno, A., Margolies, P., Kipnis, S., Bonneau, P., Marnell, S., & Killar, B. (2010). *Wellness self-management plus: Personal workbook.* New York, NY: New York State Office of Mental Health, New York State Office of Alcoholism and Substance Abuse Services, & Center for Practice Innovations at Columbia Psychiatry of the New York State Psychiatric Institute.

Segal, Z. V., Williams, J.M.G., & Teasdale, J. D. (2002). *Mindfulness-based cognitive therapy for depression: A new approach to preventing relapse.* New York, NY: Guilford Press.

Stanhope, V., Videka, L., Thorning, H., & McKay, M. (2015). Moving toward integrated health: An opportunity for social work. *Social Work in Health Care, 54,* 383–407. doi: 10.1080/00981389.2015.1025122

Straus, S. E., Richardson, W. S., Glasziou, P., & Haynes, R. B. (2011). *Evidence-based medicine: How to practice and teach it* (4th ed.). New York, NY: Churchill Livingstone Elsevier.

Straussner, S.L.A., & Calnan, A. J. (2014). Trauma through the life cycle: A review of current literature. *Clinical Social Work Journal, 42,* 323–335. doi: 10.1007/s10615-014-0496-z

Substance Abuse and Mental Health Services Administration. (2014a). *SAMHSA's concept of trauma and guidance for a trauma-informed approach* (HHS Pub. No. SMA 14-4884). Rockville, MD: Substance Abuse and Mental Health Services Administration. Retrived from http://store.samhsa.gov/shin/content/SMA14-4884/SMA14-4884.pdf

Substance Abuse and Mental Health Services Administration. (2014b). *A treatment improvement protocol: Trauma-informed care in behavioral health services* (HHS Pub. No. SMA 14-4816, TIP Series 57). Rockville, MD: Substance Abuse and Mental Health Services Administration.

Substance Abuse and Mental Health Services Administration. (2015, August 14). Trauma-informed approach and trauma-specific interventions. Retrieved from http://www.samhsa.gov/nctic/trauma-interventions

Substance Abuse and Mental Health Services Administration. (n.d.). SAMHSA's National Registry of Evidence-based Programs and Practices [NREPP]. Retrieved from http://nrepp.samhsa.gov/AllPrograms.aspx

Wahab, S. (2005). Motivational interviewing and social work practice. *Journal of Social Work, 5,* 45–60. doi: 10.1177/1468017305051365

Weathers, F. W., Litz, B. T., Keane, T. M., Palmieri, P. A., Marx, B. P., & Schnurr, P. P. (2013). The PTSD Checklist for DSM-5 (PCL-5). Retrieved from http://www.ptsd.va.gov/professional/assessment/adult-sr/ptsd-checklist.asp

Wiechelt, S. A. (2014). Intersection between trauma and substance misuse: Implications for trauma-informed care. In S. L. A. Straussner (Ed.), *Clinical work with substance-abusing clients* (3rd ed., pp. 179–201). New York, NY: Guilford Press.

Wyatt, C., Harper, B., & Weatherhead, S. (2014). The experience of group mindfulness-based interventions for individuals with mental health difficulties: A meta-synthesis. *Psychotherapy Research, 24,* 214–228. doi: 10.1080/10503307.2013.864788

CHAPTER 12

TRANSITIONAL CARE

Helle Thorning

Life consists of countless transitions. These natural challenges are often multiplied and amplified by chronic illnesses, which introduce immense complications for affected individuals and also for their family members and natural supporters (Stanhope, Videka, Thorning, & McKay, 2015). Health care reform has focused attention on the estimated 17% of U.S. adults who have comorbid mental, physical, and substance use disorders (Goodell, Druss, & Walker, 2011). Due to a systematic lack of primary and behavioral health care integration, individuals who are challenged with co-occurring disorders rarely receive adequate treatment and must resort to seeking emergency care for a physical or psychiatric crisis. On delivering treatment for the acute problem, standard practice for the emergency department staff is to provide a community referral for ongoing treatment. However, there is often a substantial delay between visiting the emergency department and receiving follow-up care in the community (Jackson et al., 2015). If too much time has elapsed between treatments, people with co-occurring disorders often disengage from treatment altogether, and the opportunity to enroll them in ongoing care is lost (Pope, Smith, Wisdom, Easter, & Pollock, 2013).

As social workers strive to integrate health care for people with co-occurring conditions, it is essential to calibrate care at different stages of life. Transitions from one setting to another are vulnerable exchange points (Naylor, Aiken, Kurtzman, Olds, & Hirschman, 2011; Stanhope et al., 2015). A system that is flexible, coordinated, and targeted is required to address the developmental needs of individuals and their family members. The Chronic Care Model (CCM) provides one such framework. The CCM seeks to ensure that people with primary and behavioral health conditions receive ongoing care during the inevitable ebbs and flows of chronic illness (Wagner, Austin, & Von Korff, 1996). The model offers a way to structure the health delivery system through organizational support, clinical information systems, decision support, and self- management support (see Chapter 2).

By moving away from interventions that primarily take place during acute and one-time events, the CCM shifts toward a system of care in which services are continuous and uniquely tailored according to an individual's preferences and needs during his or her current stage of life. The CCM's basic principles reflect the importance of mobilizing community resources in collaboration with the formal treatment system to create an environment that promotes safe and high-quality care for people with long-term conditions. Family and natural support systems play significant roles in empowering and preparing people to manage their own health and health care (Thorning & Dixon, 2016). By applying the CCM, individuals will be able to receive and participate in seamless care, thereby receiving the right level of care at the right time.

This chapter introduces the transitional care framework, which provides a conceptual plan for practice strategies that can be operationalized within the CCM. Two clinical models are introduced that focus on transition: critical time intervention (CTI) and peer bridging. A case study demonstrates how the transitional care framework promotes intensive to less intensive care that is fully supported by the family and integrated with local community resources.

THE TRANSITIONAL CARE FRAMEWORK

The term *transitional care* refers to a broad range of practice strategies that are designed to enable safe and timely movement from one setting or level of care to another, ensuring that the right setting and level of care are employed for the right amount of time. The objective is to ensure smooth transitions and continuity of care, promoting health and behavioral health integration while fostering an environment in which the service user can pursue his or her personal life goals. The transitional care framework expands what is often referred to as *discharge planning*. Traditionally, this has taken place during the conclusion of treatment in an acute care setting and has focused narrowly on the immediate needs after discharge; the individual's life goals have rarely been taken into account. Using the transitional care framework, the clinician engages with the individual about what is important to him or her in the present moment and in the long-term. This person-centered, future-oriented engagement strategy individualizes discharge planning in the context of the person's overall life goals.

Changing behaviors is hard, and staying on task to reach a goal requires motivation, perseverance, and personal investment. The charge for the clinician, therefore, is not to simply engage in a specific intervention or deliver certain kinds of help after discharge. Rather, it is to use interventions with the purpose of supporting the individual in reaching a personal goal while managing his or her chronic conditions along the way (Adams & Grieder, 2004).

The transitional care framework was originally developed for a New York State program called assertive community treatment (ACT), which was converted to time-limited services (Thorning, 2014). ACT is a community-based, mobile team intervention that is designed for people with complex primary and behavioral health conditions and uses assertive community outreach as its main strategy. The transitional care framework was developed to organize the work of the ACT team, and it is structured in three overlapping dimensions that are addressed simultaneously:

1. Engaging and envisioning life goals
2. Practicing wellness self-management
3. Integrating with the community (see Figure 12.1).

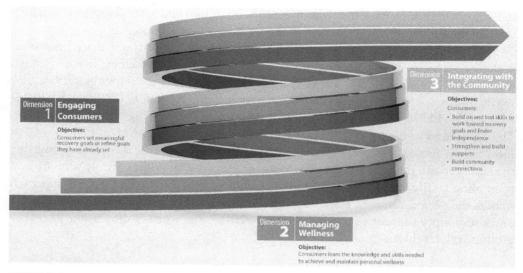

FIGURE 12.1: The transitional care framework. From "ACT Transition Curriculum, Unit 1-ACT: On the Road to Recovery," by Center for Practice Innovations, 2016 (https://rfmh.csod.com/client/rfmh/default.aspx). Copyright 2016 by Center for Practice Innovations.

The transitional care framework is grounded in the recovery model and person-centered care. Implicit in this idea is the notion that people's needs change as they progress through life. A flexible treatment approach is necessary to adapt to the presenting need at a given time. Core evidence-based practices and tools can facilitate and support growth as the individual moves across levels of care.

DIMENSION 1: ENGAGEMENT

The first dimension of the transitional care framework is *engagement*. A person-centered approach is used from the first time the clinician meets the individual. The objective for this dimension is for the individual to set or refine personal goals and establish personal preferences regarding engagement in treatment and involvement of family members and other natural supports. Two core clinical practices are person-centered care planning (PCCP) (see Chapter 10) and recovery-oriented decisions for relatives' support (REORDER), which offers a method for individuals and their families to discuss concrete ways in which the family can provide support (Cohen et al., 2013).

Primary physical and behavioral health problems are often disruptive, stressful, and challenging for individuals, families, and significant others. Family members can experience the impact of health problems in a multitude of ways. Initially, families may be puzzled by the personality and behavioral changes they observe in their relative and not know how to go about accessing available services. Families and natural supports also may have experienced problematic and difficult interactions with the mental health and criminal justice systems. Families can feel reluctant or unable to provide support. Similarly, individuals may not have a clear idea of how their families and natural supports can help them in their recovery.

REORDER is an innovative, manualized intervention that uses a shared decision-making process to determine the appropriate level of family involvement in care (Cohen et al., 2013; Dixon & Swartz, 2014). It first explores whether and how the service user would like to involve any family members or natural supports. REORDER then facilitates a dialogue with the individual about the pros and cons of involving others in treatment. The decision to involve a service user's family includes providing the family with written information about the relevant mental, physical, and substance use disorders, permitting the family to call the treatment team when concerns arise, providing family support, and promoting family attendance at educational support groups. The REORDER approach honors the person-centered component of the CCM and shows how to enhance family and community support (Thorning & Dixon, 2016). The work in dimension 1 lays the groundwork for that of dimension 2.

DIMENSION 2: MANAGING WELLNESS

Dimension 2 focuses on the collaborative process among the individual, his or her natural support systems, and clinicians. It fosters an environment in which a service user can acquire the knowledge and skills necessary to achieve and maintain wellness during the time of transition and beyond. Pat Deegan (2005) refers to the power of developing *personal medicine* or a *personal toolbox* with which the individual can identify specific care activities (e.g., listening to music, maintaining a garden, practicing yoga). Such activities are self-initiated and aimed at decreasing symptoms; improving mood, thoughts and behaviors; and enhancing the overall sense of wellbeing (Deegan, 2005).

Several workbooks are available to help cultivate personal preferences for managing wellness, such as Wellness Self-Management (Salerno et al., 2011) and the Wellness Recovery Action Plan (WRAP) (Cook et al., 2012). These plans can be used individually, in groups, or with families.

Assisting an individual in the discovery of personal wellness strategies should not wait until he or she has transitioned to the next level of care. The work in this dimension provides opportunities to identify and practice new behaviors and tackle potential barriers while planning for the next steps to be taken within the community. This dimension informs clinicians' understanding of service users' health knowledge needs, uses non-directive interviewing, explains risks and probabilities, personalizes the care planning process, and provides self-management supports (Larson, 2014). In particular, interventions that promote health literacy and elicit service user choice and decision-making can improve person-centered care and general treatment outcomes (Berkman et al., 2011; Elwyn et al., 2014).

Two broad skill sets have been recommended to assist clinicians in promoting the engagement, health literacy, and involvement of individuals, families, and community supports. They are risk-communication skills—being aware of the evidence, communicating information about benefits and harms, discussing uncertainties, clearly presenting probabilities, and using decision aids—and interpersonal or relational competencies—active listening, negotiated agenda setting and prioritizing, demonstrating empathy and emotional intelligence, facilitating involvement, clarifying the decisions that need to be made, respecting values and preferences, and supporting deliberation.

Motivational interviewing and shared decision-making can be applied sequentially. Individuals are first motivated to desire change and are then engaged in decision-making to identify a preferred approach for bringing about that change (Elwyn et al., 2014). These methods can be integrated as an ongoing process in which, for example, clinicians first provide information about options and elicit a service user's preferences and then proceed with supporting behavior change based on the service user's level of ambivalence.

Peer providers have increasingly gained recognition for facilitating sustained engagement in care. Peers empathically understand a person's situation because of shared life experiences and having encountered challenges and strengths in many wellness dimensions. Wellness-oriented approaches delivered by peer-support specialists and wellness coaches can play an important role in integrated health care models (Swarbrick, 2013). Peers can work as part of multidisciplinary care teams, helping service users and fellow team members in shifting the focus from illness treatment to wellness and recovery. Peer interventions can include assistance and modeling for meeting the challenges of lifestyle changes (e.g., diet, exercise), medication choices, and illness management through self-monitoring. These interventions can help individuals acquire the self-management skills necessary to sustain their overall health.

Social support provided by peers can help people overcome problems associated with social isolation. In a study of peer specialists hired in an emergency department to assist with discharge planning, the peers were able to successfully advocate for service user needs, help solve problems before the first follow-up appointment, and assist service users when future care arrangements fell through (Nossel et al., 2016). The peer specialists were involved in all aspects of community integration and provided a safety net by working intensively with service users after discharge until stable plans were in place (Nossel et al., 2016).

Knowledge about wellness and illness is important for informed decision-making. Psychoeducation is an intervention that has been applied with families in a variety of practice contexts, including services for diabetes management, bone marrow transplantation, restorative justice, substance use disorders, and at-risk youth (Lukens, 2015). It has also been recommended as an evidence-based practice for the treatment of severe mental illnesses (Dixon et al., 2010). Psychoeducation consists of an array of educational and therapeutic interventions directed at increasing awareness of risk and preventive factors, building on formal supports (i.e., social work and medical services) and natural supports (i.e., family and community resources) and enhancing resiliency among all family members (Lukens & Thorning, 2010).

Psychoeducation can be delivered effectively in various formats, including individual and group sessions, and can range in duration from a single meeting to many sessions over several years. Formats that use family groups can help participants share ideas and experiences and build coping and problem-solving skills through feedback from others (Lukens & Thorning, 2010).

The third dimension of the transitional care framework focuses on extending the work of the previous two dimensions such that the individual is integrating and receiving support from the community. The goal of this dimension is to solidify the gains made in the first two dimensions while actively working on the transition to formal and informal care and support within the community.

The objective is to test and hone skills that are needed to connect with the next step of care and wellness practices identified in the second dimension. All activities are focused on helping the individual work toward his or her life goals, which were identified and refined in the first dimension. Although coordination activities involving other community services should exist from the beginning, this dimension includes *linkages* to the community and *tryouts*, which are critical activities to prepare for the final transfer of care and connection with community activities. The term *linkage and tryouts* refers to a set of activities and discussions among the individual, his or her family and natural supporters, and the next level of care providers needed for a successful transition.

In the third dimension, the individual begins to implement the identified steps toward his or her recovery goals in the community. The focus is on building linkages to providers in the formal care system and to support systems for the personal wellness strategies identified in the second dimension. The third dimension provides an opportunity to assess the strength of the overall treatment plan, identified supporters, and any challenges and barriers encountered, allowing adjustments to be made before the plan is finalized. Potential challenges and barriers include lack of transportation, inadequate insurance coverage, and lack of language and culturally appropriate services.

Transfer of care refers to the follow-up appointment with new providers and personal medicine activities. While finalizing the plan, it is important to celebrate achievements, hold a formal pretransfer meeting, and arrange a final transfer of care appointment with all stakeholders to iron out wrinkles.

It is also important to monitor an individual's progress after the transition of care. This allows troubleshooting of any barriers associated with switching providers. At each step along the way, the clinician should be mindful of the need to provide a warm handoff as service users connect to new care providers and should offer support for the personal medicine practices of the individual (Deegan, 2005) (see Chapter 8).

Endings can evoke painful feelings for the individual, the family, and the clinician. When confronted with saying good-bye, both the clinician's and the individual's personal histories of endings can trigger powerful reactions. These reactions may have multilayered reverberations that can complicate the process of ending and impair the clinician's ability to facilitate the transition. Although the decision to end the relationship and carry out the transition may have been mutually agreed on, it can be difficult to relinquish a relationship that has become highly personal (Webb, 1985). Webb suggested that endings are best understood from a developmental perspective—that is, as a crisis of separation. Depending on the perceptions of the clinician and the individual, the process can feel like a loss. The individual may be unsure of his or her ability to function without the previous level of care, considering the separation to be a threat to the gains he or she has achieved. The anticipated loss of contact with a meaningful person or team may provoke a sense of grief and loss despite the excitement of moving on. To foster successful endings in all aspects of transition, it is important to attend to the following tasks throughout each dimension:

1. Celebrate gains.
2. Work through the meaning of the relationship for the individual, family, and clinician.
3. Address concerns about the future.
4. Plan ahead to maintain achieved gain.

TRANSITIONAL CARE MODELS

CRITICAL TIME INTERVENTION

Critical Time Intervention (CTI) is a program designed to prevent recurrent homelessness of people with severe mental illnesses after discharge from hospitals, shelters, prisons, and other institutions. The two goals of CTI are to prevent individuals from becoming homeless and to reduce the damaging effects of homelessness. CTI strives to facilitate continuity of care when a person is transitioning from an institutional to a community living arrangement. It targets the *critical time* of transition to keep individuals on track and provide them with support.

CTI was derived from the ACT model. ACT is an evidenced-based treatment that was designed to assist individuals who were experiencing the revolving door of psychiatric hospitalization. Its purpose is to facilitate community stabilization and mitigate the risks of homelessness, substance misuse, and incarceration. ACT was originally conceptualized as an intervention model that used a team-based approach, similar to that of a hospital unit but within the community. It was viewed as a hospital without walls that focused on community stabilization without a specified time duration.

Although CTI is based on the ACT model, it delivers care at a specific point in time and is highly focused and time limited. The model has three distinct, three-month phases: transition to the community, tryout, and transfer of care. There is also a pre-CTI period in which the service user, his or her family, the institutional staff, and the CTI worker collaborate before the individual is discharged.

The CTI worker is highly involved in the first phase, providing specialized support and implementing the transition plan. During phase 2, the CTI worker tests the integration of the individual into the community and gradually reduces involvement. The third phase occurs when the CTI worker begins to terminate services after the service user's external support network is safely in place.

Priority areas of intervention include life skills training (such as the ability to do laundry, cook, and clean), psychiatric treatment and medication management, money management, substance use and medical issues, housing stability, and engagement with family members. The CTI worker must have a limited caseload due to the high level of involvement during early stages. Before the start of each new phase, the worker and the service user develop a specialized treatment plan. A study involving 96 men discharged from a homeless shelter in New York City that used the CTI model found that postdischarge homelessness and symptom severity were greatly reduced (Herman, Conover, & Draine, 2010). Later, the model was adapted for people reentering the community from prison or jail and for women exiting prostitution or domestic violence environments. Based on success of the CTI model, ACT, which was previously thought of as a long-term service, eventually moved to time-limited services.

PEER BRIDGING

Peer support is based on "respect, shared responsibility, and mutual agreement of what is helpful" (Mead, Hilton, & Curtis, 2001, p. 134). A growing body of evidence suggests that support from those with common life experiences can enhance engagement (Dixon, Holoshitz, & Nossel, 2016); promote a culture of health and ability; increase feelings of empowerment, self-esteem, and confidence; and improve community integration and social functioning (Trachtenberg et al., 2013). Evidence suggests that services provided by peers can be as effective as or even more effective than those provided by clinicians who are not peers (Gates & Akabas, 2007).

The services provided by peer specialists may include advocacy, mentoring, role modeling, education, support, connection to natural supports and community resources, and assistance with building daily life skills. Peers can instill a sense of hope in service users, who often internalize stigmas regarding their mental health diagnoses. Service users in professional roles serve as examples that recovery is possible. Although peers work alongside and in tandem with other behavioral health professionals in a variety of settings, their main function is to act as an extension of community supports rather than as another member of the traditional framework and power dynamics of the professional caretaking model.

One promising peer-led transition model is peer bridging, which was developed by the New York Association of Psychiatric Rehabilitation Services (NYAPRS). The NYAPRS Peer Bridging program involves collaboration between community mental health centers and state psychiatric facilities, using peer support to help individuals undergoing frequent or long hospital stays with their transitions back into the community. Peer bridging offers voluntary services to hospital residents, who are often self-referred.

Certified Peer Support Specialists provide positive, supportive relationships before and after discharge, host weekly Peer Support meetings in the hospital and in the community, connect individuals to community-based services and natural supports, and assist service users with community adjustment and wellness self-management. Individuals are matched with Peer Bridgers through a mutual selection process that takes place during regular meetings with the entire peer team. They then complete peer agreements, which outline the goals, roles, and responsibilities of each party. Bridgers typically work with three to six people at a time and begin the relationship two to three months before discharge. Services last for an average of 12 months after discharge but can be longer or shorter, depending on the individual, the services needed, and the availability of resources. Individuals can participate in Peer Support meetings without referrals for as long as they would like. The Peer Bridger is not expected to take on the role of a case manager or to be a part of the treatment team, although his or her work can complement the treatment team's approach.

The following case vignette exemplifies how the transitional care framework assists the clinician in moving a service user from isolation to integration within the community.

CASE VIGNETTE

Clarisse is a 32-year-old African-American woman who works as a baker. She has been involved with her intensive case manager for almost two years after a 5-year period of frequent hospitalizations and emergency department visits due to a combination of paranoid ideations, fainting episodes, and anger outbursts. Clarisse had her first psychotic break when she was 24 years old, after a breakup with her boyfriend, whom she discovered was heavily involved with gambling. When the boyfriend moved out, Clarisse became fearful that people who had lent her boyfriend money would come after her. Over the course of several months, she became unable to leave her apartment and subsequently lost her job. She acquired two dogs to help her feel safe but had trouble taking care of them.

Her sister helped her as best as she could, called the police when she thought Clarisse needed help, took care of her dogs when she was in the hospital, and supported her when she was referred for Social Security Disability benefits. However, Clarisse was angry with her sister for hospitalizing her and often confronted her sister at her home and workplace. Eventually, Clarisse was no longer invited to holiday and family events.

Clarisse was referred to the intensive case management (ICM) team by the hospital social worker, who engaged her in ongoing outpatient treatment focused on her goals, which included living in her apartment, taking care of her dogs, finding employment, and improving her relationship with her sister (see Figure 12.2). During the course of her participation with Susan, the ICM social worker, Clarisse was diagnosed with diabetes; this

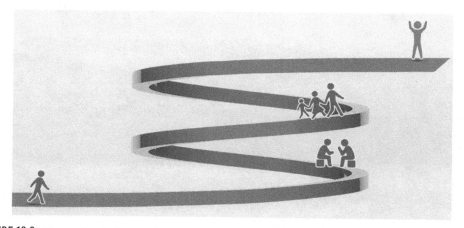

FIGURE 12.2: Dimension 1 of transitional care: engagement around life goals. From "ACT Transition Curriculum, Unit 1-ACT: On the Road to Recovery," by Center for Practice Innovations, 2016 (https://rfmh.csod.com/client/rfmh/default.aspx).

was suspected to be associated with the substantial weight gain that she experienced during the past year and was related to her use of psychiatric medication. The weight gain has bothered Clarisse, and she added a goal to tend to this part of her health.

Since her work with Susan, Clarisse has been in the apartment with her two dogs. She has had only one brief hospitalization, and her emergency department visits have greatly decreased. She now calls Susan if she has any questions or concerns about her diabetes, the care of her dogs, or issues with her landlord or neighbors. Although Clarisse is stabilizing in her community, she still relies on Susan to keep her on track. However, Clarisse would like to be more independent and is therefore moving more actively into the work of dimension two: discovering wellness tools.

Susan has referred Clarisse to the local recovery center. Tim, the peer specialist and a recovery coach, introduced Clarisse to WRAP. In doing so, she identified what activities help her stay well, such as walking her dogs. This activity brings her out of her apartment, provides exercise, helps her to meet people, and makes her feel connected to her community (see Figure 12.3). By modeling his own living and working while coping with a behavioral health condition, Tim was able to offer hope for Clarisse, her sister, and at times, Susan.

Through working on her WRAP, Clarisse identified ways in which she would like her sister to be involved in her life. This provided an opportunity for Susan to use the REORDER intervention and reinstate a dialogue between Clarisse and her sister. Initially, Clarisse and Susan conducted all of their conversations while walking Clarisse's dogs. Clarisse's sister joined in these walks whenever possible, and, using psychoeducation, the social worker promoted an exchange of knowledge among the three of them about mental illness and diabetes. They were then able to collaborate and collectively identify problem-solving strategies when issues arose. Clarisse now attends all family events. She has also reconnected with her skills as a baker and contributes to the holiday season with her specialty pies.

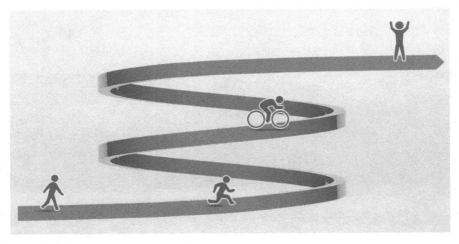

FIGURE 12.3: Dimension 2 of transitional care: managing wellness. From "ACT Transition Curriculum, Unit 1-ACT: On the Road to Recovery," by Center for Practice Innovations, 2016 (https:// rfmh.csod.com/client/rfmh/default.aspx).

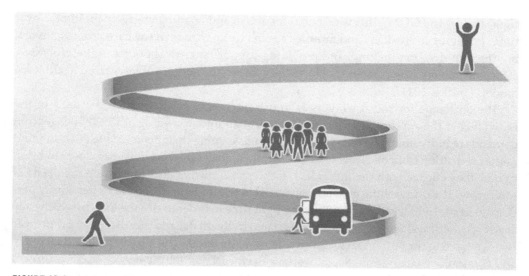

FIGURE 12.4: Dimension 3 of transitional care: integrating with the community. From "ACT Transition Curriculum, Unit 1-ACT: On the Road to Recovery," by Center for Practice Innovations, 2016 (https://rfmh.csod.com/client/rfmh/default.aspx).

Through these wellness activities, Clarisse was able to move into dimension 3 of the transitional care framework. The emphasis was on solidifying her community connections (see Figure 12.4). Other dog owners, knowing that she has a flexible schedule, sometimes ask her to walk their dogs. This makes her feel that she is needed and a part of her community and also earns her extra money. With Susan's help, Clarisse has become involved with the local animal shelter, where she volunteers between 5 and 10 hours per week in exchange for getting free care for her dogs. Volunteering at the animal shelter is a source of great pride for Clarisse, and she is thinking about pursuing a job in which she can work with animals.

With the help from Susan and Tim, Clarisse met many of her goals through formal and informal support and care in the community. A person-centered approach that fostered connecting and reconnecting to new and existing resources was critical to the success of Clarisse's transition. Clarisse's work with an ICM worker and a Peer Specialist was one step in her journey to recovery. Now, she is looking forward to new opportunities in reaching her goal of employment and beyond.

IMPLICATIONS FOR SOCIAL WORK

Encouraging families and peers to suggest strategies and resources for recovery is an essential element in transitional care and the overall recovery process. Social workers should link individuals to community resources that offer peer supports, such as self-help groups, senior centers, youth centers, exercise facilities, and other community programs. In this way, peers, families, and social supporters act as extensions to the community, as suggested by the CCM. This is essential for active and ongoing engagement in care over time. Engaging individuals and families as effective partners in the care process, involving them in decision-making, and providing support at critical points in the process—especially during care transition—have been key to the success of integrated health care models (Burke, 2011).

The challenge for social workers is to use interventions that match the need of the individual at the appropriate time. This requires an understanding of the challenges and demands of individuals' chronic conditions while keeping their personal life goals in mind as they transition from one level of care to another. Social workers must pay close attention to how they engage with the individual in the present while also addressing the needs of tomorrow. The overarching goal is to ensure that the individual and his or her family participate in the right level of care at just the right time in order to live the lives to which they aspire. Sometimes, tensions among clinicians, individuals, and families may erupt over issues related to the individual's readiness to move on or take the next step toward recovery and community integration. Social workers may worry about the service user's readiness to work, live independently, and pursue other life goals; they are often concerned about failure and subsequent setbacks. Clinicians must manage risk and community integration while promoting the dignity of risk and supporting personal choice. Because a protective stance can impede the individual's pursuit of personal goals, it is imperative that social workers be competent in managing their own personal feelings in this regard.

CONCLUSIONS

It is important for social workers to identify the three dimensions of the transitional care framework and to use evidence-based strategies along the way to engage individuals in their treatment, foster the development of wellness strategies, and ensure integration within the community. Although the three dimensions of the framework overlap, the focus of intervention varies over time, depending on where the individual is in the process of transition. As community extenders, family members, peers, and other allies form vital support networks for people in recovery.

The three dimensions of the transitional care framework help to structure the work social workers do as people move between different levels of care. Clinicians, service users, and natural supporters can together use evidence-based practices and tools with linkages to the community to pave a new road toward recovery. The values of integrated practice are exemplified in the transition process by interventions that promote and foster the partnership of individuals, families, and clinicians to cultivate hope and support.

ACKNOWLEDGMENT

I would like to thank Samantha Shaffer, Social Work Intern with the ACT Institute (2015–2016), who assisted in conducting the research on transitional practices and peer bridging.

RESOURCES

Center for Practice Innovations at Columbia University http://practiceinnovations.org/

Center for Advancement of Critical Time Intervention www.criticaltime.org

European Assertive Outreach Foundation http://www.eaof.org/

New York State Association for Psychiatric Services http://www.nyaprs.org/

Recovery to Practice http://www.samhsa.gov/recovery-to-practice

REFERENCES

Adams, N., & Grieder, D. M. (2004). *Treatment planning for person-centered care: The road to mental health and addiction recovery.* Waltham, MA: Academic Press.

Berkman, N. D., Sheridan, S. L., Donahue, K. E., Halpern, D. J., Viera, A., Crotty, K., . . . Viswanathan, M. (2011). *Health literacy interventions and outcomes: An updated systematic review* (Evidence Report/Technology Assessment No. 199). Rockville, MD: Agency for Healthcare Research and Quality.

Burke, G. (2011). *The patient-centered medical home: Taking a model to scale in New York State.* New York, NY: United Hospital Fund. Retrieved from http://www.chhs.ca.gov/InnovationPlan/PCMH-Taking%20the%20Model%20to%20Scale%20in%20NYS%20-%202011.pdf

Center for Practice Innovations. (2016). ACT transition curriculum, unit 1-ACT: On the road to recovery. Available from https://rfmh.csod.com/client/rfmh/default.aspx

Cohen, A. N., Drapalski, A. L., Glynn, S. M., Medoff, D., Fang, L. J., & Dixon, L. B. (2013). Preferences for family involvement in care among consumers with serious mental illness. *Psychiatric Services, 64,* 257–263. doi: 10.1176/appi.ps.201200176

Cook, J. A., Copeland, M. E., Jonikas, J. A., Hamilton, M. M., Razzano, L. A., Grey, D. D., . . . Boyd, S. (2012). Results of a randomized controlled trial of mental illness self-management using Wellness Recovery Action Planning. *Schizophrenia Bulletin, 38,* 881–891. doi: 10.1093/schbul/sbr012

Deegan, P. E. (2005). The importance of personal medicine: A qualitative study of resilience in people with psychiatric disabilities. *Scandinavian Journal of Public Health, 33*(Suppl. 66), 29–35. doi: 10.1080/14034950510033345

Dixon, L. B., Dickerson, F., Bellack, A. S., Bennett, M., Dickinson, D., Goldberg, R. W., . . . Kreyenbuhl, J. (2010). The 2009 Schizophrenia PORT psychosocial treatment recommendations and summary statements. *Schizophrenia Bulletin, 36,* 48–70. doi: 10.1093/schbul/sbp115

Dixon, L. B., Holoshitz, Y., & Nossel, I. (2016). Treatment engagement of individuals experiencing mental illness: Review and update. *World Psychiatry, 15,* 13–20. doi: 10.1002/wps.20306

Dixon, L. B., & Swartz, E. C. (2014). Fifty years of progress in community mental health in US: The growth of evidence-based practices. *Epidemiology and Psychiatric Sciences, 23,* 5–9. doi: 10.1017/S2045796013000620

Elwyn, G., Dehlendorf, C., Epstein, R. M., Marrin, K., White, J., & Frosch, D. L. (2014). Shared decision making and motivational interviewing: Achieving patient-centered care across the spectrum of health care problems. *The Annals of Family Medicine, 12,* 270–275. doi: 10.1370/afm.1615

Gates, L. B., & Akabas, S. H. (2007). Developing strategies to integrate peer providers into the staff of mental health agencies. *Administration and Policy in Mental Health and Mental Health Services Research, 34*(3), 293–306.

Goodell, S., Druss, B. G., & Walker, E. R., (2011). *Mental disorders and medical comorbidity* (Policy Brief No. 21). Princeton, NJ: Robert Wood Johnson Foundation. Retrieved from http://www.rwjf.org/content/dam/farm/reports/issue_briefs/2011/rwjf69438

Herman, D., Conover, S., & Draine, J. (2010). Critical Time Intervention. In A. Rubin, D. W. Springer, & K. Trawver (Eds.), *Psychosocial treatment of schizophrenia* (pp. 253–282). Hoboken, NJ: John Wiley & Sons.

Jackson, C., DuBard, A., Swartz, M., Mahan, A., McKee, J., Pikoulas, T., . . . Lancaster, M. (2015). Readmission patterns and effectiveness of transitional care among Medicaid patients with schizophrenia and medical comorbidity. *North Carolina Medical Journal, 76,* 219–226. doi: 10.18043/ncm.76.4.219

Larson, T. (Ed.). (2014). Parterning with patients, families, and communities to link interprofessional practice and education: Proceedings of a conference chaired by Terry Fulmer and Martha (Meg) Gaines. New York, NY: Josiah Macy Jr. Foundation. Retrieved from http://macyfoundation.org/docs/macy_pubs/JMF_PartneringwithPFC.pdf

Lukens, E. (2015). *Psychoeducation: An annotated bibliography.* New York, NY: Oxford University Press.

Lukens, E., & Thorning, H. (2010). Psychoeducational family groups. In A. Rubin, D. W. Springer, & K. Trawver (Eds.), *Psychosocial treatment of schizophrenia* (pp. 89–144). Hoboken, NJ: John Wiley & Sons.

Mead, S., Hilton, D., & Curtis, L. (2001). Peer support: A theoretical perspective. *Psychiatric Rehabilitation Journal, 25,* 134–141. doi: 10.1037/h0095032

Naylor, M. D., Aiken, L. H., Kurtzman, E. T., Olds, D. M., & Hirschman, K. B. (2011). The importance of transitional care in achieving health reform. *Health Affairs, 30,* 746–754. doi: 10.1377/hlthaff.2011.0041

Nossel, I. R., Lee, R. J., Isaacs, A., Herman, D. B., Marcus, S. M., & Essock, S. M. (2016). Use of peer staff in a critical time intervention for frequent users of a psychiatric emergency room. *Psychiatric Services, 67,* 479–481. doi: doi:10.1176/appi.ps.201500503

Pope, L. G., Smith, T. E., Wisdom, J. P., Easter, A., & Pollock, M. (2013). Transitioning between systems of care: Missed opportunities for engaging adults with serious mental illness and criminal justice involvement. *Behavioral Sciences & the Law, 31*(4), 444–456. doi: 10.1002/bsl.2074

Salerno, A., Margolies, P., Cleek, A., Pollock, M., Gopalan, G., & Jackson, C. (2011). Best practices: Wellness Self-Management: An adaptation of the Illness Management and Recovery program in New York State. *Psychiatric Services, 62,* 456–458. doi: 10.1176/ps.62.5.pss6205_0456

Stanhope, V., Videka, L., Thorning, H., & McKay, M. (2015). Moving toward integrated health: An opportunity for social work. *Social Work in Health Care, 54,* 383–407. doi: 10.1080/00981389.2015.1025122

Swarbrick, M. A. (2013). Integrated care: Wellness-oriented peer approaches: A key ingredient for integrated care. *Psychiatric Services, 68,* 723–726. doi: 10.1176/appi.ps.201300144

Thorning, H. (2014). On the road to recovery: ACT and beyond. In New York State Office of Mental Health (Ed.), *September 2014 newsletter.* New York, NY: New York State Office of Mental Health. Retrieved from https://www.omh.ny.gov/omhweb/resources/newsltr/2014/september/september-omh-newsletter.pdf

Thorning, H., & Dixon, L. (2016). Caregiving for individuals with serious mental illness: A life cycle perspective. In L. D. Burgio, J. E. Gaugler, & M. M. Hilgeman (Eds.), *The spectrum of family caregiving for adults and elders with chronic illness* (pp. 173–211). New York, NY: Oxford University Press.

Trachtenberg, M., Parsonage, M., Shepherd, G. & Boardman, J. (2013). *Peer support in mental health care: is it good value for money?* London, UK: Centre for Mental Health.

Wagner, E. H., Austin, B. T., & Von Korff, M. (1996). Organizing care for patients with chronic illness. *The Milbank Quarterly, 74,* 511–544. doi: 10.2307/3350391

Webb, N. B. (1985). A crisis intervention perspective on the termination process. *Clinical Social Work Journal, 13,* 329–340. doi: 10.1007/BF00755368

CHAPTER 13

INTEGRATED HEALTH CARE FOR CHILDREN AND ADOLESCENTS

Diane M. Mirabito, Aminda Heckman Chomanczuk, and Judith P. Siegel

As described by Horevitz and Manoleas (2013), an integrated health care approach "attempts to address the full biopsychosocial spectrum of needs" (p. 753) of youth and their families in a wide range of health, school, and community-based agency settings. The coordinated, integrated, and prevention-focused approach to care among allied health professionals provides an ideal way to comprehensively address the wide range of physical, mental, educational, and psychosocial needs of youth and their families and to provide them with a combination of education, prevention, and intervention services (Horevitz & Manoleas, 2013).

This chapter provides an overview of key concepts, skills, and knowledge about integrated health care approaches that can be used with children, adolescents, parents, and families in a variety of practice settings, including primary care, school-based health clinics, and community-based health and mental health agencies. The discussion includes attention to key components of integrated health care with youth and families, including access to and continuity of care, prevention and wellness, and interprofessional practice. Foundational concepts and specialized practice strategies are provided, including use of screening and assessment tools and preventive and evidence-based interventions for youth and their families. Prevention and wellness strategies include psychoeducation and health promotion. Evidence-based intervention strategies include cognitive-behavioral therapy (CBT), motivational interviewing (MI), mindfulness, and trauma-focused approaches and family-focused interventions for youth who have experienced internalizing or externalizing problems, trauma, or substance misuse (Suarez, Belcher, Briggs, & Titus, 2012). A case example of social work practice with youth in a school-based health clinic highlights the key themes of the chapter. The multifaceted roles of social workers are discussed along with the essential clinical and collaborative skills they need for effective practice with youth and families in integrated health care settings.

HEALTH NEEDS AND HEALTH CARE DISPARITIES FOR CHILDREN AND ADOLESCENTS

Despite significant changes in health care policy resulting from the Patient Protection and Affordable Care Act (ACA), children and adolescents in low-income households remain disproportionately affected by a variety of health problems. The medical and mental health needs of children and adolescents living in poverty can directly result from or be exacerbated by the convergence of detrimental influences on child and adolescent development, including exposure to extreme stress related to poverty, violence, and trauma. Children and adolescents who live in poor families are more than twice as likely to be at high risk for developmental, behavioral, and social delays compared with children and adolescents in families with higher incomes (Children's Defense Fund, 2014), and they are also less likely to receive preventive medical and dental care (Children's Defense Fund, 2014; Mirabito & Lloyd, 2017).

Adolescent health includes a broad spectrum of physical, emotional, and mental health concerns, including acne, weight, depression, school performance, family problems, and use of tobacco, alcohol, and drugs. Adolescents with the largest health care expenses incur costs from injury, mental health issues, substance use problems, and pregnancy (Newacheck, Wong, Galbraith, & Hung, 2003). Studies have shown that stress during adolescence leads to risky behaviors such as poor dietary choices, sexual risk taking, and alcohol, drug, and tobacco use (Rew, Johnson, & Young, 2014). Adolescent mortality results not only from illness but also from preventable social, environmental, and behavioral factors. Behavioral factors are particularly important in adolescent health because they affect morbidity and mortality. Economically disadvantaged adolescents who are homeless; lesbian, gay, bisexual, transgendered, and queer or questioning (LGBTQ); living in or aging out of foster care; or in the juvenile and criminal justice systems are particularly vulnerable because they are at high risk for serious health problems and are likely to have insurance coverage only in those states that have expanded Medicaid (English, Scott, & Park, 2014). Many of these youth experience complex behavioral health difficulties and frequently engage in risky, health-compromising behaviors, but they receive no services to meet their needs (Horowitz, McKay, & Marshall, 2005; McKay, Lynn, & Bannon, 2005).

INTEGRATED HEALTH CARE PRACTICE SETTINGS

The goals of integrated health care are to provide continuity of care, prevention, and treatment or intervention for medical and behavioral health concerns. To achieve these goals, health care models can be coordinated, co-located, or integrated, depending on the level of communication between medical and behavioral health care providers and the integration of treatment plans (Marlowe, Hodgson, Lamson, White, & Irons, 2012) (see Chapter 8). Settings that are co-located and integrated (Marlowe et al., 2012) are considered to have the highest level of integration because medical and behavioral health care providers practice in the same location, share referrals, and have opportunities for in-person communication and collaboration about services and treatment plans. Examples of these settings include hospital and community-based primary care clinics, school-based health clinics, and comprehensive community-based health and mental health clinics. It is anticipated that the ACA will bring previously uninsured families with extensive psychosocial needs into primary care settings (Lynch & Franke, 2013). In these settings, medical providers address the physical symptoms presented by young people, and behavioral health care providers address their concurrent psychosocial issues (Marlowe et al., 2012).

Historically, school-based health clinics located in elementary and secondary public schools have been a model of care for integrated health approaches for children and adolescents. In support of this approach, Manning (2009) maintained that the "physical and mental health of children and adolescents are not separate issues and need to be addressed together" (p. 48). Manning described the ways in which four major physical health issues (obesity, diabetes, asthma, and teen pregnancy) and five key mental health issues (suicide, depression, attention-deficit hyperactivity disorder [ADHD], aggression, and violence) significantly affect children's overall health, wellbeing, and school functioning.

Behavioral health care settings, such as inpatient, outpatient, day, and residential treatment programs, are considered coordinated services, characterized by telephone or email communication between medical and behavioral health care providers. Although medical services may not be provided on site in these settings, there are often opportunities for on-site individual and team consultations with a range of other health care and educational professionals, including psychiatrists, psychologists, occupational and speech therapists, social workers, teachers, and school staff.

INTERPROFESSIONAL PRACTICE IN INTEGRATED HEALTH CARE SETTINGS

Interprofessional practice, which includes ongoing collaboration and consultation among allied health care professionals and behavioral health care providers, is a key component of integrated health care and a core skill that is used by all professionals across diverse settings. Interprofessional practice teams composed of diverse professionals work together to provide a range of health, behavioral health, and health education services. For example, an interdisciplinary team in a school-based health clinic, hospital, or community-based primary care clinic may include a medical doctor or nurse practitioner, a social worker, and a health educator, providing a full range of medical, behavioral health, and health education services to children, adolescents, and their families. In community-based, comprehensive, multiservice centers, such teams may also include dental providers, attorneys, drug counselors, and outreach workers, who provide dental, behavioral health, legal, and youth development services. As suggested by Charles and Alexander (2014), an intensive family support outreach team consisting of a social worker, a psychologist, a nurse, and a child care worker can travel to rural communities to provide children and their families with needed health and mental health services.

Interprofessional practice skills promote effective collaboration among interdisciplinary team members through strategies of mutual respect, shared knowledge of various professionals' expertise, and communication among professionals about their areas of proficiency (Charles & Alexander, 2014). Lynch and Franke (2013) observed that for settings in which medical and behavioral health services are in different locations, strategies such as shared electronic health records can be used to increase communication and mitigate the disadvantages of distance between social workers and pediatricians.

SCREENING AND ASSESSMENT TOOLS

Promoting a comprehensive treatment approach in integrated health care encourages the formation of multidisciplinary teams (Horevitz & Manoleas, 2013; Mechanic, 2012) and the use of screening tools that can be administered in interdisciplinary settings, such as community health centers or school-based health clinics. For children and adolescents, it is essential that these screening tools promote prevention and early detection of risk-taking behaviors (Kuhlthau et al., 2011) as well as health, mental health, and behavioral issues (Anderson, Chen, Perrin, & VanCleave, 2015). This is especially germane for teens because 75% of adolescent morbidity and mortality results from risky behaviors such as unprotected sex, poor diet, or drug abuse (Salerno, Marshall, & Picken, 2012), and early identification can result in risk reduction (Michigan Department of Health and Human Services, n.d.). The following sections discuss examples of three relevant screening tools that can be used in integrated health care settings.

BRIGHT FUTURES NATIONAL CENTER

The Bright Futures National Center (BFNC) was originally created by an interdisciplinary team convened by the U.S. Maternal and Child Health Bureau (MCHB), Health Resources and Services Administration (HRSA), and the Medicaid Bureau. For the past 25 years, BFNC has provided guidelines for child and adolescent wellness care; it is now under the auspices of the American Academy of Pediatrics (AAP; 2016). Although the educational information and screening tools from *Bright Futures: Guidelines for Health Supervision of Infants, Children, and Adolescents* (Hagan, Shaw, & Duncan, 2008) have primarily been used in pediatricians' offices, BFNC's main goal is for the material to be implemented in integrated health settings such as school-based health centers, public health clinics, community health centers, Indian Health Service clinics, and other primary care facilities. The ACA includes a provision to ensure that children receive the standard of preventive care screenings and services recommended by its guidelines (AAP, 2016).

Packets of information focus on wellness (e.g., nutrition, exercise) and mental health (e.g., depression, anxiety) and are separated into appropriate age groups. Parents are asked to fill out the forms for younger children, and adolescents are offered self-administered questionnaires. For example, the Pediatric Symptom Checklist (PSC) is a 35-item survey that screens for emotional and behavioral problems. The same questionnaire is provided to youth 11 years of age or older (PSC-Youth Report) and is completed by them. BFNC provides advisors to assist organizations in implementing BFNC screening tools and information into practice. Most of the materials are available in Spanish, and there are interactive apps for both practitioners and parents (AAP, 2016).

RAPID ASSESSMENT FOR ADOLESCENT PREVENTIVE SERVICES

The Rapid Assessment for Adolescent Preventive Services (RAAPS) was built on the American Medical Association's Guidelines for Adolescent Preventive Services (GAPS), which consisted of four pages with 60 to 71 questions (Yi, Martyn, Salerno, & Darling-Fisher, 2009). To make the assessment more time efficient (about 5 to 7 minutes) but still maintain its comprehensive nature, the questionnaire was reduced to about 21 questions that can be completed by individuals between 9 and 24 years of age on paper or by tablet. RAAPS also offers short forms based on age groups. It is a risk-assessment tool that provides a screening snapshot for eating disorders, emotional and behavioral concerns, substance misuse, safety, and violence (RAAPS, n.d.), and it has good face validity and reliability (Salerno et al., 2012). Example items include the following:

- In the past 12 months, have you ever taken diet pills or laxatives, vomited, or used starvation to lose weight?
- Do you eat some fruits and vegetables every day?
- Do you always wear a lap or seat belt when in a car, truck, or van?
- Have you ever carried a weapon (e.g., gun, knife, club) to protect yourself?

CRAFFT SCREENING TOOL

The CRAFFT was created by The Center for Adolescent Substance Abuse Research (CeASAR) at Boston Children's Hospital and is recommended by AAP's Committee on Substance Abuse (CeASAR, n.d.). It is a screening tool for youth substance misuse that can be self-administered and completed in less than 10 minutes, and it is available in 12 languages, including Chinese, Russian, and Spanish. It has been validated for youth between 12 and 18 years of age (Harris et al., 2015) and has been shown to reduce underage drinking (Clark, Gordon, Ettaro, Owens, & Moss, 2010). The acronym CRAFFT stands for the following screening items:

- **C**ar: "Have you ever ridden in a car driven by someone (or yourself) who was high or had been using alcohol or drugs?"
- **R**elax: "Do you ever use alcohol or drugs to relax, feel better about yourself, or fit in?"

- **A**lone: "Do you ever use alcohol or drugs while you are by yourself or alone?"
- **F**orget: "Do you ever forget things you did while using alcohol or drugs?"
- **F**riends: "Do your family or friends ever tell you that you should cut down on your drinking or drug use?"
- **T**rouble: "Have you ever gotten into trouble while you were using alcohol or drugs?"

The complete CRAFFT screening toolkit and instructions are available free of charge at http://www.childrenshospital.org/ceasar/crafft.

EVIDENCE-BASED INTERVENTIONS

Of particular interest for integrated health care providers is the ACA's emphasis on using evidence-based interventions and therapeutic modalities. Among them are CBT, MI, mindfulness, and trauma-focused and family-focused interventions.

COGNITIVE-BEHAVIORAL THERAPY

Cognitive behavioral therapy (CBT) has a strong evidence base for treatment and relapse prevention in adults with unipolar depression and anxiety and in adolescents with unipolar depression (Rupke, Blecke, & Renfrow, 2006). Further evidence suggests that CBT can also be effectively used with children and adolescents to treat anxiety disorders, anger issues, and cannabis and tobacco addictions (Hofmann, Asnaani, Vonk, Sawyer, & Fang, 2012). Trauma-focused CBT (TF-CBT) has reduced symptoms of posttraumatic stress disorder and depressive and behavioral problems in children who have experienced trauma (Cary & McMillen, 2012).

What makes CBT an ideal modality for children and adolescents is its "here and now" approach, which connects coping skills to concrete actions (Friedberg & McClure, 2002) with considerable evidence in favor of modeling, coaching, and practicing new skills between sessions (Landolt & Kenardy, 2015). Although age is sometimes a factor in determining the appropriateness of a CBT intervention, the clinician should also consider the social and cognitive developments of young people, including language acquisition, perspective-taking ability, reasoning capacity, and verbal regulation skills (Friedberg & McClure, 2002). The use of CBT in primary care settings has grown in popularity.

Clabby (2006) offered a menu of CBT techniques designed for use in busy settings. For example, the technique described by the acronym BATHE helps the practitioner get to the heart of what is most concerning the service user during the first interview while also identifying psychosocial issues that need to be addressed. The acronym stands for the following:

- **B**ackground: "What else is going on in your life?"
- **A**ffect: "How did you (or do you) feel about this?"

- **T**rouble: "What troubles you the most about this?"
- **H**andle: "How are you handling this?"
- **E**mpathy: "That sounds really hard . . ."

Another technique Clabby described is CARL: "**C**hange it, **A**ccept it, **R**eframe it, or **L**eave it" (2006). This intervention helps service users take credit for the decisions that were already made in a particular troubling situation but then allows them to think of their options and choose their next steps. Other effective interventions suggested by Clabby (2006) include journaling, homework, and completion of handouts.

MOTIVATIONAL INTERVIEWING

Motivational interviewing (MI) has been established as an effective intervention for substance misuse and smoking cessation in teens because the method relies on strongly engaging the service user to facilitate change for himself or herself (Barnett, Sussman, Smith, Rohrbach, & Spruijt-Metz, 2012; Colby et al., 1998). A hallmark of MI treatment is to emphasize the service user's choice and support self-efficacy. Clinicians are reminded to "stop, drop, and roll" when working with resistance: stop and reflect on the child's experience, drop the issue and let go of counterarguments, and roll with the resistance (Naar-King & Suarez, 2011).

Other evidence supports MI's usefulness for reducing sexually risky behavior and encouraging a healthy diet and physical activity (Cushing, Jensen, Miller, & Leffingwell, 2014). Walpole and colleagues (2013) found that MI in conjunction with diet and exercise helped overweight and obese adolescents lose weight. They attributed part of its effectiveness to increasing a youth's awareness of unhealthy behaviors, showing how those behaviors are inconsistent with personal values, and helping the individual to envision change. This finding is similar to that of Channon, Smith, and Gregory (2003), who reported positive outcomes using MI for adolescents diagnosed with diabetes. They found it to be a strong tool for glycemic control because the clinician works with the youth to build awareness, find alternatives, solve problems, make choices, and set goals while refraining from challenging resistance or engaging in confrontation with the service user.

MI has a strong evidence base for substance misuse, and group MI has been used to decrease substance use and recidivism rates for adolescents with a first-time alcohol or drug offense. The Free Talk program is a six-session MI group that is publicly available (Group MI for Teens, n.d.). Participants in Free Talk groups reported feeling respected by the leader and responded well to change talk and open-ended questions; this encouraged them to more readily accept the treatment (D'Amico et al., 2015; D'Amico, Hunter, Miles, Ewing, & Chan Osilla, 2013).

As with CBT, language skills and reasoning capacity must be considered when weighing the use of MI as a treatment modality for children and adolescents. Youth who are older than 11 years of age are more capable of discussing ambivalence and identifying personal principles (Naar-King & Suarez, 2011). However, MI generally appears to be highly effective in promoting self-efficacy and enacting change in adolescents (Erickson,

Gerstle, & Feldstein, 2005). MI strategies can also be used to improve adherence to CBT (Naar-King & Suarez, 2011).

MINDFULNESS INTERVENTIONS

Mindfulness is a state of consciousness that focuses on the present experience and includes mechanisms of focused attention, observation of one's experience in a nonreactive and nonjudgmental manner, and emotional regulation. There is a strong movement throughout the country to provide mindfulness interventions for children and adolescents, particularly as a universal intervention with students in preschool through high school settings, to increase attention and achieve positive psychological and academic outcomes. A meta-analysis of 20 studies with youth between the ages of 6 and 21 years, implemented from 2004 to 2011, suggested that mindfulness might be particularly effective with clinical populations in settings such as hospitals and mental health clinics and nonclinical populations in settings such as community-based youth programs and schools (Zoogerman, Goldberg, Hoyt, & Miller, 2015).

Mindfulness-based cognitive therapy (MBCT) and mindfulness-based stress reduction (MBSR) are widely used for a range of physical and mental health concerns such as depression, anxiety, and stress. They were originally designed for adult populations but have since been adapted for use with children and adolescents. For example, MBCT has been used with youth age 13 to 18 years who have ADHD and their parents to reduce the adolescents' inattention, conduct, and peer problems and the parents' care-giving stress (Haydicky, Shecter, Wiener, & Ducharme, 2015). MBCT for children (MBCT-C), implemented for 8- to 14-year-olds, has been modified by involving parents and shortening the length and number of sessions. MBSR for teens (MBSR-T), used with youth 14 to 18 years of age, focuses on stress reduction relevant to the social and interpersonal developmental challenges of adolescence (Zoogerman et al., 2015).

Mindfulness-based approaches have been used effectively to decrease impulsivity and improve emotional regulation for adolescents with substance use problems, who often have difficulties regulating impulses and emotions. Mindfulness strategies have been used to help adolescents develop and accept awareness of triggers and urges to use substances and to aid in the process of repairing and reversing neuronal changes associated with substance misuse and relapse (Wittenauer, Ascher, Briggie, Krieter, & Chavez, 2015).

Like mindfulness, yoga (which is considered a mind-body medicine) focuses on the interactions between the body and the mind and on the ways in which physical, emotional, and spiritual factors affect health. Yoga has been used effectively to help adolescents with substance use problems develop the mindfulness needed to remain in the present moment with focused attention, instead of diverting attention and awareness to escape from the present, which is often typical with substance misuse. Although studies have suggested that yoga can be effective in treating anxiety and depression in children and adolescents by reducing stress, further empirical research is needed to extend knowledge and application of these findings (Wittenauer et al., 2015).

TRAUMA-FOCUSED INTERVENTIONS

Identification and assessment of trauma in children and adolescents is often complicated and prolonged because they frequently have behavioral and emotional dysregulation problems that can develop into a range of physical, emotional, cognitive, developmental, and behavioral difficulties if left unaddressed. Trauma-focused, evidence-based treatment approaches used with adults, such as CBT and dialectical behavior therapy (DBT), have been adapted to meet the developmental needs of children and adolescents (Racco & Vis, 2015).

CBT, which is the most researched and most evidence-based approach to treatment for traumatized children and adolescents, focuses on addressing and changing dysfunctional thoughts, behaviors, and emotions. DBT is a specialized form of CBT that uses individual psychotherapy and group skill building to teach four core skills:

1. Mindfulness
2. Emotion regulation
3. Distress tolerance
4. Interpersonal effectiveness

Interventions that include both the mind and the body, such as physically based relaxation strategies, are more beneficial in the early stages of treatment, compared with cognitive processing strategies. Research suggests that it is important for children and adolescents to first master body and sensory awareness before they can make effective use of cognitive and behavioral interventions (Racco & Vis, 2015).

Trauma-focused CBT (TF-CBT) is a specialized trauma approach that is appropriate and has demonstrated efficacy for youth between 3 and 18 years of age who have experienced a wide range of traumatic events. TF-CBT, which uses individual sessions with youth and joint sessions with their parents over a period of 12 to 16 sessions, includes modules focused on psychoeducation, relaxation and affect modulation, cognitive processing, development of trauma narratives, safety planning, in vivo practice, and parent skill development (Racco & Vis, 2015). Cary and McMillen (2012) reported that the most helpful TF-CBT techniques for youth and their families were psychoeducation about trauma-related symptoms, modulation skills for physiological and emotional distress, and the creation of a trauma narrative.

FAMILY-FOCUSED INTERVENTIONS

Although the family context is relevant to all users of integrated health services, it is of utmost importance for children and adolescents. As McKay and Bannon (2004) pointed out, mental health problems in children are particularly common in low-income urban communities, where the prevalence of children with mental health care needs may be as high as 40%. At the same time, these children are the least likely to receive mental health care due to lack of access to services and high rates of disengagement, even when treatment is available.

Research suggests that parental attitudes about services and providers are one of the strongest barriers to continued involvement in mental health treatment. Consequently, it is vital that service providers become aware of strategies that are most likely to encourage parents to participate in recommended services. To do so, it is important to consider the past and current life circumstances of the parents who play such critical roles in their children's lives. Too often, they have grown up in families with violence or neglect, leading to higher incidences of health and mental health problems and difficulties in the parenting role (Steele et al., 2016). Many parents whose children are in need of services are themselves struggling with stressors related to poverty and family instability. It is not uncommon for the mothers of children at risk to be suffering from symptoms of depression or posttraumatic stress disorder (PTSD). In addition to health and mental health problems, parents who live under extreme stress and who have been exposed to potentially traumatic events often develop substance use disorders. Adolescents whose parents misuse substances are at high risk for early use and have higher levels of mental health symptoms (Siegel, 2015).

Given the likelihood that parents of high-risk children are struggling with their own stressors and health and mental health problems, an integrated health care perspective that addresses the needs of all family members may be most beneficial. As Lindsey, Chambers, Pohle, Beall, and Lucksted (2013) suggested, it is important to not blame the parents for their child's problems but to instead recognize the struggles they have in parenting their child. A non-blaming, supportive stance is essential in developing a collaborative relationship. It is also important to stress the benefits of integrated services to improve functioning in several areas and to help the parents identify goals that may increase motivation. Rather than viewing the parents as being deficient or causing the child's problems, service providers should make every effort to empathize with the adults in the family and should strive to establish a relationship that builds on compassion, empowerment, and cultural acknowledgment (Becker, Buckingham, & Brandt, 2015).

The decision to engage in services often runs contrary to the norms held by extended family members and friends, who may distrust service providers or view mental health symptoms as personal weaknesses (Lindsey et al., 2013). Engaging families allows for a comprehensive understanding of the families' needs and concerns. In this way, the social worker and other providers are better able to offer preventive measures by raising awareness of concerns (e.g., teen pregnancy, diet, depression, anxiety, nutrition) and can create pathways that help all family members improve their health.

Working with parents may also provide opportunities to build on existing strengths and help family members develop the skills that are commonly associated with resilience. Given the multiplicity of family kinship arrangements and cultural diversity, there are advantages to considering a family resilience framework rather than family assessment approaches that tend to be static, pathology focused, and specific to white, intact, two-parent families (Hawley, 2013). Walsh (2013) suggests that identifying areas that contribute to family resilience can guide assessment and intervention. Themes include the importance of belief systems, communication, problem solving, and organizational patterns such as flexibility and connection.

In addition to an approach built on principles of resilience, there are dozens of evidence-supported family therapy models that have been developed to work with specific problem areas in children and adolescents, including depression, substance misuse, and PTSD (Kaslow, Broth, Smith, & Collins, 2012). Other models have been established to strengthen families with multiple problems and enlist parental involvement in response to behavioral or emotional concerns. They include proactive sexual education that may protect children against sexual exploitation, unwanted pregnancy, and HIV infection (Prado et al., 2012; Timm, 2013). Several of these approaches stress the importance of building attachment between parent and child. Evidence-based models that have proved successful in working with high-risk populations emphasize flexibility, collaborative processes through engagement, responsiveness to youth and parental perspectives and concerns, services that fit the family's needs and are perceived as relevant, and strategies to overcome obstacles to continuing treatment (Bruns et al., 2014). In response to the needs of families, multiple models have been developed that include psychoeducation, multifamily groups, and parental empowerment (Hoagwood et al., 2014).

CASE VIGNETTE

Tanya is a 14-year-old Haitian girl in her first year at a large urban public high school in Los Angeles, California. Despite a strong record of academic achievement in elementary and junior high school, Tanya is at risk for failing several classes in this school due to poor attendance, inattention in the classroom, and failure to complete homework assignments. Although Tanya enjoyed school in the past, she lost interest this year as she became involved with her first boyfriend, Malcolm, who is a junior in the same school. Tanya has found herself spending most of her time with Malcolm and, as a result, has not been investing the time and attention to schoolwork that she did previously.

Tanya has been worried about her continually declining school performance and is particularly concerned that the school guidance counselor will be sending a notice home regarding her multiple absences. She has also been increasingly distressed about constant fights she has with both her mother and her boyfriend. She has missed her period for almost two months and worries that she may be pregnant.

As she became more and more upset, Tanya finally confided all of these concerns to her best friend, Wanda, who suggested that she go to the health clinic in their school and offered to go with her. Tanya had recently learned about the school-based health clinic when the social worker and health educator from the clinic gave a presentation to her advisory class about the clinic's services. Wanda highly recommended the clinic's services because she had gone to the school-based health clinic at the beginning of the school year to obtain a medical and sports evaluation and to update her immunizations. Because Tanya was very scared and did not know what else she could do, she took Wanda's advice and went with her to the clinic.

ASSESSMENT AND INTERVENTIONS

Tanya made an appointment to talk the next day with Janet, one of the social workers at the school-based health clinic. In conducting her initial meeting with Tanya, Janet assessed that Tanya's primary concerns were her fear of being pregnant, the tension she was experiencing with her boyfriend and her mother, and her fears about failing several classes. During the first visit, she arranged for Tanya to have a pregnancy test at the clinic. Because the pregnancy test result was positive, Tanya was offered social work options counseling—a brief, one- to three-session, crisis-focused intervention offered to all young women with positive pregnancy tests at the clinic to help them consider all of their options and develop plans regarding pregnancy. The social worker arranged for Tanya to have a gynecological examination with the nurse practitioner and a risk-reduction counseling session with the health educator (both at the school-based health clinic) to provide further information and develop risk-reduction and contraceptive strategies related to sexually transmitted infections (STIs) and future pregnancy.

In her initial assessment, the social worker learned that Tanya lived with her mother, maternal grandmother, and four siblings (ages 3, 6, 8, and 10 years). The family had immigrated from Haiti seven years ago. Tanya's father, who had lived in Haiti and had been estranged from the family since Tanya was five years old, died of AIDS two years ago. Although they were estranged for many years, Tanya and her father had reconnected a year before his death. Tanya, who had previously been very close to her mother and grandmother, described ongoing struggles with them regarding her limits, freedoms, responsibilities, and choice of friends. Moreover, she described increasing feelings of depression about the estrangement with her family and her conflict and guilt about becoming sexually active without her family's knowledge.

During the focused options counseling session, the social worker engaged Tanya in a lengthy discussion about the pros and cons of each side of her decision and presented her with information about the three options she had—keeping the baby, having an abortion, or arranging for adoption of the baby. In exploring her reactions to the pregnancy, the social worker learned that Tanya was quite conflicted about making a decision. Although she was able to acknowledge that she was too young to have a child, she felt compelled to consider doing so as a result of the significant pressure she experienced from her boyfriend, her lack of interest in school, her hope that having a child would bring her closer to her family, and her strong religious prohibitions against abortion. On the social worker's further exploration regarding feelings of depression, Tanya expressed unresolved feelings of loss and sadness related to recent changes in the family, including her father's death from AIDS and the loss of her previously close relationships with her mother and grandmother.

The social worker further explored depression, suicidality, and other risk factors and behaviors, including unprotected sex and STIs. She discussed with Tanya the benefits of having an opportunity to engage in counseling to address the feelings of loss and conflict that she was experiencing about her relationships with family members and to discuss the pressures of starting high school, becoming sexually active, and navigating the many challenges of adolescence. The social worker was knowledgeable about policies in California, which provided Tanya the right to make a confidential decision about her reproductive health care choices without parental involvement. The social worker suggested that Tanya take a few days to think over her options and consider whether she wanted to involve her boyfriend or her mother in a further discussion.

In a follow-up appointment four days later, Tanya discussed with the social worker her decision to have an abortion. Although she was somewhat ambivalent about this choice, she also felt relieved that the social worker had helped her to conclude that this was the best decision for her at this time in her life. Guided by the California state law protecting adolescents' confidentiality regarding reproductive health care, the social worker helped Tanya arrange an appointment to have an abortion at a high-quality abortion clinic. She provided Tanya with psychoeducation regarding the feelings of loss and potential depression that are common after abortion. She also discussed with her the value of continued counseling to address those feelings, highlighting the importance of continued follow-up with medical, social work, and health education services. Tanya decided not to have a joint meeting with her boyfriend; instead, she chose to work with Janet to decide how she would inform her boyfriend about her decision and how she could discuss, negotiate, and implement strategies for safe sex with him in the future.

The social worker also indicated that she was available to help Tanya with her overall adjustment to school, her family relationships, and other personal concerns. In addition to providing continued individual counseling, the social worker conducted a home-school meeting with Tanya, her mother, and several of her teachers to plan for ways to better support Tanya's academic progress. The social worker held several conjoint sessions with Tanya and her mother to address ways to improve their communication and support Tanya's development.

DISCUSSION

This case illustrates the range of roles assumed by social workers who practice from an integrated health perspective in school-based health clinics. In this practice setting, the social worker and other health care providers were able to provide integrated medical, social work, and health education services to Tanya that focused on prevention, education, and intervention for physical and mental health, school, and family concerns. Although the social worker explored Tanya's desire to involve her mother, she was not surprised to hear that Tanya did not feel ready to involve her regarding the pregnancy. The social worker provided focused options counseling to help Tanya handle the immediate crisis of her pregnancy, engaged Tanya in risk-reduction counseling to help her with ongoing decision-making regarding safe sex, and thoroughly assessed Tanya's medical, mental health, school, interpersonal, and health education needs.

After helping Tanya handle the initial crisis of her pregnancy, the social worker actively worked with Tanya to engage school staff and her mother to address other pressing school and family concerns. In conjoint counseling sessions, the social worker provided psycho-education and support to Tanya and her mother to address the changes in their relationship and to help them handle the typical challenges of adolescence. The social worker was also cognizant of the cultural differences between Tanya, who is growing up in Los Angeles, and her mother, who was raised in Haiti, and helped them to manage their differences. To help Tanya and her family access services, the social worker engaged in interprofessional practice with interdisciplinary health care professionals in the school-based clinic, teachers and other school staff within the school, and service providers at community-based agencies.

IMPLICATIONS FOR SOCIAL WORK PRACTICE

Social workers who practice in integrated health care settings with children, adolescents, and their parents or families need to possess a wide range of clinical practice skills for assessment and intervention and interprofessional practice skills to effectively consult and collaborate with interdisciplinary professionals. The needed clinical practice skills include a solid foundation in culturally competent person-in-environment and biopsychosocial approaches to assessment and the use of assessment and screening tools, brief behavioral interventions, and evidence-based practices (e.g., MI, CBT). Training in family systems is essential to develop effective engagement, assessment, and intervention skills with parents, caretakers, and other family members (Horevitz & Manoleas, 2013). Social workers also must be knowledgeable about chronic illness, psychotropic medications, and sexuality and skilled in relaxation and mindfulness techniques, the provision of psychoeducation, and advocacy with interprofessional staff regarding behavioral health and medical needs (Horevitz & Manoleas, 2013).

Social workers who practice in integrated health care settings need to develop an understanding of and genuine appreciation for the specific roles and functions of other professionals and be able to clearly articulate and model the social work role within interprofessional collaborative relationships and teams. Professional colleagues in settings with children and adolescents include medical doctors, nurse practitioners, nurses, physician assistants, drug counselors, and health educators; psychiatrists and psychologists; principals, teachers, and other school staff; and occupational, speech, and art therapists. Pecukonis et al. (2013) maintained that all professionals need to learn to recognize and challenge hierarchical structures that present obstacles to effective collaboration. They recommended that social workers develop skills in communication, problem solving, and conflict management to collaborate effectively in interdisciplinary teams. They emphasized that social workers potentially have expertise in "tolerance for conflict, negotiation of boundaries, and willingness to confront competitiveness" in interprofessional teams (Pecukonis et al., 2013, p. 630). In addition to team-based skills, social workers also can benefit from having effective skills in so-called curbside consultations—brief, informal consultations with medical providers to help facilitate treatment (Horevitz & Manoleas, 2013).

CONCLUSIONS

Integrated health services for youth address a wide range of physical, mental health, substance use, psychosocial, educational, and family needs. These prevention, intervention, and education services are delivered to youth and their families in a range of settings, including hospitals, social service or mental health agencies, and schools. As a result of the ACA, social workers who work with youth and their families need a broad set of skills in clinical and interprofessional practice (Mason, 2013; Morgan, Kuramoto, Emmet, Stange, & Nobunaga, 2014). Clinical skills are required to provide screening, assessment, and evidence-based interventions, and skills in interprofessional practice are needed to engage in ongoing collaboration and consultation with diverse health care, educational, legal, and health education professionals who are involved in the lives of children, adolescents, and their families.

RESOURCES

American Academy of Child & Adolescent Psychiatry (AACAP) http://www.aacap.org

Bright Futures, American Academy of Pediatrics (AAP) https://brightfutures.aap.org/about/Pages/About.aspx

The CRAFFT Screening Tool, The Center for Adolescent Substance Abuse Research (CeASAR) http://www.childrenshospital.org/ceasar/crafft

Free Talk, Group MI for Teens https://groupmiforteens.org/programs/freetalk

The National Child Traumatic Stress Network (NCTSN), Center for Mental Health Services (CMHS), Substance Abuse and Mental Health Services Administration (SAMHSA), U.S. Department of Health and Human Services (DHHS) http://www.nctsnet.org/

National Institute of Mental Health (NIMH), National Institutes of Health (NIH), U.S. Department of Health and Human Services (DHHS) https://www.nimh.nih.gov/index.shtml

Provider Guide—Adolescent Screening, Brief Intervention, and Referral to Treatment for Alcohol and Other Drug Use: Using the CRAFFT Screening, Massachusetts Department of Public Health Bureau of Substance Abuse Services http://www.ncaddnj.org/file.axd?file=2014%2F7%2FProvider+Guide+-+CRAFFT+Screening+Tool.pdf

Quick Guide to Clinical Techniques for Common Child and Adolescent Mental Health Problems, Center for School Mental Health Analysis and Action (CSMHA), University of Maryland (UMD), Baltimore http://www.schoolmentalhealth.org/Resources/Clin/QuickGuide.pdf

Relaxation Downloads, Student Wellness Center, Dartmouth College http://www.dartmouth.edu/~healthed/relax/downloads.html

Screening Recommendations, Rapid Assessment for Adolescent Preventive Services (RAAPS) https://www.raaps.org/recommendations.php

Trauma Institute (TI) & Child Trauma Institute (CTI) http://www.childtrauma.com/

REFERENCES

American Academy of Pediatrics (AAP). (2016). About Bright Futures. Retrieved from https://brightfutures.aap.org/about/Pages/About.aspx

Anderson, L. E., Chen, M. L., Perrin, J. M., & VanCleave, J. (2015). Outpatient visits and medication prescribing for U.S. children with mental health conditions. *Pediatrics, 136,* e1178–e1185. doi: 10.1542/peds.2015-0807

Barnett, E., Sussman, S., Smith, C., Rohrbach, L. A., & Spruijt-Metz, D. (2012). Motivational interviewing for adolescent substance use: A review of the literature. *Addictive Behaviors, 37,* 1325–1334. doi: 10.1016/j.addbeh.2012.07.001

Becker, K. D., Buckingham, S. L., & Brandt, N. E. (2015). Engaging youth and families in school mental health services. *Child and Adolescent Psychiatric Clinics of North America, 24,* 385–398. doi: 10.1016/j.chc.2014.11.002

Bruns, E. J., Walker, J. S., Bernstein, A., Daleiden, E., Pullmann, M. D., & Chorpita, B. F. (2014). Family voice with informed choice: Coordinating wraparound with research- based treatment for children and adolescents. *Journal of Clinical Child & Adolescent Psychology, 43*, 256–269. doi: 10.1080/15374416.2013.859081

Cary, C. E., & McMillen, J. C. (2012). The data behind the dissemination: A systematic review of trauma-focused cognitive behavioral therapy for use with children and youth. *Children & Youth Services Review, 34*, 748–757. doi: 10.1016/j.childyouth.2012.01.003

Center for Adolescent Substance Abuse Research (CeASAR). (n.d.). The CRAFFT screening tool. Retrieved from http://www.childrenshospital.org/ceasar/crafft

Channon, S., Smith, V. J., & Gregory, J. W. (2003). A pilot study of motivational interviewing in adolescents with diabetes. *Archives of Disease in Childhood, 88*, 680–683. doi: 10.1136/adc.88.8.680

Charles, G., & Alexander, C. (2014). An introduction to interprofessional concepts in social and health care settings. *Relational Child & Youth Care Practice, 27*(3), 51–55. Available from http://www.rcycp.com/

Children's Defense Fund. (2014). *The State of America's Children 2014*. Washington, DC: Children's Defense Fund. Retrieved from http://www.childrensdefense.org/library/state-of-americas-children/2014-soac.pdf?utm_source=2014-SOAC-PDF&utm_medium=link&utm_campaign=2014-SOAC

Clabby, J. F. (2006). Helping depressed adolescents: A menu of cognitive-behavioral procedures for primary care. *Primary Care Companion for CNS Disorders, Journal of Clinical Psychiatry, 8*, 131–141. doi: 10.4088/PCC.v08n0302

Clark, D. B., Gordon, A. J., Ettaro, L. R., Owens, J. M., & Moss, H. B. (2010). Screening and brief intervention for underage drinkers. *Mayo Clinic Proceedings, 85*, 380–391. doi: 10.4065/mcp.2008.0638

Colby, S. M., Monti, P. M., Barnett, N. P., Rohsenow, D. J., Weissman, K., Spirito, A., . . .Lewander, W. J. (1998). Brief motivational interviewing in a hospital setting for adolescent smoking: A preliminary study. *Journal of Consulting and Clinical Psychology, 66*, 574–578. doi: 10.1037/0022-006X.66.3.574

Cushing, C. C., Jensen, C. D., Miller, M. B., & Leffingwell, T. R. (2014). Meta-analysis of motivational interviewing for adolescent health behavior: Efficacy beyond substance use. *Journal of Consulting and Clinical Psychology, 82*, 1212–1218. doi: 10.1037/a0036912

D'Amico, E. J., Houck, J. M., Hunter, S. B., Miles, J.N.V., Chan Osilla, K., & Ewing, B. A. (2015). Group motivational interviewing for adolescents: Change talk and alcohol and marijuana outcomes. *Journal of Consulting and Clinical Psychology, 83*, 68–80. doi: 10.1037/a0038155

D'Amico, E., Hunter, S., Miles, J., Ewing, B., & Chan Osilla, K. (2013). A randomized controlled trial of a group motivational interviewing intervention for adolescents with a first time alcohol or drug offense. *Journal of Substance Abuse Treatment, 45*, 400–408. doi: 10.1016/j.jsat.2013.06.005

English, A., Scott, J., & Park, M. J.; Center for Adolescent Health and the Law & National Adolescent and Young Adult Health Information Center. (2014). Implementing the Affordable Care Act: How much will it help vulnerable adolescents & young adults? Retrieved from http://nahic.ucsf.edu/wp-content/uploads/2014/01/VulnerablePopulations_IB_Final.pdf

Erickson, S. J., Gerstle, M., & Feldstein, S. W. (2005). Brief interventions and motivational interviewing with children, adolescents, and their parents in pediatric health care settings: A review. *Archives of Pediatric Adolescent Medicine, 159*, 1173–1180. doi: 10.1001/archpedi.159.12.1173

Friedberg, R. D., & McClure, J. M. (2002). *Clinical practice of cognitive therapy with children and adolescents: The nuts and bolts*. New York, NY: The Guilford Press.

Group MI for Teens. (n.d.). Free talk. Retrieved from https://groupmiforteens.org/programs/freetalk

Hagan, J. F., Shaw, J. S., & Duncan, P. M. (Eds.). (2008). *Bright futures: Guidelines for health supervision of infants, children, and adolescents* (3rd ed.). Elk Grove Village, IL: American Academy of Pediatrics.

Harris, S. K., Knight, J. R., Jr., Van Hook, S., Sherritt, L., Brooks, T. L., Kulig, J. W., . . . Saitz, R. (2015). Adolescent substance use screening in primary care: Validity of computer self-administered versus clinician-administered screening. *Substance Abuse, 37*, 197–203. doi: 10.1080/08897077.2015.1014615

Hawley, D. R. (2013). The ramifications for clinical practice of a focus on family resilience. In D. S. Becvar (Ed.), *Handbook of family resilience* (pp. 51–64). New York, NY: Springer. doi: 10.1007/978-1-4614-3917-2

Haydicky, J., Shecter, C., Wiener, J., & Ducharme, J. M. (2015). Evaluation of MBCT for adolescents with ADHD and their parents: Impact on individual and family functioning. *Journal of Child and Family Studies, 24,* 76–94. doi: 10.1007/s10826-013-9815-1

Hoagwood, K. E., Olin, S. S., Horwitz, S., McKay, M., Cleek, A., Gleacher, A., . . . & Hogan, M. (2014). Scaling up evidence-based practices for children and families in New York State: Toward evidence-based policies on implementation for state mental health systems. *Journal of Clinical Child & Adolescent Psychology, 43,* 145–157.

Hofmann, S. G., Asnaani, A., Vonk, I. J., Sawyer, A. T., & Fang, A. (2012). The efficacy of cognitive behavioral therapy: A review of meta-analyses. *Cognitive Therapy and Research, 36,* 427–440. doi: 10.1007/s10608-012-9476-1

Horevitz, E., & Manoleas, P. (2013). Professional competencies and training needs of professional social workers in integrated behavioral health in primary care. *Social Work in Health Care, 52,* 752–787. doi: 10.1080/00981389.2013.791362

Horowitz, K., McKay, M., & Marshall, R. (2005). Community violence and urban families: Experiences, effects, and directions for intervention. *American Journal of Orthopsychiatry, 75,* 356–368. doi: 10.1037/0002-9432.75.3.356

Kaslow, N. J., Broth, M. R., Smith, C. O., & Collins, M. H. (2012). Family-based interventions for child and adolescent disorders. *Journal of Marital and Family Therapy, 38,* 82–100. doi: 10.1111/j.1752-0606.2011.00257.x

Kuhlthau, K., Jellinek, M., White, G., VanCleave, J., Simons, J., & Murphy, M. (2011). Increases in behavioral health screening in pediatric care for Massachusetts Medicaid patients. *Archives of Pediatric Medicine, 165,* 660–664. doi: 10.1001/archpediatrics.2011.18

Landolt, M. A., & Kenardy, J. A. (2015). Evidence-based treatments for children and adolescents. In U. Schnyder & M. Cloitre (Eds.), *Evidence based treatments for trauma-related psychological disorders: A practical guide for clinicians* (pp. 363–380). Cham, Switzerland: Springer International Publishing. doi: 10.1007/978-3-319-07109-1

Lindsey, M. A., Chambers, K., Pohle, C., Beall, P., & Lucksted, A. (2013). Understanding the behavioral determinants of mental health service use by urban, under-resourced black youth: Adolescent and caregiver perspectives. *Journal of Child and Family Studies, 22,* 107–121. doi: 10.1007/s10826-012-9668-z

Lynch, S., & Franke, T. (2013). Communicating with pediatricians: Developing social work practice in primary care. *Social Work in Health Care, 52,* 397–416. doi: 10.1080/00981389.2012.750257

Manning, A. R. (2009). Bridging the gap from availability to accessibility: Providing health and mental health services in schools. *Journal of Evidence-Based Social Work, 6,* 40–57. doi: 10.1080/15433710802633411

Marlowe, D., Hodgson, J., Lamson, A., White, M., & Irons, T. (2012). Medical family therapy in a primary care setting: A framework for integration. *Contemporary Family Therapy, 34,* 244–258. doi: 10.1007/s10591-012-9195-5

Mason, S. (2013). The Affordable Care Act and social work. *Families in Society: The Journal of Contemporary Social Services, 94,* 67–68. doi: 10.1606/1044-3894.4297

McKay, M. M., & Bannon, W. M., Jr. (2004). Engaging families in child mental health services. *Child & Adolescent Psychiatric Clinics of North America, 13,* 905–921. doi: 10.1016/j.chc.2004.04.001

McKay, M. M., Lynn, C. J., & Bannon, W. M., Jr. (2005). Understanding inner city child mental health need and trauma exposure: Implications for preparing urban service providers. *American Journal of Orthopsychiatry, 75,* 201–210. doi: 10.1037/0002-9432.75.2.201

Mechanic, D. (2012). Seizing opportunities under the Affordable Care Act for transforming the mental and behavioral health system. *Health Affairs, 31,* 376–382. doi: 10.1377/hlthaff.2011.0623

Michigan Department of Health and Human Services. (n.d.). Child and Adolescent Health Center Program: Overview. Retrieved from http://www.michigan.gov/mdhhs/0,5885,7-339-73971_4911_4912-342503--,00.html

Mirabito, D., & Lloyd, C. (2017). Health issues affecting urban children. In N. K. Phillips & S. L. A. Straussner (Eds.), *Children in the urban environment: Linking social policy and clinical practice* (pp. 169-189, 3rd. ed.). Springfield, IL: Charles C. Thomas.

Morgan, O., Kuramoto, F., Emmet, W., Stange, J. L., & Nobunaga, E. (2014). The impact of the Affordable Care Act on behavioral health care for individuals from racial and ethnic communities. *Journal of Social Work in Disability & Rehabilitation, 13*, 139–161. doi: 10.1080/1536710X.2013.870518

Naar-King, S., & Suarez, M. (Eds.). (2011). *Motivational interviewing with adolescents and young adults.* New York, NY: Guildford Press.

Newacheck, P. W., Wong, S. T., Galbraith, A. A., & Hung, Y.-Y. (2003). Adolescent health care expenditures: A descriptive profile. *Journal of Adolescent Health, 32*(S6), 3–11. doi: 10.1016/S1054-139X(03)00064-8

Pecukonis, E., Doyle, O., Acquavita, S, Aparicio, E., Gibbons, M., & Vanidestine, T. (2013). Interprofessional leadership training in MCH social work. *Social Work in Health Care, 52*, 625–641. doi: 10.1080/00981389.2013.792913

Prado, G., Pantin, H., Huang, S., Cordova, D., Tapia, M. I., Velazquez, M.-R., . . . Estrada, Y. (2012). Effects of a family intervention in reducing HIV risk behaviors among high-risk Hispanic adolescents: A randomized controlled trial. *Archives of Pediatrics and Adolescent Medicine, 166*, 127–133. doi: 10.1001/archpediatrics.2011.189

Racco, A., & Vis, J.-A. (2015). Evidence based trauma treatment for children and youth. *Child and Adolescent Social Work Journal, 32*, 121–129. doi: 10.1007/s10560-014-0347-3

Rapid Assessment for Adolescent Preventive Services (RAAPS). (n.d.). Retrieved from https://www.raaps.org/

Rew, L., Johnson, K., & Young, C. (2014). A systematic review of interventions to reduce stress in adolescence. *Issues in Mental Health Nursing, 35*, 851–863. doi: 10.3109/01612840.2014.924044

Rupke, S. J., Blecke, D., & Renfrow, M. (2006). Cognitive therapy for depression. *American Family Physician, 73*, 83–86. Retrieved from http://www.aafp.org/journals/afp.html

Salerno, J., Marshall, V. D., & Picken, E. B. (2012). Validity and reliability of the Rapid Assessment for Adolescent Preventive Services adolescent health risk assessment. *Journal of Adolescent Health, 50*, 595–599. doi: 10.1016/j.jadohealth.2011.10.015

Siegel, J. P. (2015). Emotional regulation in adolescent substance use disorders: Rethinking risk. *Journal of Child & Adolescent Substance Abuse, 24*, 67–79. doi: 10.1080/1067828X.2012.761169

Steele, H., Bate, J., Steele, M., Dube, S. R., Danskin, K., Knafo, H., . . . Murphy, A. (2016). Adverse childhood experiences, poverty, and parenting stress. *Canadian Journal of Behavioural Science, 48*, 32–38. doi: 10.1037/cbs0000034

Suarez, L. M., Belcher, H. M. E., Briggs, E. C., & Titus, J. C. (2012). Supporting the need for an integrated system of care for youth with co-occurring traumatic stress and substance abuse problems. *American Journal of Community Psychology, 49*, 430–440. doi: 10.1007/s10464-011-9464-8

Timm, T. M. (2013). Family resilience and sexuality, In D. S. Becvar (Ed), *Handbook of family resilience* (pp. 515–530). New York, NY: Springer-Verlag. doi: 10.1007/978-1-4614-3917-2

Walpole, B., Dettmer, E., Morrongiello, B. A., McCrindle, B. W., & Hamilton, J. (2013). Motivational interviewing to enhance self-efficacy and promote weight loss in overweight and obese adolescents: A randomized controlled trial. *Journal of Pediatric Psychology, 38*, 944–953. doi: 10.1093/jpepsy/jst023

Walsh, F. (2013). Community-based practice applications of a family resilience framework. In D. S. Becvar (Ed), *Handbook of family resilience* (pp. 65–82). New York, NY: Springer.

Wittenauer, J., Ascher, M., Briggie, A., Kreiter, A., & Chavez, J. (2015). The role of complementary and alternative medicine in adolescent substance use disorders. *Adolescent Psychiatry, 5*, 96–104. doi: 10.2174/2210676605666150311224407

Yi, C. H., Martyn, K., Salerno, J., & Darling-Fisher, C. S. (2009). Development and clinical use of Rapid Assessment for Adolescent Preventive Services (RAAPS) questionnaire in school-based health centers. *Journal of Pediatric Health Care, 23*, 2–9. 10.1016/j.pedhc.2007.09.003

Zoogerman, S., Goldberg, S. B., Hoyt, W. T., & Miller, L. (2015). Mindfulness interventions with youth: A meta-analysis. *Mindfulness, 6*, 290–302. doi: 10.1007/s12671-013-0260-4

CHAPTER 14

INTEGRATED HEALTH CARE ROLES FOR SOCIAL WORKERS

Lynn Videka, Brenda Ohta, Anna M. Blackburn,
Virgen T. Luce, and Peggy Morton

Changes in the U.S. health care system over the past several years were spurred by the Patient Protection and Affordable Care Act (ACA), which was enacted to address the interacting factors of high costs and mediocre outcomes of the nation's health care system. Underlying factors that drove these features were social inequality and inadequate care for chronic and disabling health conditions, including behavioral health conditions (Kovner & Knickman, 2015). People with low incomes and low educational levels have more health problems and less access to preventive care and early intervention, resulting in disability and advanced care costs. The expenses of serving people with disabilities and advanced chronic illnesses account for 86% of the total health care expenses in the United States—17 times higher than average the average population (Gerteis et al., 2014; Goodell, Bodenheimer, & Berry-Millet, 2009).

Behavioral health care needs have grown in the United States, and parity for behavioral and physical health care is part of the ACA. People with chronic health conditions have substantial rates of behavioral health comorbidities (Dangremond, 2015; Honey, Emerson, Llewellyn, & Kariuki, 2010; Lucas, 2007; McClure, Teasell, & Salter, 2015; Treharne, Lyons, Booth, & Kitas, 2007; Walker & Gonzales, 2007). Misuse of and addiction to prescription medications is an increasing problem. Substance misuse is credited as the cause of an alarming rise in death rates in the U.S. population, especially for middle-aged men (Case & Deaton, 2015; Vital Statistics Rapid Release Program, 2016). Aging of the U.S. and global populations and the resulting changes in health care needs, including multiple chronic conditions, are poorly served by the standard, specialist-driven, unintegrated health care service system of the United States.

Over the past 30 years, there has been a call for more integration of physical and behavioral health services, especially for older adults and people with disabilities. Early integrated health programs were developed in the 1980s and 1990s in the Veterans

Administration (VA) health care system, Federally Qualified Health Centers (FQHCs) such as the Cherokee Health System, and health maintenance organizations (HMOs) such as Kaiser Permanente (Collins, Hewson, Munger, & Wade, 2010). These innovative approaches stimulated interest in integrated health care models and influenced health care policy reform and passage of the ACA. Integrated health services address the psychosocial determinants of health that account for more than 70% of visits to primary care providers (Collins et al., 2010). Renewed attention to the integration of body and mind in health care services creates new and exciting opportunities for social workers in health care.

The ACA changes reimbursement strategies and access to improve the experienced quality of health services, reduce costs, and improve health outcomes for all Americans. The strategies to achieve this Triple Aim include new roles focused on linkages and integration in the health care system that also break down barriers to collaboration among health professionals (see Chapter 1).

This chapter discusses enduring and newly transformed roles for social workers in health care. Social work and integrated health competencies for professional practice in health care social work are compared. Examples of programs with innovative social work roles in interprofessional, integrated health services are provided. The chapter concludes with recommendations for social work education and workforce development.

WORKFORCE GROWTH FOR SOCIAL WORK IN HEALTH CARE

The social work profession has grown over the past 25 years. The U.S. Department of Labor projects a growth rate of 12% for the profession between 2014 and 2024 (Bureau of Labor Statistics, 2015). This is almost double the 7% growth rate projected for all occupations. Employment growth for child and family social workers is projected to be 6% during the same period, and health care and behavioral health care social work is expected to grow at a rate of 19%. This is the highest growth rate for any social work specialty. A total of 331,000 social workers (45% of all social workers in the United States) are employed in health and behavioral health settings, making health the largest employment setting for the profession. This means that there will be many new health sector jobs for licensed social workers, especially those with a master's degree in social work (MSW). Pay is also comparatively higher in the health and behavioral health sectors; hospitals and government-funded agencies are the highest-paying social work settings (Bureau of Labor Statistics, 2015). Consequently, social work in integrated health care is not only a growing employment sector, but also one of the better-paying sectors in social work.

New and differently defined roles will become available for social workers in integrated health care settings. Between considering the social determinants of health, reducing health disparities, improving the quality of care, and containing the costs of care, social work practitioners are in a position to educate people about health care in a multidisciplinary, integrated system and to guide access to services among the complexities of health insurance and benefit programs. To understand the importance and function of the new roles, it is essential to understand health care services from the perspective of a social-ecological model.

ECOLOGICAL VIEW OF HEALTH SERVICES

In traditional models of health care services, service user–provider interactions were viewed as dyadic, and communication between the service user and his or her provider was considered central. Although family, culture, and other external influences were recognized, they were considered to be interfering factors when they clashed with service user–provider communications and were largely ignored or taken for granted when they facilitated these interactions.

In the ecological model, a person is viewed as living in a nested set of interrelated environments. The individual is nested in family, cultural, and community environments that influence health, lifestyle behaviors, and experiences with specialty and primary health care services. The ecological perspective is consistent with the ACA's recognition of the social determinants of health and health care delivery (Andrews, Darnell, McBride, & Gehlert, 2013) (see Chapter 1).

Using an ecological lens, health services are no longer based on one-to-one models of care but instead must explicitly recognize family, community, and cultural effects on individual behaviors and outcomes and on the health care system as a whole. The ecological model also recognizes the complex financial, organizational, and service delivery interactions among insurers, primary care services, and specialty care services. These multidirectional and complex influences must be considered in delivering health care. The transactional, boundary-spanning view creates much potential and many roles for social workers in integrated health and behavioral health.

NEW SOCIAL WORK ROLES
IN INTEGRATED HEALTH CARE

New roles designed to span service user and health care systems and environments are listed in Table 14.1. There are four major categories of roles for social workers under the ACA: traditional behavioral health specialist roles, roles that address care coordination, leadership roles, and community practice roles that address service users' cultural and neighborhood environments and health disparities.

Every social work role is focused on spanning boundaries between the person's life environment and his or her health care. The boundary spanned may be between the individual and the family or between the individual and community resources. A common family bridging role is that of a provider of psychoeducation about health conditions. For example, after a stroke, families need to know about cardiovascular disease, the rehabilitation process, and the emotional demands of rehabilitation. Psychoeducation and preparation of family members to support the service user is useful for many chronic or disabling health conditions.

TABLE 14.1: Roles in Integrated Health

Role	Description
Behavioral Health	
Behavioral health provider	Provides mental health and health care services in traditional, carved out, or integrated settings.
Behavioral health consultant	Provides assessment, screening, referral, and brief behavioral health intervention in primary care or acute care settings.
Peer counselor	Provides counseling, advocacy, and fellowship exchange based on his or her lived experience with someone going through a similar experience.
Care Coordination	
Care coordinator	Provides a person-centered, cost-effective, interdisciplinary, assessment-based approach to integrating social supports and health care. This results in a comprehensive care plan that is managed and monitored.
Care manager	Helps patients and caregivers effectively manage their health care plans and associated psychosocial situations.
Disease manager	Responsible for the management of health care for members of a patient population with a chronic illness who need help with health care management.
Case manager	Acts as a patient advocate and resource manager who provides critical information and recommendations to the interprofessional care team.
Community Practice	
Patient navigator	Helps patients establish eligibility, apply, and enroll in health insurance and access health care. Provides outreach and education about medical care and insurance.
Family navigator	Focuses on family-level health care and insurance needs.
Community organizer	Builds collective action within a community to achieve designated community goals.
Community health worker	Promotes community health by providing guidance, liaison services, culturally and linguistically appropriate communication, advocacy, follow-up, and proactive identification.
Community integrator	Responsible for integrating health and behavioral health care for people with chronic health conditions.
Leadership	
Implementation specialist	Responsible for adoption, implementation, and sustainment of evidence-based practices in an organization.
Supervisor	Oversees, directs, and guides the work of another professional or paraprofessional worker.
Program director	Plans, directs, and supervises the operation of a program in a health care setting.
Care line director	Serves a major management role of a major division of care in a health care organization.
Executive leader	Acts as chief executive officer of a health care organization, such as a hospital or clinic.

Adapted from "Moving Toward Integrated Health: An Opportunity for Social Work," by V. Stanhope, L. Videka, H. Thorning, and M. McKay, 2015, *Social Work in Health Care, 54,* p. 396. Copyright 2015 by Taylor & Francis.

Boundaries among health providers also need to be spanned, such as when the individual is transitioning from acute care to rehabilitation or to home. For example, a person with a mobility disorder needs planning and attention to the physical and emotional details of his or her environment during the transition from rehabilitation to home. The discharge-planning role typically considers these boundary-spanning challenges for service user safety and wellbeing. Examples later in this chapter illustrate boundary-spanning approaches that assist people with transitions from community to hospital and hospital to home environments.

Many roles for social workers under the ACA—especially outside of the traditional behavioral health provider roles—are not designated as social work positions and are not reserved for those with social work credentials. This means that social workers must compete for jobs with other professionals. Because licensing laws usually protect only the behavioral health dimensions of social work practice, they are of limited relevance in care coordination and community practice roles for social workers in health care.

BEHAVIORAL HEALTH SPECIALIST ROLES

Traditional roles for social workers under the ACA include providing mental health and substance misuse health care services. Social workers have specialized skills in these areas and are licensed to provide insurance-reimbursable services. In a systematic review, Harkness and Bower (2009) found that primary care services that included specialized mental health providers produced modest but positive effects in terms of fewer visits to primary care providers, lower prescription costs, and fewer referrals to specialists.

What is new about behavioral health care roles under the ACA is that they are integrated with person-centered care, primary health care, and wellness self-management. The behavioral health care provider is no longer operating in a separate and largely unconnected sector of the health care system. The ACA provides incentives for health care services to be linked through accountable care organizations and other integrated approaches to health care delivery, especially for people with chronic, co-occurring, and complicated health problems. These policies have altered behavioral health care roles.

The changes include working in faster-paced and nontraditional environments. For example, behavioral health specialists are working in primary care health clinics and school health clinics, and they are serving as consultants in rehabilitation, acute care, and long-term care settings. The social work role has also changed in that several new dimensions have been added. The social work role is explicitly interprofessional, and skills are needed to work with physicians, nurses, pharmacists, and peer or community workers. Collaboration sometimes occurs through the electronic health record (EHR). Clear, concise recording and technical skills are needed to use the EHR optimally. Notes must be entered promptly in specific technical language so that the information can be useful to other practitioners. Social work behavioral health care providers also use the EHR for referral and screening prompts.

Another difference is the emphasis on evidence-based, brief interventions instead of long-term services in specialized settings. Behavioral health specialists are part of the larger health care team and are evaluated for their contributions to the quality and efficiency of service users' care. At a Federally Qualified Health Center (FQHC), the social work role may be that of a depression specialist who is on call and joins the requesting primary care provider during primary health care visits (see Chapter 8). The consulting depression specialist screens the service user for behavioral health needs and delivers evidence-based interventions such as SBIRT (i.e., screening, brief intervention, and referral to treatment)—a 20-minute, structured protocol for reducing harmful drinking (see Chapter 9). The depression specialist may also conduct a warm handoff, which is an in-person referral to another health provider. The emphasis is on harm reduction, medication, exercise, meditation, and interpersonal relationships rather than traditional, long-term therapy.

For primary behavioral health populations, including people with diagnosed substance use disorders or psychiatric disabilities, primary health and behavioral health services are provided as part of supported living environments. Some specialized behavioral health agencies have created primary care clinics in addition to their existing behavioral health services. In other cases, the specialized behavioral health agency has an explicit care coordination relationship with an organization providing primary care. Behavioral health clinicians are expected to provide psychoeducation about the importance of primary and oral health care. They are expected to deliver wellness self-management services that are based on the service user's taking charge and making choices about his or her health lifestyle and health care—especially for some of the known health risks that psychotropic medications create, such as type 2 diabetes, weight gain, and neuro-motor disorders. Behavioral health specialists are increasingly expected to have a holistic approach to the health of service users in behavioral health settings.

CARE COORDINATION ROLES

Most health care dollars are spent on people with chronic and multiple comorbid conditions (Stanton & Rutherford, 2006). This population includes Medicaid and Medicare dually eligible older adults, people with significant disabilities, and people with multiple chronic conditions who also have multiple prescription medications with behavioral health and physical health side effects. Care coordination provides health services across environmental settings.

Care coordination promotes communication and holistic care among multiple providers who are not otherwise explicitly working together. In the traditional approach of specialist-driven medical care, these populations of service users were not efficiently cared for because there was no requirement that specialists communicate with each other in providing care, no shared record of treatment, no communication of test results, and the persistence of a financing system that rewarded more treatment with more payment—even if treatment was duplicated. The Guided Patient Services (GPS) and the Visiting Nurse Services (VNS) programs (discussed later) are coordinated care programs.

Evidence for the effectiveness of coordinated care includes better health outcomes and reduced health care costs. The Cochrane Stroke Group found that coordinated inpatient stroke care resulted in a reduced likelihood of service user death and an increased likelihood of living independently at home one year after the stroke event (Stroke Unit

Trialists' Collaboration, 2013). Patient-oriented, coordinated, interprofessional care was found to improve diabetes management and service user compliance with treatment regimens (Renders et al., 2000). Gomes, Calanzani, Curiale, McCrone, and Higginson (2013) found that home-based, palliative, coordinated care resulted in individuals' more often passing away at home with reduced symptom loads; there were no negative effects on caregivers but mixed evidence on cost reduction. Reilly et al. (2015) found that case management for people with dementia delayed admittance to a nursing home by 12 months and increased access to community services during that period.

Other studies have found mixed or inconclusive evidence of the effectiveness of coordinated care. Aubin et al. (2012) found no consistent evidence that coordinated care improved cancer treatment or survival. Coordinated care programs for adults with asthma have been shown to improve asthma-related quality of life, but results have been inconclusive in terms of health services use, costs, and quality-of-life outcomes (Peytremann-Bridevaux, Arditi, Gex, Bridevaux, & Burnand, 2015). Campbell et al. (2016) found that coordinated care that focused on the transition from pediatric care to adult care for youth with chronic conditions led to modest improvements in health care self-management and readiness to transfer to adult health services, but there were no differences in success of the transfer or long-term outcomes.

One challenge in drawing conclusions about coordinated care is that it is a broad and varied service approach. Although systematic reviews about coordinated care have found some positive programs, few have isolated key characteristics of effective care coordination programs (Institute of Medicine, 2015). Better program specification and strong, multimethod research studies are needed to draw firm conclusions about the effectiveness of coordinated care. Even with mixed results on effectiveness, however, coordinated care continues to be developed to treat the growing number of people seeking better and more comprehensive care for chronic health conditions.

Social workers are often involved in care coordination efforts, but care coordination roles are not by any means reserved for social workers. The most traditional care coordination role for social workers is that of case management. In case management, health care is coordinated with respect to the person but not necessarily in relation to the health or other care systems. Contemporary care coordination roles rely on interprofessional communication and collaboration; services that span the boundaries of home, hospital, and discharge settings; and clear communication with the service user and family. There are jobs for social workers in case management and care coordination. However, nurses and peer providers also provide care coordination and case management services, and social workers must compete with other workers for these roles. This is especially concerning in that peer mental health care providers have been found to provide case management services with equivalent effectiveness in mental health outcomes and service user satisfaction when compared with professionals (Pitt et al., 2013).

COMMUNITY PRACTICE ROLES

Community practice roles typically span service user, cultural, health care, and community environments. Newly defined roles, such as service user navigator and family navigator, span the boundaries between service users and health care financing, regulatory, and service delivery systems to overcome barriers to accessing health insurance and health care services. Under the ACA, these roles have enabled people—particularly the 25% of Americans who previously did not have health insurance—to obtain insurance and navigate the complex insurance system options, including the computer glitches that plagued the early days of the state and federal insurance exchanges and the ongoing changes in insurance vendors in the exchange insurance market. Service user and family navigator roles have helped African-American women with positive breast cancer test results to seek and sustain care as a remedy to the breast cancer mortality disparities between African-American women and women of other races. Service user navigators have also assisted minority families with children whose parents were uninsured (Jia et al., 2014).

A peer navigator program was created to help people with psychiatric disabilities more fully use primary health care to reduce the morbidity and mortality disparities that this population faces (Kelly et al., 2014). Although MSW social workers typically do not serve as service user navigators, they do create, supervise, and ensure quality in service user navigation programs. Working with peer providers is often omitted from discussions of interprofessional practice. However, peers—people with lived experience of health conditions—increasingly play a role in health care services and should be viewed as part of the interprofessional team.

MANAGEMENT AND LEADERSHIP ROLES

Social workers have increased opportunities for leadership roles in health care. They can be leaders in staff positions, such as supervisors or program directors, and they often hold executive roles, such as vice president or chief executive officer. One conceptualization of the leadership function is that of *adaptive leadership*—the possibility of leadership in any role, whether in the private or public sector (Heifetz, Grashow, & Linsky, 2009). Heifetz et al. (2009) asked why anyone would want to take on the challenges, tests, and trials of leadership. According to these authors, "our work begins with the assumption that there is no reason to exercise leadership . . . unless you care about something deeply" (Heifetz et al., 2009, p. 3). They define that something as a "collective purpose that goes beyond your own individual ambition" (Heifetz et al., 2009, p. 3).

Social work leadership is guided by a collective purpose because the profession is value-based and principle-driven. For example, social workers in health care may be motivated by the desire to reduce health care disparities and achieve health care equity, or by the goal to optimize outcomes for every person they work with, or by an understanding of the profound difference that culture makes in shaping a person's response to a health care treatment plan. These values inform the greater good that motivates social work leadership. There are leadership opportunities for social workers in every aspect of their work. Leadership requires openness and motivation to do things better—to serve individuals better or more humanely, to experiment and test potentially more effective approaches to serving a population with a particular health condition, to improve evidence-based practices within a health care service, or to improve care coordination to better serve a unique population.

Martin and Rogers (2004) discussed the requirements of social work leadership in interprofessional health care organizations:

> Leaders are required to set a proactive agenda. They have a key role in developing a shared and compelling vision of better services and then aligning this vision with the direction and objectives of the organisation to clarify purpose and strategies so that the desired change can be achieved. (pp. 4–5)

A staff social worker can also be a leader. Flexible and adaptive leadership in social work is needed at every level (Yukl & Mahsud, 2010). Social workers can lead by ensuring that health care is person-centered—that is, the individual service user's preferences and cultural perspective are at the center of health care service delivery. Leadership is also expressed in designated roles, such as supervisor or program manager. In these roles, social work leadership includes creating program innovations; inspiring, motivating, and guiding the work of others; and leading organizations toward better performance and increased efficiency.

Formal leadership roles also garner higher compensation than other social work roles. A 2011 workforce study conducted by the National Association of Social Workers (NASW) showed that the median compensation of an administrative social work position in the health sector was $92,000 per year, compared with the compensation of all social workers in health care, which was $60,000 per year (Center for Workforce Studies, 2011).

New leadership roles under the ACA include that of implementation specialist. The implementation specialist social worker is responsible for adopting and sustaining the use of evidence-based practices in health care organizations. This role helps to bring the best scientific evidence to health care practices. For example, prior research showed that, despite the technological prompts found in the VA's sophisticated EHRs, problem drinking, a common behavioral health care issue among veterans, was not being addressed even after positive screening results (Claiborne et al., 2010). The cause of this situation was a culture that considered a certain level of alcohol misuse as normative. Strong leadership is needed to overcome cultural barriers to adapting contemporary evidence-based practice. In a Cochrane review of implementation of evidence-based practice, support was found for the hypothesis that opinion leaders have more success than non–opinion leaders in causing organizations to adopt more evidence-based practices (Flodgren et al., 2011). To be viewed as an opinion leader in an organization is a reflection of leadership. Respected leaders in the workplace in a variety of roles can influence innovation and the selection of the best available practice methods. Becoming an opinion leader creates leadership opportunities for social workers.

Social work's strong tradition of clinical supervision creates an opportunity for leadership that sustains continuous improvement-oriented health services. Supervised practice is required for advanced social work licensure in many states. Supporting learning by practitioners and performance through supervision is one of the proudest traditions in social work. However, many social workers think that supervision is under attack by the need to maximize billable services hours and by other health care financing policies. Supervision and case consultation are features of professional practice that all social workers should sustain. Increasingly, social workers supervise paraprofessional workers, including service user navigators, community health workers, and peer counselors. In an interprofessional collaboration course that focuses on professional–peer collaboration, peer providers have described the disrespect and dismissiveness with which their presence on health care teams is received by many professionals. Social workers with skills in cultural competence and respect for all persons should lead the integration of these helpers into health care service teams.

In advanced leadership roles, such as director or vice president of a health care service or chief executive officer of a health organization, social workers have the power and authority to change health care systems and achieve better health care through innovation in institutions and structures. The need for clear pathways to leadership is discussed later in this chapter.

COMPETENCIES NEEDED FOR NEW ROLES

Education for health professionals is based on acquiring competency, which is considered essential for effective professional practice. Social work competencies are defined by the Council on Social Work Education (CSWE). Competencies for practice in integrated health care are defined by the Center for Integrated Health Solutions (CIHS). The CSWE and CIHS competencies are compared in Table 14.2.

TABLE 14.2: Competencies for Social Work Integrated Health Care

SAMHSA/CIHS Competencies	CSWE Competencies
Interpersonal communication	Engagement with individuals, families, groups, organizations, and communities
Collaboration and teamwork	Demonstration of ethical and professional behavior
Screening and assessment	Assessment of individuals, families, groups, organizations, and communities
Care planning and care coordination	Evaluation of practice with individuals, families, groups, organizations, and communities
Intervention	Intervention with individuals, families, groups, organizations, and communities
Cultural competence and adaptation	Engagement of diversity and difference in practice
Systems-oriented practice	Engagement in practice-informed research and research-informed practice
Evidence-based practice and quality improvement strategies	Advancement of human rights and social, economic, and environmental justice
Informatics	Engagement of policy practice

Column 1 adapted from *Core Competencies for Integrated Behavioral Health and Primary Care* (pp. 8-9), by M. A. Hoge, J. A. Morris, M. Laraia, A. Pomerantz, and T. Farley, 2014, Washington, DC: Center for Integrated Health Solutions. Copyright 2014 by Substance Abuse and Mental Health Services Administration-Health Resources and Services Administration. Column 2 adapted from *Educational Policy and Accreditation Standards* (p. 8), by Council on Social Work Education., 2015, Alexandria, VA: Council on Social Work Education. Copyright 2015 by Council on Social Work Education.

The CSWE defines competencies that are needed for practitioners to fulfill the purpose of the profession, which is to "promote human and community well-being":

> Guided by a person-in-environment framework, a global perspective, respect for human diversity, and knowledge based on scientific inquiry, the purpose of social work is actualized through its quest for social and economic justice, the prevention of conditions that limit human rights, the elimination of poverty, and the enhancement of the quality of life for all persons, locally and globally" (Council on Social Work Education, 2015, p. 5).

Competency-based education does not set curriculum; it instead focuses on educational outcomes of graduates. CSWE requires nine competencies of all MSW graduates. MSW educational programs can include additional, program-specific competencies at the foundational or advanced specialization level and are required to define one or more advanced specializations of practice.

Competencies for integrated health social work practice have been developed by the SAMHSA-HRSA Center for Integrated Health Solutions (CIHS) (Hoge, Morris, Laraia, Pomerantz, & Farley, 2014). These standards were designed to fill the gap in defining skills for the emerging integrated health workplace. They are relevant to primary care providers and behavioral health specialists, but they are not mandated for health program accreditation. They serve as a skill performance benchmark and as a resource for creating job descriptions in integrated health. They are designed to apply across service user populations and settings. They apply to professionals, paraprofessionals, practitioners, direct care staff, and peers with lived experience who are employed in health service roles (e.g., peer counselors, community health workers, service user navigators).

The competencies presume a workplace in which there is "close or full collaboration and one of three organizational models: some systems integration, integrated practice, or transformed/merged practice" (Hoge et al., 2014, p. 5). The CIHS competencies were based on structured interviews with experts, an integrated health literature review, and a review and analysis of other competency statements.

There is a considerable amount of correspondence between the two sets of competencies, especially in the areas of interpersonal communication, assessment, intervention (e.g., systems-oriented intervention), cultural competence, and evidence-based practice. However, there is a lack of correspondence between CIHS and CSWE in a few competency areas. For example, CSWE places a heavier emphasis on ethical practice, social justice, and practice that is influenced by and influences social policy, while the CIHS competencies focus on some areas that are omitted in the CSWE competencies, such as collaborative teamwork, care coordination, care planning, and informatics.

Through its integrated health initiative, CSWE encourages social work educational programs to embrace interprofessional education (CSWE et al., 2013). Workforce training grants funded by the Health Resources and Services Administration (HRSA) have stimulated universities to create integrated care specializations for social workers. However, it is unclear how many schools of social work—beyond those with HRSA-funded initiatives—invest in interprofessional education. Techniques such as shared decision-making are not taught at many schools of social work despite the scientific evidence for their effectiveness (Légaré et al., 2014). Case management is a staple course in social work education, but it is unclear to what extent the care coordination approach is taught. There is also a need for more research on the effectiveness of interprofessional education and practice. Systematic reviews in 2009 and 2013 found that although interprofessional education is effective in changing organizational practices and attitudes of providers in health care settings, there is only limited evidence that it produces better health outcomes (Reeves, Perrier, Goldman, Freeth, & Zwarenstein, 2013; Zwarenstein, Goldman, & Reeves, 2009). The absence of a social work competency on the use of technology raises questions about the extent to which social work leverages technology's potential to advance the profession. Some student field internship evaluations include critiques of students' abilities to effectively use EHRs. Although electronic recording is a fact of life for reimbursement and quality improvement in many agencies, it has not yet been a focus of social work education.

NEW ROLES: INNOVATION IN PRACTICE SETTINGS

The following three programs are examples of innovation and social work role potential in integrated health care practice. They illustrate social work roles in behavioral health care practice, care coordination, community-focused practice, and leadership. They illustrate the importance of spanning boundaries, breaking barriers, and thinking creatively about the contributions that social work can make in health care service organizations. They illustrate shared roles and interprofessional practice that involve negotiating fluid and sometimes overlapping roles with other health professionals. Finally, they show how the social worker's knowledge about cultural diversity, social justice, ethics, and behavioral health improve health care for vulnerable populations.

PROGRAM 1: GUIDED PATIENT SERVICES

Guided Patient Services (GPS) is sponsored by a major urban medical center and addresses the need for enhanced care transitions for high-risk individuals (https://www.gpscolumbus.com/). It uses a three-pronged approach for care integration across time and settings:

1. Preadmission screening to identify individuals at risk for readmission and adverse health outcomes, including those with multiple chronic health conditions or co-occurring substance use or mental health morbidities
2. Social work–nurse collaborative case management teams for care/discharge planning
3. Postdischarge transitional care follow-through for up to 90 days

Social workers and nurses work in teams with physicians and other clinicians (e.g., physical therapists, pharmacists, primary care nurses, home health care, skilled nursing facility care providers). Hospital clinicians from surgical preadmission areas or the emergency department also collaborate.

The GPS preadmission protocol begins with telephone outreach, assessment, and risk screening for patients undergoing elective surgery (e.g., orthopedic surgery, cardiac surgery) and with emergency room assessment for nonelective patients (e.g., those with congestive heart failure). A risk screening questionnaire is administered. Responses are used to formulate a plan to lower the risk for readmission. Early care planning maximizes service user and family engagement to develop mutually acceptable goals, set expectations for the clinical course of care and discharge, advance directives, and review service user wishes and cultural preferences.

An MSW or a registered nurse (RN) provider completes the care plan. MSW and RN roles in this model overlap and require a high degree of interprofessional communication and collaboration. Service users with highly complex behavioral and environmental situations may require more time with an MSW provider, whereas service users with complex and chronic medical needs may require more time with an RN provider. In the hospitalization phase, the MSW and RN providers continue to work together as an integrated team, incorporating the preadmission plan, reassessing and revising as needed, and facilitating communication with all involved stakeholders.

The final phase of GPS occurs during the transition from hospital to home or to another postacute setting, and it may last up to 90 days. The frequency of contact with an MSW or RN provider during this time is based on the service user's level of risk and includes follow-up calls regarding medication management, physician follow-through, in-home services, family support, and other interventions based on illness, recovery, and service needs.

In GPS, the integrated health care social work role requires a licensed professional with an MSW degree. Essential social work competencies include the following:

1. Critical thinking
2. Responsiveness to diversity and the ability to identify social factors that drive variation in service user health behavior and use
3. Ability to work in multiple practice contexts to meet the challenge of following the service user across time and settings
4. Ability to communicate using new technologies available in the EHR

The GPS MSW role is multifaceted. Primary responsibilities encompass high-risk screening using evidence-based criteria; securing service user and family care and support; facilitating oral and written communication among stakeholders (e.g., service users, families, clinical professionals) for person-centered care; ensuring clinical understanding of the medical conditions, including potential adverse outcomes; providing medications and other therapies; offering rehabilitation and recovery, including options for safe discharge and care transitions; guiding service user progression through system transition points, including coordinating with physicians, other clinical professionals, post-hospital providers, and insurers; conducting crisis assessments and brief interventions to address the impact on health outcomes and barriers to service that are created by service users' psychosocial stressors; advocating on behalf of service users; and coordinating services to provide full comprehensive care for each service user.

The GPS program supports interprofessional practice through consistent protocols; active physician and department leadership; daily communication among team members regarding individual care, team progress, and group dynamics; and a well-documented care plan that incorporates person-centered, clinical, psychosocial, safety, and educational elements. In the GPS model, social workers must acquire a basic understanding of medical conditions, treatments, and skills to clarify roles with the nurse counterpart. The shared competencies between the two disciplines gives rise to opportunities for overlap, redundancy, and confusion between the roles of the MSW and RN providers and in how the MSW and RN providers are perceived by service users, families, and other team members. Delineation of roles, clarity regarding who will take the lead for which individuals, collegiality, and professional respect are necessary to ameliorate these challenges. GPS outcomes include reduced hospital length of stay, reduced readmission rates, improved individual experience scores related to discharge and care transitions, and improved rates of discharge directly to home rather than to a subacute nursing or rehabilitation facility.

PROGRAM 2: CASE MANAGEMENT AT UNIVERSITY HOSPITALS

University Hospitals' (UH) case management model is delivered by a department of more than 40 social workers, whose primary responsibility is to coordinate safe and efficient discharge plans for all individuals (n.d.). The service user population consists of a wide range of people with medical and psychiatric diagnoses, including those with geriatric needs. There is at least one social worker assigned to every medical and surgical unit in the hospital, including neurology, cardiovascular care, oncology, orthopedics, and trauma. The interdisciplinary team for each unit consists of physicians, nurses, nurse practitioners, pharmacists, psychiatrists, physical and occupational therapists, and nutritionists. Social workers function as team leaders, conducting hospital rounds daily with the interdisciplinary team to discuss service users' treatment plans. Full assessments are done for individuals with psychosocial needs. Social workers use crisis intervention skills, strong communication skills, and advocacy to provide an efficient intervention for the service user. Social workers also participate in hospital-wide committees and initiatives that support cost-saving measures and quality improvement.

The team social worker creates a comprehensive discharge plan that includes a thorough psychosocial assessment of the service user and his or her home environment, family support system, insurance coverage and other financial resources, medical diagnosis, daily functioning level, and discharge plan needs. Discharge planning includes the service user's ability to access continued health care services and medications. Discharge planning may require arranging home health care services, including treatments and nursing interventions; arranging a rehabilitation transfer; arranging nursing home placement; accessing state and federal programs, including the Department on Aging, to help the individual obtain needed services; and identifying psychiatric follow-up care, including inpatient, outpatient, and intensive outpatient programs. Social workers are responsible for providing education to the team and the service user regarding appropriate postacute placement options. Social workers are the experts on helping an individual find the most appropriate rehabilitation setting, which may range from inpatient acute to subacute skilled nursing care to in-home and outpatient rehabilitation. Social workers also provide information on accessing continued health care and medication follow-up. Social workers consult with service users to access their health care benefits through their insurance and to advocate for posthospital needs. Because insurance coverage determines when an individual is discharged, social workers collaborate with the inpatient team to ensure a safe plan that balances medical safety and insurance benefits. Social workers use crisis intervention skills, strong communication skills, and team advocacy to ensure that the most effective discharge plans are created.

In creating effective and safe discharge plans, social workers are knowledgeable and mindful of hospital-wide cost-savings initiatives. Hospitals strive to meet internal financial goals by preventing readmissions and excessive stays in hospitals and postacute rehabilitation facilities. Well-organized discharge plans keep individuals in their communities and prevent readmissions. Individuals who lack safe discharge plans due to limited financial resources or a lack of insurance are identified early during an admission. Social workers use hospital charitable funds and federal programs to prevent these individuals from having lengthy and costly admissions.

University Hospital participates in a payment program bundled with the Centers for Medicare and Medicaid Services (CMS), which waives the "3-day stay rule" for individuals undergoing a joint replacement operation. The 3-day stay rule, detailed in section 1861(i) of the Social Security Act of 1935, states that Medicare Part A will cover postacute services in a skilled nursing facility or subacute rehabilitation facility if the individual stays in the hospital for a qualifying 3-day inpatient stay. The waiver program is used to reduce hospital length of stay for individuals who do not require a 3-day acute hospital stay. The social worker provides education on this program to help individuals identify whether they can use the waiver. In general, social workers focus on creating effective discharge plans and facilitating smooth transitions from hospitals to postacute settings including nursing homes, rehabilitation centers, and the individual's home with proper home health care services.

PROGRAM 3: VISITING NURSE SERVICE

Social work interns participate in interprofessional, integrated primary care with medically frail older adults who have complex medication regimens. This HRSA-funded demonstration was implemented at Visiting Nurse Service (VNS), a large home health organization that provides postacute care to dually eligible Medicare-Medicaid populations with multiple chronic conditions (https://www.vnsny.org/). Service users are older adults with multiple chronic conditions and numerous prescribed medications. The primary care team includes nurse practitioners, social workers, and pharmacists. The team calls in other professionals (e.g., physicians, physical therapists, occupational therapists) as required for each case. The team operates virtually, using the EHR to communicate, coordinate, and collaborate in providing person- and family-centered care.

Interprofessional practice at VNS is supported by monthly case seminars; these case presentations deepen understanding of each profession's approach and role. Social workers created a resource booklet on social insurance (i.e., Medicaid and Medicare) benefits and limits and presented it at the seminar. The booklet was enthusiastically received by the other health professionals, who lacked understanding of the policies and regulations regarding reimbursement and service policies of the payors.

Team-based care is delivered in individuals' homes and involves their family members. Social work interns use a short-term, structured, and focused assessment tool that enables them to conceptualize and communicate biopsychosocial issues and needed interventions. The social workers assess individuals' understanding of and adherence to medication regimens and medical care plans by exploring their thoughts, feelings, and concerns. They evaluate service users' attitudes toward their treatment plans and their overall functioning, the barriers to medical compliance, and how to best assist individuals in accessing care. The social workers make weekly home visits to the service users and report their status, including health and medication problems, to the team. The following case example highlights a typical service user.

CASE VIGNETTE

Andrea is a single, 80-year-old, white woman who has been diagnosed with diabetes, atherosclerotic heart disease, and gastroesophageal reflux; she has a medication regimen of more than 10 prescriptions. Andrea lives with her adult daughter in a two-bedroom apartment and was referred due to noncompliance with attending her primary care medical appointments and nonadherence to her medication regimen. Andrea had full-range affect and good long-term memory but had deficient short-term memory. She denied symptoms of depression but admitted to feeling overwhelmed with her medication regimen.

The social worker successfully engaged Andrea with a person- and family-centered care approach, recognizing the importance of all parties' participation in care and decision-making. Andrea had cancelled some medical appointments due to lack of access to transportation. Applying an ecological perspective, the social worker worked with Andrea and her daughter to develop a plan that included referral to Access-a-Ride, which provides transportation for people with disabilities or health conditions who are unable to use public transportation. This allowed Andrea to attend her medical appointments, become less socially isolated, and increase her connection to her community because Access-a-Ride also provided rides to the local church and senior center.

The second issue addressed was Andrea's medication adherence. The VNS team used an assessment tool called Medication Regimen Complexity Index (MRCI), which provided a score for Andrea's medication complexity. Based on Andrea's MRCI score, the pharmacist organized her medications in a monthly blister pack. Every team member observed and reported on the packs when visiting Andrea. Team members used the EHR to report her increasing compliance with her medication and medical appointments.

Andrea's medical adherence and social functioning improved, and the inpatient team honored Andrea and her family's choices, which were consistent with their cultural values and belief systems. The program reduced unnecessary medications and repeat hospitalizations. The social work role on the team expanded over time due to regular home visits and the worker's knowledge of programs and policies that affected Andrea's eligibility for care.

IMPLICATIONS FOR SOCIAL WORK

Health care reform and passage of the ACA have increased attention to the integration of physical and mental health and the consideration of service users in their natural social environments. The place for social work in health care has expanded, and new roles have been defined, as illustrated in the three program examples. However, the place of social work in the health care workforce is still ambiguous. Although the Bureau of Labor Statistics (2015) reported that more than 300,000 social workers were employed in the health workforce, major health care texts and reports omit social work from the list of health care professions (Kovner & Knickman, 2015). The three programs previously described provide positive examples of progressive roles for social work in integrated health care. However, this level of progressive innovation is not found across the health care sector.

Social work continues to have an ambivalent identity as a health profession. On some university campuses, social work remains outside of the extensive interprofessional education initiatives. Social work roles also overlap with nursing and peer roles, especially in case management and care coordination. The lack of emphasis in social work education on health and health care creates a disadvantage for social workers competing for positions in the health sector and is likely related to the advancement of nurses in many case management and care coordination positions.

The well-established emphasis on the inclusion of social work in Public Health Service Title VII funding and the recent CSWE emphasis on integrated health and the role for social work have resulted in workforce development training programs sponsored by HRSA and have improved the commitment of social work to health care; however, work is still needed to ensure recognition of the importance of including social work as a health care profession. There is a great opportunity for the profession to create pathways for competitive preparation for social work practice in the health sector, which is a major economic sector in the United States.

Social work education also needs to improve its emphasis on organizational practice and direct practice skills. Many dimensions of competencies are needed. For example, social workers need to be competent in interprofessional practice in health care settings. Social workers need to articulate how they can use negotiation and conflict management skills to resolve individual–family conflicts or conflicts between providers. Social workers can contribute a great deal to ensuring an ethical lens on practice, given the emphasis in social work education on ethics and values. Social workers need to be able to assertively articulate a clear definition of the social work role and what social work services can contribute to service users' health. In most health care settings, other professionals do not understand what social workers can contribute, and it is up to the social worker to be able to assertively communicate how their profession can advance health care goals.

Social workers also need to understand innovation and the process for implementing successful innovations. To be prepared to be innovation leaders and to thrive in the health sector, social workers need a much better understanding of the relevance of organizational and business practices in advancing clinical outcomes. They need to understand how policies and regulations affect practices and create constraints on services. The three program examples all emphasized social workers' knowledge of insurance, public policy, and program and financing systems. This knowledge bolstered the social workers' influence and role in interprofessional teams. This was demonstrated in the VNS programs when the nurse and pharmacist partners wanted social workers' help in understanding health care policies and reimbursement guidelines. It is not sufficient for the health care social worker to provide clinical services to individuals. Social workers need to be able to articulate how they contribute to the achievement of the organization's goals and can do so in ways that maximize resources for the organization as well as service user outcomes. They need to understand how to exert leadership and define their special contribution to interprofessional health care teams and health care organizations.

Competency for technology in practice is strikingly absent in social work education. Consequently, social workers are underprepared to use and develop the increasingly sophisticated technology in health care. This is worrisome for the leadership of the profession due to the growing need to harness technology for social good instead of viewing technology as a threat. The three program examples illustrated the role of EHRs in facilitating interprofessional communication to benefit service users.

Understanding the policy and business aspects of practice is also important for social workers who are private practitioners and those who provide contract services to health organizations (a growing proportion of the workforce). It is important to have business knowledge to compete with professionals from public health, public administration, and business schools for the leadership roles in health care.

Education beyond the master's degree can provide an important workforce preparation strategy. Several schools of social work, including those at New York University, the University of Michigan, the University of Pittsburgh, Hunter College, and Simmons College, host post–master's degree certificate programs to prepare social workers for practice and leadership in integrated health care settings. There are also interprofessional postprofessional degree programs at universities such as Drexel University and the University of Massachusetts.

CONCLUSIONS

The Triple Aim creates new and expanding roles for social workers in health care. There is tremendous opportunity for social work to strengthen its role in integrated health care. Social work education prepares social workers to integrate social and behavioral determinants of health with medical care. A rich ethics tradition and value-based education, which address social justice and cultural and other forms of diversity, position the social worker to be a leader in person-centered care that reduces health disparities for vulnerable and oppressed populations.

To take full advantage of the expanded psychosocial roles for social workers in health care, more programs need to create an integrated health advanced specialization. They need to address strategies for more thoroughly preparing social workers to work in interprofessional teams, provide an understanding of effective evidence-based strategies for person-centered care coordination, and use modern health technologies to support interprofessional practice and benefit individual care through accurate and timely information sharing across service system boundaries.

RESOURCES

Bureau of Labor Statistics—Social Workers, U.S. Department of Labor http://www.bls.gov/ooh/community-and-social-service/social-workers.htm

Center for Workforce Studies (the Center), National Association of Social Workers (NASW) http://workforce.socialworkers.org

Collaborative Care Implementation Guide, AIMS Center, University of Washington https://aims.uw.edu/resource-library/collaborative-care-implementation-guide

Education and Training Resources, Center for Integrated Health Solutions, SAMHSA-HRSA http://www.integration.samhsa.gov/workforce/education-training

Health Resources and Services Administration (HRSA) http://bhw.hrsa.gov/index.html

National Association of State Mental Health Program Directors (NASMHPD) http://www.nasmhpd.org

Social Work and Integrated Behavioral Healthcare Project, Council on Social Work Education (CSWE) http://www.cswe.org/CentersInitiatives/DataStatistics/IntegratedCare.aspx

Web-Based Certificate in Integrated Behavioral Health and Primary Care, School of Social Work, University of Michigan http://ssw.umich.edu/offices/continuing-education/certificate-courses/integrated-behavioral-health-and-primary-care

REFERENCES

Andrews, C. M., Darnell, J. S., McBride, T. D., & Gehlert, S. (2013). Social work and implementation of the Affordable Care Act. *Health & Social Work, 38,* 67–71. doi: 10.1093/hsw/hlt002

Aubin, M., Giguère, A., Martin, M., Verreault, R., Fitch, M. I., Kazanjian, A., & Carmichael, P-H. (2012). Interventions to improve continuity of care in the follow-up of patients with cancer. *Cochrane Database of Systematic Reviews, 7,* Article No. CD007672. doi: 10.1002/14651858.CD007672.pub2

Bureau of Labor Statistics, U.S. Department of Labor. (2015, December 17). Occupational outlook handbook (2016-17 ed.), Social workers. Retrieved from http://www.bls.gov/ooh/community-and-social-service/social-workers.htm

Campbell, F., Biggs, K., Aldiss, S. K., O'Neill, P. M., Clowes, M., McDonagh, J., . . . Gibson, F. (2016). Transition of care for adolescents from paediatric services to adult health services. *Cochrane Database of Systematic Reviews, 4*, Article No. CD009794. doi: 10.1002/14651858.CD009794.pub2

Case, A., & Deaton, A. (2015). Rising morbidity and mortality in midlife among white non-Hispanic Americans in the 21st century. *Proceedings of the National Academy of Sciences of the United States of America, 112*, 15078–15083. doi: 10.1073/pnas.1518393112

Center for Workforce Studies. (2011). *Social workers in hospitals & medical centers: Occupational profile*. Washington, DC: Center for Workforce Studies, National Association of Social Workers. Retrieved from http://workforce.socialworkers.org/studies/profiles/Hospitals.pdf

Claiborne, N., Videka, L., Postiglione, P., Finkelstein, A., McDonnell, P., & Krause, R. D. (2010). Alcohol screening, evaluation, and referral for veterans. *Journal of Social Work Practice in the Addictions, 10*, 308–326. doi: 10.1080/1533256X.2010.500963

Collins, C., Hewson, D. L., Munger, R., & Wade, T. (2010). *Evolving Models of Behavioral Health Integration in Primary Care*. New York, NY: The Milbank Memorial Fund. Retrieved from http://www.milbank.org/uploads/documents/10430EvolvingCare/EvolvingCare.pdf

Council on Social Work Education (CSWE). (2015). *Educational policy and accreditation standards, 2015*. Alexandria, VA: Council on Social Work Education. Retrieved from http://www.cswe.org/File.aspx?id=81660

Council on Social Work Education, The Center for Integrated Health Solutions, Substance Abuse and Mental Health Services Administration–Health Resources and Services Administration. (2013). Advanced clinical social work practice in integrated healthcare. Retrieved from http://www.cswe.org/File.aspx?id=62697

Dangremond, C. K. (2015). A visual overview of health care delivery in the United States. In A. R. Kovner & J. R. Knickman (Eds.), *Jonas and Kovner's health care delivery in the United States* (pp. 13–28, 11th ed.). New York, NY: Springer.

Flodgren, G., Parmelli, E., Doumit, G., Gattellari, M., O'Brien, M. A., Grimshaw, J., Eccles, M. P. (2011). Local opinion leaders: Effects on professional practice and health care outcomes. *Cochrane Database of Systematic Reviews, 8*, Article No. CD000125. doi: 10.1002/14651858.CD000125.pub4

Gerteis, J., Izrael, D., Deitz, D., LeRoy, L., Ricciardi, R., Miller, T., & Basu, J. (2014). *Multiple chronic conditions chartbook: 2010 medical expenditure panel survey data* (AHRQ Pub. No. 14-0038). Rockville, MD: Agency for Healthcare Research and Quality, U.S. Department of Health & Human Services.

Gomes, B., Calanzani, N., Curiale, V., McCrone, P., & Higginson, I. J. (2013). Effectiveness and cost-effectiveness of home palliative care services for adults with advanced illness and their caregivers. *Cochrane Database of Systematic Reviews, 6*, Article No. CD007760. doi: 10.1002/14651858.CD007760.pub2

Goodell, S., Bodenheimer, T., & Berry-Millet, R. (2009). *Care management of patients with complex health care needs* (Policy Brief No. 19). Princeton, NJ: Robert Wood Johnson Foundation. Retrieved from http://www.rwjf.org/content/dam/farm/reports/issue_briefs/2009/rwjf49853

Guided Patient Services. (n.d.). Retrieved from https://www.gpscolumbus.com/

Harkness, E. F., & Bower, P. J. (2009). On-site mental health workers delivering psychological therapy and psychosocial interventions to patients in primary care: Effects on the professional practice of primary care providers. *Cochrane Database of Systematic Reviews, 1*, Article No. CD000532. doi: 10.1002/14651858.CD000532.pub2

Heifetz, R., Grashow, A., & Linsky, M. (2009). *The practice of adaptive leadership: Tools and tactics for changing your organization and the world*. Boston, MA: Harvard Business School.

Hoge, M. A., Morris, J. A., Laraia, M., Pomerantz, A., & Farley, T. (2014). *Core competencies for integrated behavioral health and primary care*. Washington, DC: Center for Integrated Health Solutions, Substance Abuse and Mental Health Services Administration-Health Resources and Services Administration. Retrieved from http://www.integration.samhsa.gov/workforce/Integration_Competencies_Final.pdf

Honey, A., Emerson, E., Llewellyn, G., & Kariuki, M. (2010). Mental health and disability. In J. H. Stone & M. Blouin (Eds.), *International encyclopedia of rehabilitation*. Buffalo, NY: Center for International Rehabilitation Research Information and Exchange. Retrieved from http://cirrie.buffalo.edu/encyclopedia/en/pdf/mental_health_and_disability.pdf

Institute of Medicine. (2015). *Measuring the impact of interprofessional education on collaborative practice and patient outcomes*. Washington, DC: The National Academies Press. doi: 10.17226/21726

Jia, L., Yuan, B., Huang, F., Lu, Y., Garner, P., Meng, Q. (2014). Strategies for expanding health insurance coverage in vulnerable populations. *Cochrane Database of Systematic Reviews, 11*, Article No. 008194. doi: 10.1002/14651858.CD008194.pub3

Kelly, E., Fulginiti, A., Pahwa, R., Tallen, L., Duan, L., & Brekke, J. S. (2014). A pilot test of a peer navigator intervention for improving the health of individuals with serious mental illness. *Community Mental Health Journal, 50*, 435–446. doi: 10.1007/s10597-013-9616-4

Kovner, A. R., & Knickman, J. R. (Eds.). (2015). *Jonas and Kovner's health care delivery in the United States* (11th ed.). New York, NY: Springer.

Légaré, F., Stacey, D., Turcotte, S., Cossi, M.-J., Kryworuchko, J., Graham, I. D., ... Donner-Banzhoff, N. (2014). Interventions for improving the adoption of shared decision making by healthcare professionals. *Cochrane Database of Systematic Reviews, 9*, Article No. CD006732. doi: 10.1002/14651858.CD006732.pub3

Lucas, R. E. (2007). Long-term disability is associated with lasting changes in subjective well-being: Evidence from two nationally representative longitudinal studies. *Journal of Personality and Social Psychology, 92*, 717–730. doi: 10.1037/0022-3514.92.4.717

Martin, V., & Rogers, A. (2004). *Leading interprofessional teams in health and social care*. New York, NY: Routledge.

McClure, A., Teasell, R., & Salter, K. (2015). Psychosocial issues educational supplement. In R. Teasell, N. Hussein, N. Foley, & A. Cotol (Eds.), *Evidence-based review of stroke rehabilitation* (16th ed). London, Ontario, Canada: Heart & Stroke Foundation, Canadian Partnership for Stroke Recovery. Retrieved from http://www.ebrsr.com/sites/default/files/F_Psychosocial_Issues_(Questions_and_Answers).pdf

Peytremann-Bridevaux, I., Arditi, C., Gex, G., Bridevaux, P.-O., & Burnand, B. (2015). Chronic disease management programmes for adults with asthma. *Cochrane Database of Systematic Reviews, 5*, Article No. CD007988. doi: 10.1002/14651858.CD007988.pub2

Pitt, V., Lowe, D., Hill, S., Prictor, M., Hetrick, S. E., Ryan, R., & Berends, L. (2013). Consumer-providers of care for adult clients of statutory mental health services. *Cochrane Database of Systematic Reviews, 3*, Article No. CD004807. doi: 10.1002/14651858.CD004807.pub2

Reeves, S., Perrier, L., Goldman, J., Freeth, D., & Zwarenstein, M. (2013). Interprofessional education: Effects on professional practice and healthcare outcomes (update). *Cochrane Database of Systematic Reviews, 3*, Article No. CD002213. doi: 10.1002/14651858.CD002213.pub3

Reilly, S., Miranda-Castillo, C., Malouf, R., Hoe, J., Toot, S., Challis, D., & Orrell, M. (2015). Case management approaches to home support for people with dementia. *Cochrane Database of Systematic Reviews, 1*, Article No. CD008345. doi: 10.1002/14651858.CD008345.pub2

Renders, C. M., Valk, G. D., Griffin, S. J., Wagner, E., van Eijk, J. T., & Assendelft, W. J. J. (2000). Interventions to improve the management of diabetes mellitus in primary care, outpatient and community settings. *Cochrane Database of Systematic Reviews, 4*, Article No. CD001481. doi: 10.1002/14651858.CD001481

Social Security Act of 1935, 42 U.S.C. § 1861(i) (1982).

Stanton, M. W., & Rutherford, M. (2006). *The high concentration of U. S. health care expenditures* (AHRQ 06-0060, Research in Action Issue 19). Rockville, MD: Agency for Healthcare Research and Quality, U.S. Department of Health & Human Services. Retrieved from https://meps.ahrq.gov/data_files/publications/ra19/ra19.pdf

Stroke Unit Trialists' Collaboration. (2013). Organised inpatient (stroke unit) care for stroke. *Cochrane Database of Systematic Reviews, 9*, Article No. 000197. doi: 10.1002/14651858.CD000197.pub3

Treharne, G. J., Lyons, A. C., Booth, D. A., & Kitas, G. D. (2007). Psychological well-being across 1 year with rheumatoid arthritis: Coping resources as buffers of perceived stress. *British Journal of Health Psychology, 12,* 323–345. doi: 10.1348/135910706X109288

University Hospitals. (n.d.). Case management. Retrieved from http://www.uhhospitals.org/compcare/about-us/our-services/case-management

Visiting Nurse Service of New York. (n.d.). Retrieved from https://www.vnsny.org/

Vital Statistics Rapid Release Program, National Vital Statistics System, National Center for Health Statistics. (2016). Quarterly provisional estimates for selected causes of death: United States, 2014–Quarter 4, 2015.

Walker, I. D., & Gonzalez, E. W. (2007). Review of intervention studies on depression in persons with multiple sclerosis. *Issues in Mental Health Nursing, 28,* 511–531. doi: 10.1080/01612840701344480

Yukl, G., & Mahsud, R. (2010). Why flexible and adaptive leadership is essential. *Consulting Psychology Journal: Practice and Research, 62,* 81–93. doi: 10.1037/a0019835

Zwarenstein, M., Goldman, J., & Reeves, S. (2009). Interprofessional collaboration: Effects of practice-based interventions on professional practice and healthcare outcomes. *Cochrane Database of Systematic Reviews, 3,* Article No. CD000072. doi: 10.1002/14651858.CD000072.pub2

CHAPTER 15

INTERPROFESSIONAL PRACTICE

Janna C. Heyman

A key element of integrated health care is the adoption of a person-centered approach, which focuses on respecting an individual's values, preferences, and belief systems. The paradigm shift to person-centered care started with the report published in 2001 by the Institute of Medicine (IOM) on the value of this perspective (Epstein & Street, 2011). This approach is an organizing principle for the interprofessional team, which has been defined as a collection of "different health or social care professionals who share a team identity and work together closely in an integrated and interdependent manner to solve problems, deliver services, and enhance health outcomes" (IOM, 2015, p. xii).

Interprofessional practice can help to reduce fragmentation in the service delivery system and provide significant benefits to individuals and their families. In interprofessional practice, members of the care team listen to individuals, respect their wishes, identify and assess their needs, and follow-through with their care. Interprofessional practice focuses on improving outcomes, providing necessary services, and ensuring access to and continuity of care (Archer et al., 2012; IOM, 2015). Involving multiple perspectives in person-centered care offers individuals and their families the benefits of applying diverse knowledge and experience on shared goals, decisions, and treatments. The Council on Social Work Education (2014) stresses the importance of including social workers in the interprofessional team and promoting integrated team-based care as an effective and efficient way to improve health and coordinate care.

This chapter addresses the values and practices of interprofessional teams across settings and populations, illustrating the challenges and opportunities that involved professionals face. Interprofessional principles and strategies that social workers contribute to integrated health care are discussed, and future ways that interprofessional team members can influence integrated health care are explored. The importance of interprofessional education (IPE) across disciplines and in the context of discipline-specific education is highlighted.

INTERPROFESSIONAL PRACTICE
IN DIFFERENT SETTINGS

Interprofessional collaboration is critical in promoting person-centered care and building an effective plan to address an individual's needs (see Chapter 10). One of the advantages of employing a variety of professional perspectives is the synergy of knowledge that is available to inform assessment and treatment. In 2009, a national group of health professions formed the Interprofessional Education Collaborative (IPEC). The IPEC's Expert Panel provided a detailed report underscoring the four core competency domains of interprofessional education:

1. Values and ethics, emphasizing the importance of acting with honesty and integrity and respecting the dignity and privacy of individuals
2. Roles and responsibilities, including the disclosure of roles and responsibilities to all individuals, family members, and professionals
3. Communication, with a focus on how to effectively communicate and provide feedback
4. Teamwork, consisting of team-based care that engages other professionals and enriches team performance (IPEC Expert Panel, 2011).

These core competencies highlight some of the key elements for effective interprofessional practice. Although the IPEC provides valuable guidelines about practice, it is also important to recognize that "the implementation of integrated care can vary by setting, target service population, interest in collaboration, financial implementations, training, referral resources, practice resources, and the level of investment in the belief that collaboration can be impactful for improved patient outcomes" (Curtis & Christian, 2012, p.14).

Studies have explored differences in interprofessional practice among urban, suburban, and rural settings. Croker and Hudson (2015) described the nature of interprofessional relationships in rural settings, emphasizing that professionals often already know each other and that these established relationships provide opportunities for effective collaboration. Other authors have cited rural settings as rich sources for growth in interprofessional practice due to more intimate workplaces and communities (Hays, 2008; Thistlethwaite, 2007). Urban settings can also provide opportunities for enhanced collaboration among members of the interprofessional team through a rich array of available settings and resources.

Ko, Murphy, and Bindman (2015) examined various approaches and challenges to bridging the differences in integrated health care programs between hospitals and community health centers in five cities. They found that the duration of a site's integration was positively related to the level of trust among its service providers. The study also found that some of the successful information exchange included access to medical records and collaboration over care plans.

Interprofessional partnerships and approaches to care may also differ by a site's level of integration. This has been measured by the degree of collaboration among team members, ranging from minimal collaboration to full integration (Doherty, McDaniel, &

Baird, 1996; Heath, Wise Romero, & Reynolds, 2013). Heath et al. (2013) separated integrated health care into six levels of collaboration/integration, with three main categories:

1. Coordinated
2. Co-located
3. Integrated

Each category comprises two levels: *coordinated* care consists of minimal collaboration (level 1) and basic collaboration at a distance (level 2); *co-located* care includes basic collaboration on site (level 3) and close collaboration on site with some system integration (level 4); and *integrated* care consists of close collaboration approaching full integration (level 5) and full collaboration within a transformed/merged practice (level 6) (see Chapter 8).

Based on the type of model, the interprofessional team's functional capacity may vary. For example, if all professionals are on site, they may be able to hold face-to-face case consultations, host regular team meetings, and access shared records. In an organization that is considered to be level 6, a "fuller collaboration between providers has allowed antecedent system cultures (whether from two separate systems or from one evolving system) to blur into a single transformed or merged practice. Providers and patients view the operation as a single health system treating the whole person" (Heath et al., 2013, p. 6).

The manner in which the interprofessional team functions is also based on team members' prior levels of experience and training. Ko, Bailey-Kloch, and Kim (2014) explored the diverse experiences of social workers and other health care professionals with respect to their attitudes toward health care teams. They found that "female students, older adult students, and students with longer interprofessional practice experience had more positive attitudes toward interprofessional practice" (Ko et al., 2014, p. 552). The type of setting may further affect the function of an interprofessional team, necessitating unique roles of its members with respect to their use of educational and training material, referral processes, and methods of medical record exchange. Although most settings serve the general population, some concentrate on specific populations (e.g., children, older adults, veterans), and still others define themselves by their niche service provisions, such as trauma care or emergency care.

INTERPROFESSIONAL PRACTICE PRINCIPLES AND STRATEGIES

The IOM report prepared by Mitchell et al. (2012) identified the core principles and values of team-based health care (see Table 15.1). The authors underscored the changing health care system and described the "urgent need for high functioning teams" (Mitchell et al., 2012, p. 2). These teams must focus on ways to improve communication and address fragmentation of services and must be prepared to continually assess their roles and responsibilities. All members of the interprofessional team bring different assets to the table.

TABLE 15.1: Principles of Team-Based Health Care

Principle	Explanation
Shared goals	The team, including the service user, family members, and other support people, works to establish shared goals that reflect service user and family priorities and can be clearly articulated, understood, and supported by all team members.
Clear roles	There are clear expectations for each team member's functions, responsibilities, and accountabilities, which optimize the team's efficiency and often make it possible for the team to take advantage of division of labor, thereby accomplishing more than the sum of its parts.
Mutual trust	Team members earn each other's trust, creating strong norms of reciprocity and greater opportunities for shared achievement.
Effective communication	The team prioritizes and continuously refines its communication skills. It has consistent channels for candid and complete communication, which are accessed and used by all team members across all settings.
Measurable processes and outcomes	The team agrees on and implements reliable and timely feedback on successes and failures in both the functioning of the team and achievement of the team's goals. These are used to track and improve performance immediately and over time.

Data from *Core Principles & Values of Effective Team-Based Health Care* (Discussion Paper, p. 6), by P. H. Mitchell, M. K. Wynia, R. Golden, B. McNellis, S. Okun, C. E. Webb, . . . and I. Von Kohorn, 2012 (https://www.nationalahec.org/pdfs/VSRT-Team-Based-Care-Principles-Values.pdf). Copyright 2012 by the National Academy of Sciences.

The assets need to be maximized by ensuring role clarity, identifying responsibilities, and ensuring that trust and respect are given to all members of the team (Oyama, 2015).

The guiding principles laid out in the 2012 report delineate six functional areas in which interprofessional teams need to be actively engaged (see Figure 15.1):

1. Ensuring holistic and person-centered care
2. Providing education regarding health, behavior, and disease prevention
3. Establishing shared goals and engaging in shared decision-making
4. Developing treatment and intervention plans
5. Evaluating and reassessing performance
6. Building system capacity and advocating for change

ENSURING HOLISTIC PERSON-CENTERED CARE

The term *holistic* refers to caring for the whole person. This view is essential to person-centered care in integrated systems because it focuses on the individual's wellbeing. With this approach, the care team (including the individual and the family) can play an active part in focusing on a service user's needs. Epstein and Street (2011) asserted that "helping patients to be more active in consultations changes centuries of physician-dominated dialogues to those that engage patients as active participants" (p. 100). As

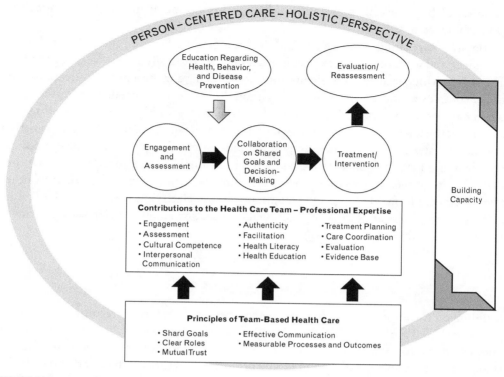

FIGURE 15.1: Holistic perspective of person-centered care.

important members of the interprofessional team, social workers play a significant role in the engagement, assessment, and validation of service users' voices. Social workers can contribute through their knowledge and ability to conduct a biopsychosocial assessment. This assessment may identify factors affecting a service user's wellbeing, including psychosocial issues such as interpersonal stressors, depression, anxiety, and substance use problems; health and mental health risks; and access to social and community resources, such as housing and finances. Social workers can also transfer their knowledge and skills in working with diverse populations who may have different cultural and belief systems, such as those pertaining to family, religion, and spirituality. This knowledge can help in training fellow team members to recognize that a person's culture may affect his or her development of goals, decisions, and treatment options.

HEALTH, BEHAVIOR, AND DISEASE PREVENTION

In the United States, the use of routine and preventive services occurs at approximately one half of the recommended rate (Centers for Disease Control and Prevention, 2016). Individuals often seek care only during a time of crisis. When service users are in the middle of a crisis, it may be difficult for them to listen, comprehend, and integrate information provided by the care team. Whether during a routine health visit or in a crisis situation, health care literacy is critical; it is described as the ability to communicate, process, and understand basic health information, which is important to inform decision-making (Maramaldi et al., 2014).

Before establishing shared goals and decision-making for care, the individual needs to understand what the problem or condition may be. In all situations, language matters. The way in which information is communicated can have far-reaching implications. The use of complex medical terminology and jargon should be minimized. To help, the social worker and other members of the interprofessional team should provide further information about the diagnosis, behavior, or health need that is being addressed and information revealed by any conducted tests. They should identify and explore other health-related concerns and listen to concerns raised by the individual, such as those about his or her care, family, friends, or pets. Social workers can then follow-up and work with other team members to facilitate effective communication, clarifying whether the individual and family members need or want additional information about the diagnosis, treatment options, or terminology.

ESTABLISHING SHARED GOALS

Building on the importance of holistic, person-centered care, the interprofessional team develops shared goals. Mitchell et al. (2012) stated that "the team—including the patient and, where appropriate, family members or other support persons—works to establish shared goals that reflect patient and family priorities, and that can be clearly articulated, understood, and supported by all team members" (p. 6). The service user needs to fully understand his or her problem, situation, and possible care options. Through this understanding, individuals can be empowered and can partner with professionals to develop shared goals. Because people may have different definitions of "being an active participant," the interprofessional team needs to listen and respect each service user's values, preferences, and beliefs and how he or she wants to participate in the team. Through trust and respect, team members can build healthy relationships that benefit individuals and their families. Hoge, Morris, Laraia, Pomerantz, and Farley (2014) emphasized that collaboration includes understanding roles, expressing professional opinions, and resolving any differences that may arise. Addressing these issues can greatly improve health outcomes.

DEVELOPING TREATMENT PLANS

The next step in the process is the development of treatment plans based on the shared goals that have been established. Coordination of care needs—whether they are basic or complex—requires an investment of time and effort by the service user, family, and interprofessional team. For example, if an older adult is considered overweight, has high blood pressure, and feels depressed, it is essential for the interprofessional team to work with the individual to address each of these areas. If the treatment plan is for the individual to use the primary care health center but access to services is a problem because he or she lives in a distant rural area, another plan for getting to the center needs to be coordinated. The social worker can collaborate with the individual, family, and other team members to discuss the possibility of regular visits, consider the use of telehealth (if appropriate), and develop plans for on-site services in the interest of most effectively addressing the individual's unique array of health, nutritional, and behavioral health needs.

EVALUATING AND REASSESSING

As part of the process, successful outcomes require continuous evaluation and reassessment. Pivotal questions should include the following:

- How has the developed treatment plan been working for you?
- Does the treatment plan need to be refined?
- What specific changes need to be made?
- How can the interprofessional team help implement these changes?
- How can the treatment plan be reevaluated to determine if these changes have actually impacted care?

These questions can help clarify and provide valuable feedback to the individual and the care team.

BUILDING SYSTEM CAPACITY

The interprofessional team may often be confronted with issues that transcend the boundaries between care settings (e.g., inpatient acute care, inpatient and outpatient long-term care, primary care). The interprofessional team may need to advocate for system changes to strengthen access to the service delivery system. Addressing the fragmentation of services and access to care helps to reduce barriers for future care recipients.

Interprofessional team members need to advocate for change and help build capacity in their facilities or settings and in the larger community. Social workers can play an important part in shaping these activities. Actions include partnering with interprofessional team members to address problems with site administrators. Team members can participate and serve on committees in the setting to bring into the forefront the challenges and opportunities associated with the delivery of integrated health care. Workplace challenges also need to be addressed, including complications that may arise when sharing information among team members in person or via technology.

Another way to become involved is to work with city, county, state, and national organizations by giving presentations at public hearings and conferences to raise awareness about important gaps and service needs. The strategies previously described are essential to strengthening interprofessional practice in integrated health care. As depicted in Figure 15.1, all members of the interprofessional team need to work in unison to build on their practice skills and develop approaches to help individuals best address their shared goals and interventions. More research needs to be conducted to understand the importance of these advocacy strategies and their impact on outcomes.

In integrated health care contexts, team members must be flexible and ready to respond to meet the needs of the service user. In reflecting on the principles of team-based care, social workers have critical knowledge and skills that they alone can bring to the interprofessional team. These skills are transferrable to different populations and health settings. Social workers are uniquely prepared for interprofessional practice due to their knowledge of engagement, assessment, effective communication, facilitation, authenticity, advocacy, evidence-based practice, care coordination, and case management. As part of their education, it is also important to build on strategies that social workers and other health care professionals can use to strengthen collaborative practices within interprofessional team settings.

INTERPROFESSIONAL EDUCATION

IPE plays a central role in training future health care professionals. The World Health Organization (WHO) defines IPE as "students from two or more health care professions learning with, from and about each other in order to enhance collaboration in a shared learning environment and improve health outcomes" (Health Professions Networks, 2010, p. 13). Haddara and Lingard (2013) questioned the divergent goals of IPE, describing them as sometimes oscillating between promoting successful outcomes and quelling power struggles that arise among professionals in different disciplines. They challenged IPE professionals to address this discourse to improve collaboration and educational training.

Improving IPE in integrated health care can help shape the way in which future professionals draw on their knowledge and expertise when working with individuals and families. IPE is crucial for all levels of education to build capacity for health care professionals to collaborate and improve treatment outcomes. There is limited research on the impact of IPE in integrated health care settings. Mitchell et al. (2015) found that significant improvements were documented in process outcomes regarding disease control. They highlighted the role of IPE in the delivery of care but observed that further information is needed to explore the specific impact of the team on outcomes. A paucity of research remains in integrated health care regarding the differences made by IPE across diverse settings and populations. Further research is needed to determine whether interprofessional teams in integrated health care settings can strengthen teamwork and improve outcomes.

IPE is essential to preparing professionals to work in integrated health care. All health care professionals could benefit from IPE in their specific disciplines and in cross-training among a variety of disciplines. Models of IPE stress the importance of students' developing and understanding their own professional identities and learning how to build good communication skills among team members (Bridges, Davidson, Odegard, Maki, & Tomkowiak, 2011; Conigliaro et al., 2013).

CASE VIGNETTES

Role plays and case-simulated interactive sessions have been effective approaches for IPE training. Two cases are described that can be used to inspire dialogue among students, faculty, and professionals.

CASE 1: ANNA

Anna is a 15-year-old, African-American girl who has just entered her sophomore year in high school. She is in kinship foster care with her 74-year-old grandmother because her mother was recently convicted of a drug-related crime and will soon be serving a 3-year sentence. In her freshman year, Anna did well in school and was on the freshman track team. However, her grades have recently dropped, and she has been staying up late at night. Anna has repeatedly told her grandmother that she cannot sleep, complaining about back pain or tension and saying that she does not like school. Her grandmother decided to bring her to the community health care center.

Anna was seen by a physician and a nurse at the center. Her pulse was 90 beats/minute, her respiration rate was 22 breaths/minute, her blood pressure was 129/90 mm Hg, and her body mass index was 21. She stated that she had felt worried for the past 6 months. Anna appeared anxious and stated that she had difficulty concentrating at school and trouble sleeping at night. Because Anna presented with clinically significant symptoms of generalized anxiety disorder, the physician introduced a social worker into the discussion with Anna and her grandmother and asked that Anna further explain some of her concerns about school and her family.

CASE 2: ANH

Anh is a 78-year-old, Vietnamese woman who does not speak English. Anh's daughter accompanied her to the hospital clinic because she was concerned that her mother appeared sad, was not interested in her usual hobbies, and sometimes forgot things. Anh, who has lived alone since her husband passed away 4 years ago, says that she feels guilty because she is a burden to her daughter. Anh tells the physician and social worker that she has been increasingly tired lately and has experienced feelings of hopelessness. She denies suicidal thoughts.

Anh's pulse was 76 beats/minute, her respiration rate was 14 breaths/minute, her blood pressure was 140/90 mm Hg, and her body mass index was 33. Her Patient Depression Questionnaire 9 (PHQ-9) depression score was 11, and she stated that she felt "down." Anh's urine and blood screens were negative for alcohol and drugs. The physician and social worker thought that Anh's high PHQ-9 score should be further explored and that a Mini-Mental State Examination should be completed.

In both of these cases, it may be helpful for the interprofessional team to address the following questions:

- What issues should the team members discuss with the service user and her family?
- How can the team begin to engage the service user and her family?
- What information can help the service user and her family become involved in developing shared goals and engaging in shared decision-making?
- What is the role of each team member?
- What factors may impact communication between team members?

The two case vignettes can be used to stimulate discussion about the concerns raised by the interprofessional teams. Students and professionals are often quick to find solutions to the questions raised, but it is worthwhile to focus on listening and processing what is being discussed. These cases can be used to strategize different ways to focus on person-centered goals and decisions and to target approaches that improve interprofessional team practices, roles, and communication.

IMPLICATIONS FOR SOCIAL WORK PRACTICE

The Council on Social Work Education's 2015 *Educational Policy and Accreditation Standards* "recognizes a holistic view of competence; that is, the demonstration of competence is informed by knowledge, values, skills, and cognitive and affective processes that include the social worker's critical thinking, affective reactions, and exercise of judgment in regard to unique practice situations" (p. 6). Working in integrated health care settings, social workers need to be prepared to use the holistic perspective in conjunction with person-centered care. Through their participation in engagement and assessment as members of an interprofessional team, social workers can collaborate with individuals and families by applying a person-in-environment lens to address each practice situation and target each service user's unique health care needs. Social workers possess important knowledge and practice skills to bring to the interprofessional team—skills that can be used in different settings and with different populations and that translate extremely well for interprofessional work. Horevitz and Manoleas (2013) observed that although social workers often feel prepared in integrated health care settings, they can still benefit from honing their collaboration skills and receiving additional psychoeducation in areas such as psychotropic medications, chronic illnesses, and problems with substance use. Social workers need to strengthen IPE in foundational, graduate-level, and continuing education settings. IPE can foster collaborations among different disciplines within a learning institution.

University and college leaders need to be willing to foster open dialogue among various health professional schools (i.e., medical, social work, and nursing schools) to encourage IPE development. The IOM (2015) has recognized the challenges of bringing together different disciplines and health systems. If the administration and faculty develop a shared mission to encourage the development and expansion of IPE, efforts may be more collaborative. One strategy to encourage this approach is to offer innovative initiatives to build capacity for cross-school IPE. Social workers and other health care professionals need to assume leadership roles and encourage these discussions within larger university and college settings.

Faculty development is critical to the future of IPE. For some faculty, integrated health care and interprofessional practice are new concepts, and training and engagement of faculty are of the utmost importance. If the goal is to expand education to address innovative and exciting opportunities, faculty inclusion is vital. It can be achieved by modeling different approaches, such as team teaching, active learning classrooms, simulations, service-learning, and case-based learning.

CONCLUSIONS

The IPEC (2011) has recognized that "teamwork training for interprofessional collaborative practice in health professions education has lagged dramatically behind these changes in practice, continually widening the gap between current health professions training and actual practice needs and realities" (p. 5). Although education reform has not always aligned with health system redesign (Cox & Naylor, 2013; Mitchell et al., 2015), it is critical that IPE move forward to benefit service users and the greater good.

In integrated health care, interprofessional practice is a collaborative approach that focuses on person-centered care to improve individual health care outcomes. Collaboration within interprofessional teams does not simply happen; it starts with discipline-based education that recognizes the importance of IPE. Interprofessional practice is strengthened by team members' understanding that each profession brings to the table a unique set of knowledge and skills. Professional roles need to be respected by all members of the interprofessional team; the ability to communicate effectively requires commitment and effort on behalf of all parties (Oyama, 2015). The workplace setting can also foster learning opportunities between professions. IPE can prepare the health professional for team-based collaborative care. With this in mind, all professions have a shared responsibility in educating the health care professionals of tomorrow. Social workers are uniquely qualified to work within interprofessional teams in integrated health care settings and to be leaders in the field.

RESOURCES

Center for Integrated Health Solutions (CIHS), Substance Abuse and Mental Health Services–Health Resources and Services Administration (SAMHSA-HRSA) http://www.integration.samhsa.gov

Integrated Behavioral Health Partners (IBHP), Community Partners http://www.ibhp.org

Interprofessional Education Collaborative (IPEC) https://ipecollaborative.org/

National Academies of Practice www.napractice.org

National Center for Interprofessional Practice and Education, University of Minnesota https://nexusipe.org

Patient-Centered Integrated Behavioral Health Care Principles & Tasks, Advancing Integrated Mental Health Solutions (AIMS), University of Washington http://uwaims.org/files/Aims_principles_checklist_final.pdf

REFERENCES

Archer, J., Bower, P., Gilbody, S., Lovell, K., Richards, D., Gask, L., . . . Coventry, P. (2012). Collaborative care for people with depression and anxiety. *Cochrane Database of Systematic Reviews, 10,* Article No. CD006525. doi: 10.1002/14651858.CD00625.pub2

Bridges, D. R., Davidson, R. A., Odegard, P. S., Maki, I. V., & Tomkowiak, J. (2011). Interprofessional collaboration: Three best practice models of interprofessional education. *Medical Education Online, 16,* Article No. 6035. doi: 10.3402/meo.v16i0.6035

Centers for Disease Control and Prevention. (2013, June 12). Preventive health care. Retrieved from http://www.cdc.gov/healthcommunication/ToolsTemplates/EntertainmentEd/Tips/PreventiveHealth.html

Conigliaro R., Kuperstein J., Dupuis J., Welsh D., Taylor, S., Weber, D., & Jones, M. (2013). The PEEER model: Effective healthcare team-patient communications. *MedEdPORTAL, 9,* Pub. Id. 9360. doi: 10.15766/mep_2374-8265.9360

Council on Social Work Education. (2014). *The role of social work in the changing health-care landscape: Principles for public policy.* Alexandria, VA: Council on Social Work Education. Retrieved from http://www.cswe.org/File.aspx?id=78367

Council on Social Work Education. (2015). *2015 educational policy and accreditation standards for baccalaureate and master's social work programs.* Alexandria, VA: Council on Social Work Education.

Cox, M, & Naylor, M. (Eds.). (2013). Transforming patient care: Aligning interprofessional education with clinical practice redesign: Proceedings of a conference sponsored by the Josiah Macy Jr. Foundation. New York, NY: Josiah Macy Jr. Foundation. Retrieved from http://macyfoundation.org/docs/macy_pubs/JMF_TransformingPatientCare_Jan2013Conference_fin_Web.pdf

Croker, A., & Hudson, J. N. (2015). Interprofessional education: Does recent literature from rural settings offer insights into what matters? *Medical Education, 49,* 880–887. doi: 10.1111/medu.12749

Curtis, R., & Christian, E. (Eds.). (2012). *Integrated care: Applying theory to practice.* New York, NY: Routledge.

Doherty, W. J., McDaniel, S. H., & Baird, M. A. (1996). Five levels of primary care/behavioral healthcare collaboration. *Behavioral Healthcare Tomorrow, 5*(5), 25–27.

Epstein, R. M., & Street, R. L., Jr. (2011). The values and value of patient-centered care. *Annals of Family Medicine, 9,* 100–103. doi: 10.1370/afm.1239

Haddara, W., & Lingard, L. (2013). Are we all on the same page? A discourse analysis of interprofessional collaboration. *Academic Medicine, 88,* 1509–1515. doi: 10.1097/ACM.0b013e3182a31893

Hays, R. B. (2008). Interprofessional education in rural practice: How, when and where. *Rural and Remote Health, 8,* Article No. 939. Retrieved from http://www.rrh.org.au/publishedarticles/article_print_939.pdf

Health Professions Networks—Nursing & Midwifery Office. (2010). In D. Hopkins (Ed), *Framework for action on interprofessional education & collaborative practice.* Geneva, Switzerland: Department of

Human Resources for Health, World Health Organization. Retrieved from http://apps.who.int/iris/bitstream/10665/70185/1/WHO_HRH_HPN_10.3_eng.pdf

Heath, B., Wise Romero, P., & Reynolds, K. A. (2013). *A standard framework for levels of integrated healthcare.* Washington, DC: Center for Integrated Health Solutions, Substance Abuse and Mental Health Services Administration-Health Resources and Services Administration. Retrieved from http://www.integration.samhsa.gov/integrated-care-models/A_Standard_Framework_for_Levels_of_Integrated_Healthcare.pdf

Hoge, M. A., Morris, J. A., Laraia, M., Pomerantz, A., & Farley, T. (2014). *Core competencies for integrated behavioral health and primary care.* Washington, DC: Center for Integrated Health Solutions, Substance Abuse and Mental Health Services Administration-Health Resources and Services Administration. Retrieved from http://www.integration.samhsa.gov/workforce/Integration_Competencies_Final.pdf

Horevitz, E., & Manoleas, P. (2013). Professional competencies and training needs of professional social workers in integrated behavioral health in primary care. *Social Work in Health Care, 52,* 752–787. doi: 10.1080/00981389.2013.791362

Institute of Medicine. (2001). *Crossing the quality chasm: A new health system for the 21st century.* Washington, DC: National Academy Press. doi: 10.17226/10027

Institute of Medicine. (2015). *Measuring the impact of interprofessional education on collaborative practice and patient outcomes.* Washington, DC: The National Academies Press. doi: 10.17226/21726

Interprofessional Education Collaborative (IPEC). (2011). Team-based competencies: Building a shared foundation for education and clinical practice: Proceedings of a conference sponsored by Interprofessional Education Collaborative. Washington, DC: Interprofessional Education Collaborative. Retrieved from http://www.aacn.nche.edu/leading-initiatives/IPECProceedings.pdf

Interprofessional Education Collaborative (IPEC) Expert Panel. (2011). *Core competencies for interprofessional collaborative practice: Report of an expert* panel. Washington, DC: Interprofessional Education Collaborative. Retrieved from http://www.aacn.nche.edu/education-resources/ipecreport.pdf

Ko, J., Bailey-Kloch, M., & Kim, K. (2014). Interprofessional experiences and attitudes toward interprofessional health care teams among health sciences students. *Social Work in Health Care, 53,* 552–567. doi: 10.1080/00981389.2014.903884

Ko, M., Murphy, J., & Bindman, A. B. (2015). Integrating health care for the most vulnerable: Bridging the differences in organizational cultures between US hospitals and community health centers. *American Journal of Public* Health, *105*(Suppl. 5), S676–S679. doi: 10.2105/AJPH.2015.302931

Maramaldi, P., Sobran, A., Scheck, L., Cusato, N., Lee, I., White, E., & Cadet, T. J. (2014). Interdisciplinary medical social work: A working taxonomy. *Social Work in Health Care, 53,* 532–551. doi: 10.1080/00981389.2014.905817

Mitchell, G. K., Burridge, L., Jianzhen, Z., Donald, M., Scott, I. A., Dart, J., & Jackson, C. L. (2015). Systematic review of integrated models of health care delivered at the primary-secondary interface: How effective is it and what determines effectiveness? *Australian Journal of Primary Health.* 21, 391–408. doi: 10.1071/PY14172

Mitchell, P., Wynia, M., Golden, R., McNellis, B., Okun, S., Webb, C. E., . . . & Von Kohorn, I. (2012). *Core principles & values of effective team-based health care.* Washington, DC: Institute of Medicine, The National Academy of Sciences. Retrieved from https://www.nationalahec.org/pdfs/vsrt-team-based-care-principles-values.pdf

Oyama, O. (2015). Introduction to the primary care team. In M. A. Burg and O. Oyama (Eds.), *The behavioral health specialist in primary care: Skills for integrated practice* (pp. 1–20). Springer Publishing Company.

Patient Protection and Affordable Care Act, 42 U.S.C. § 18001 et seq. (2010).

Thistlethwaite, J. (2007). Interprofessional education in Australasia. *Journal of Interprofessional Care, 21* (4), 369–372. doi: 10.1080/13561820701482536

CHAPTER 16

HEALTH INFORMATION TECHNOLOGY

Elizabeth B. Matthews, Virna Little, Benjamin Clemens, and Jordana Rutigliano

Health information technology (HIT) refers to a broad set of technologies that can be used to store, analyze, and share health information (Office of the National Coordinator for Health Information Technology [ONC], 2013). HIT has the potential to benefit health and behavioral health care delivery in several ways, such as improving access to care; facilitating the exchange of information; guiding treatment-related decisions in an evidence-based, person-centered manner; and providing mechanisms to monitor and track individual and population health (President's Council of Advisors on Science and Technology, 2010). Because of this enormous potential, HIT has become centrally embedded in the efforts to reform health and behavioral health care systems.

As HIT becomes a prominent component of routine service delivery, social workers will invariably come into contact with computerized systems of some kind. This is particularly true in integrated health care settings, where medical and behavioral health care intersect. Although the scope of HIT will continue to expand as technology evolves and innovates, most technological advancements in this area revolve around the electronic health record (EHR). This chapter reviews common applications of EHR systems in integrated settings, discusses how the technology can be used to benefit care delivery, and identifies existing challenges associated with integrating various forms of HIT into routine services.

Although the term *health information technology* is primarily used to describe the electronic platforms that manage information, technology is also being used as a mechanism for delivering health and behavioral health care services. Telehealth and health-related services through mobile platforms (mHealth) leverage HIT and other forms of technology to provide direct care, deliver psychoeducation, and monitor health remotely. The adoption of HIT is deeply embedded in broader health care reform efforts, and the policies relevant to HIT adoption are summarized in the next section.

HEALTH INFORMATION TECHNOLOGY AND HEALTH CARE POLICY

Although national investment in HIT is hardly new, recent efforts to improve the quality of health and behavioral health services have dramatically accelerated the adoption of various forms of HIT. The Health Information Technology for Economic and Clinical Health (HITECH) Act, passed as part of the American Recovery and Reinvestment Act of 2009, has played a crucial role in shaping the integration of HIT into mainstream health and behavioral health systems. The goal of the HITECH Act was twofold: to strengthen the nation's HIT infrastructure and to boost adoption rates of EHRs (DesRoches, Painter, & Jha, 2015). Infrastructure development was backed by funding allocated to research, educational programs, and technical assistance and training related to HIT implementation. One of the most prominent aspects of the HITECH Act was authorization of the EHR incentive program. This program allocated more than $30 billion to the Centers for Medicare and Medicaid Services (CMS) to support the adoption and implementation of EHR systems (Buntin, Jain, & Blumenthal, 2010). In addition to the sizable financial backing of this initiative, the CMS Incentive Program is significant because of its influence on how EHR systems have been integrated into health and mental health care delivery systems.

The first component of the CMS Incentive Program offers financial support for health care providers who are planning to adopt or implement an EHR system. To qualify for these payments, eligible professionals must adopt a certified EHR system. Certified EHRs are designated systems that meet minimum standards for technological capability, functionality, and security (ONC, 2016). After adoption of a certified EHR system, the CMS Incentive Program provides opportunities for ongoing financial support for health care providers to effectively implement EHRs. This financial support is guided by *meaningful use criteria*, a set of care delivery standards designed to signify that EHR systems are being integrated into health care services in a way that improves the quality and safety of care (Federal Office of Rural Health Policy, 2015). The Meaningful Use program is composed of three progressive stages through which qualified professionals must advance to continue qualifying for payment; each signifies a more sophisticated and more optimal use of EHR systems. Starting in 2015, providers failing to demonstrate proficiency at the first stage of the Meaningful Use program will incur financial penalties in the form of reduced reimbursement rates.

The Meaningful Use program has significantly shaped the process of EHR implementation in several ways. First, the financial incentives appear to have effectively increased EHR use among health and behavioral health care providers because EHR adoption rates have risen sharply since passage of the HITECH Act (Jamoom & Hing, 2015). Second, the criteria included in the EHR Meaningful Use standards have also played an important role in influencing which functions are most commonly embedded in EHR systems and how providers are integrating these systems into care delivery processes. Overall, by strengthening the HIT infrastructure and boosting EHR adoption rates, the HITECH Act has helped establish the central role of technology in emerging models of integrated health care such as accountable care organizations,

Medicaid health homes, and patient-centered medical homes. HIT is also a central component of the Patient Protection and Affordable Care Act (ACA) and its primary goals of increasing access to quality health and behavioral health care services. In particular, efforts to enhance the quality and control the cost of services rely on tracking, monitoring, and holding organizations accountable to several quality indicators. These efforts lean heavily on the HIT infrastructure created by the HITECH Act to enable organizations and regulatory bodies to collect these data and use them to inform care decisions (Buntin, Jain, & Blumenthal, 2010).

In effect, the HITECH Act and the ACA have placed HIT at the center of efforts to innovate and improve the nation's health care system. This is particularly salient in models of coordinated care, in which information must be shared across interdisciplinary teams of professionals. The following sections describe how various forms of HIT and HIT-driven care have been integrated into delivery systems to improve the quality, safety, and accessibility of services.

ELECTRONIC HEALTH RECORDS

EHRs are computerized systems used for storing, accessing, and exchanging health information securely. EHR systems have improved the quality and safety of care by facilitating the exchange of information necessary for care coordination, providing mechanisms for guiding evidence-based clinical decisions, and creating tools for population management and tracking (Buntin, Burke, Hoaglin, & Blumenthal, 2011). Because of their enormous potential to improve the delivery of primary and mental health care, adoption rates have continued to increase dramatically in recent years. Adoption rates among medical professionals have reached as high as 80% (DesRoches, Painter, & Jha, 2015); more than half of all behavioral health organizations have implemented an EHR, and another fourth are planning to do so in the near future (National Council for Community Behavioral Healthcare, 2012). Although the exact structure and functionality of EHRs vary by system, this section summarizes common ways in which EHRs can be used to enhance care in integrated settings.

CLINICAL DECISION SUPPORT SYSTEMS

Clinical decision support systems (CDSSs) are a core function of many EHRs. CDSS tools give health and behavioral health care providers automated, person-specific recommendations that are used to guide evidence-based decision-making (Kawamoto, Houlihan, Balas, & Lobach, 2005). Ideally, a CDSS is a mechanism to deliver correct information at the correct junction to the correct provider.

CDSSs can be *active* or *passive*. Active decision supports deliver specific information that is meant to directly and immediately influence provider behavior (Bell et al., 2014). Active CDSS tools are commonly used to provide reminders of overdue assessments, screenings, or routine medical reassessments for chronic medical conditions. In the behavioral health context, a CDSS can be used to remind clinicians to complete important updates, such as annual reassessments and treatment plan reviews, or to alert psychiatric providers of essential medication management tasks, such as laboratory work to check lithium levels.

Passive decision supports can serve as a way to convey contextual information about a service user that may also be used to guide a provider's decision-making throughout the course of treatment. Examples include significant historical information and information about service users' values or preferences related to care. In contrast to prompts for specific and immediate action, passive supports are designed to provide information that may influence or inform a provider's overall approach to care or understanding of a service user. Passive decision support is offered in several ways, often appearing in functional spaces where other information is contained, such as problem lists, medication lists, and demographic sections of an EHR. Formatting, highlighting, or other methods of accentuating text may be used to bring this information to a provider's attention.

In addition to being active or passive, decision supports can be further categorized as *synchronous* or *asynchronous*. Synchronous decision supports are displayed at the time that the alert can be acted upon (McCoy et al., 2012). For example, a pop-up alert prompting a provider to order a specific test is considered an active, synchronous decision support.

Asynchronous decision supports are not tied to specific clinical actions and may be displayed at times other than when the provider is with the service user. Examples of passive, asynchronous clinical decision supports include *dashboards* and *report cards*. A dashboard provides summary information about a particular subset of a population or provider caseload. Dashboards can display statistical information to providers about quality metrics or summarize financial information stored in the record. This is a useful mechanism for monitoring populations of interest, such as service users with dual diagnoses and other high-risk groups. A provider report card consists of information about the provider's clinical practice, such as productivity or specific outcome measures for a provider panel. Provider-specific report cards can improve the quality of care by identifying areas in need of improvement or highlighting areas of success.

CDSSs play an important role in integrated health care in several ways. Active supports can alert providers across disciplines to clinically relevant actions. Because decision supports are often shared with all qualified providers, care can be effectively managed by a team of individuals. Passive CDSSs can also be an effective way of sharing information among team members by ensuring that all treating providers have common access to information that may be relevant to important care decisions. A CDSS provides useful tools to manage the quality of overall care through dashboard and provider report card features. CDSSs have improved preventive care by increasing providers' compliance with recommended clinical guidelines (Bright et al., 2012). Although CDSSs can be powerful, overburdening providers with data may increase the risk of overlooking other relevant information (Carspecken, Sharek, Longhurst, & Pageler, 2013). Therefore, the quantity of decision support should be considered, and restraint should be employed to avoid the possibility of desensitizing providers to alerts in an EHR.

DISEASE REGISTRIES

Although CDSS features are often used to inform care at the individual or subgroup level, EHRs can also track larger groups of interest through the use of disease registries. This is an important tool in meeting one of the goals of the Triple Aim: improving population health (see Chapter 3). EHRs excel at collecting structured information; however, without effective mechanisms to organize and store the data, its utility is greatly diminished. Registries function by collecting, storing, and tracking specific information of interest about a particular disease or set of problems in a separate database (Larsson et al., 2011).

When the registry is configured, EHR users can identify specific types of information to be collected and stored. Information is commonly stratified by disease, age, specific risk factors, or a combination of these conditions. After the inclusion criteria are set by a provider, the registry compiles information for all eligible service users in a format that enables reporting and summarization. Registry functions often include query tools that allow users to create custom reports or apply filters, offering flexibility in the ways providers can view or organize service user information stored in the database.

Storing information in a registry can benefit the quality of care in many ways. By allowing users to easily retrieve relevant information about specific groups of interest, registries can illuminate important patterns or characteristics that are common in a service user population. Viewing aggregated data may help providers or organizations recognize gaps in care that would be difficult to identify through individual chart reviews. This information can be tracked over time, providing a mechanism for quality monitoring and improvement. For example, high-risk service users with missed appointments can be identified for outreach, or those recently discharged from a hospital can be contacted for care management services. These benefits also extend beyond organization-level quality improvement to generate new and efficient mechanisms for larger-scale research. Because registries are designed to track data over time, they provide population-specific information that can be used to explore health outcomes longitudinally or before and after a particular intervention has been implemented.

ELECTRONIC PORTALS

As the functionality of EHRs has advanced, the prevalence of *portals* has become more mainstream. There are two main types of portals: the patient portal and the specialty provider or community portal. Patient portals are more commonly used and are offered by most EHRs. A patient portal is a personal health record attached to an EHR system. It provides service users with the ability to interact with their providers and systems of care in real time. Common features of a patient portal include the ability for service users to make and change appointments, send electronic messages to providers, and receive information such as appointment reminders or laboratory test results. Many patient portals have been expanded to include features that allow service users to receive health information related to their diagnoses or laboratory results, see their records, view details of who has accessed their records, and complete questionnaires or screening instruments that get populated in their EHRs. The addition of service user portals has transformed care in many ways, including administrative operations. Providers of all disciplines in integrated settings can receive electronic messages from service users throughout the day, often with expectations of real-time responses. The electronic messages and scheduling replace what used to exist as phone volume for the practices, allowing for a shift in resources to support more back-end functions.

By enabling individuals to easily and quickly access their health care records, patient portals help service users develop a sense of ownership of their health information and records and allow important information to be quickly located in times of emergency. Patient portals provide extensive health information opportunities with data housed inside the portals themselves and through links to outside resources. Although service users are receptive to enrolling in these portals, research and provider experiences indicate that only about 33% of those with access to patient portals use them (Irwin, 2013). There is evidence suggesting that service users who are more engaged with their providers are more likely to adopt and use a patient portal (Agarwal, Anderson, Zarate, & Ward, 2013). Therefore, providers can play an important role in leveraging this resource. Although patient portals often provide extensive information and access, they have not been shown to improve health outcomes or engagement in care among service users (Ammenwerth, Schnell-Inderst, & Hoerbst, 2012; Archer, Fevrier-Thomas, Lokker, McKibbon, & Strauss, 2011). However, because service users may be underutilizing this resource, it is possible that the true potential of patient portals has yet to be fully realized.

Maintaining the security of protected health information has been a focus of discussion as the uses and functionalities of portals have been expanded. The Health Insurance Portability and Accountability Act (HIPAA) requires that service users have access to their own records and information about others who accessed their health information. Patient portals provide a mechanism for providers to meet these guidelines (Office of the Federal Register, 2002). Initially, some behavioral health care providers in integrated settings voiced concern about the ability of service users to access providers' progress notes and see their diagnoses. However, as portal use has expanded, providers have increasingly agreed that service users have the right to access their records and individual notes. There has been acknowledgment that the delivery of person-centered care should include a service user who is informed and educated about his or her mental health diagnosis and treatment. As a result of increased transparency in health and behavioral health care records, there has been a growing shift in the way providers document their notes. Knowing that service users read their progress notes has prompted many providers to reduce professional jargon in favor of more user-friendly language and to increase the number of quotations that represent the exact thoughts or feelings of the service users.

There are many facets to building and developing portals. Organizations have developed comprehensive programs to educate and enroll service users in the use of portals by providing information in the languages and literacy levels of those they serve. Consent for sharing of information between organizations has been largely developed in a way that resembles consent forms for the health information exchanges. Organizations continue to struggle with special populations and their rights to confidential records, such as adolescents, individuals who have proxy representatives, and those in abusive relationships. These populations provide challenges to organizations that strive to expand access to health records and health care. Many organizations have figured out ways to segregate adolescents' confidential or reproductive visits or have developed proxy access, and others have chosen to exclude these populations entirely from portal access.

Whereas patient portals increase access to health information for service users, specialty provider and community portals are used to share information about mutual service users with providers outside of EHR systems. Many of these community or provider portals allow outside providers to enter information directly into EHR systems (e.g., hospital discharge summaries, test results). These community providers also have real-time access to each mutual service user's health record and the ability to see critical information relating to his or her care, such as medications, laboratory results, appointment notes, allergies, and diagnoses. Such information can be lifesaving when service users are being treated by providers who do not know their medical or behavioral health histories, such as in the emergency department. Community-based organizations, such as substance abuse programs, may also use provider portals. Portals can expedite admissions by providing the ability to view medical clearance and behavioral health assessments for an individual being referred from an integrated setting.

As the use of portals expands, many service users will seek out providers who offer portals due to the ease of access, communication, and scheduling that this technology affords. Organizations are beginning to require outside specialty and community providers to participate in their community portals. The continued advancement of service user and provider portals promises to be one of the largest transformations in the delivery of care in the near future.

COLLABORATIVE DOCUMENTATION

Although functions embedded in the EHR have the potential to significantly change the way that care is delivered in health and behavioral health settings, in many ways, the impact of these tools depends on how they are incorporated into clinical care. One mechanism for integrating EHRs meaningfully into clinical encounters is through the practice of collaborative documentation. Collaborative documentation, also known as concurrent documentation, is a model of clinical practice in which service users, in conjunction with their providers, are directly involved in the process of documenting their visits (Stanhope, Ingoglia, Schmelter, & Marcus, 2013).

The collaborative documentation model was developed in the community behavioral health care field where, historically, documentation has been a private exercise. In the past decade there has been movement toward empowering service users to engage more actively in their own recovery. This model is supported by the development of HIT, including features of the EHR that assist service users, particularly those with lower literacy levels, in reading and understanding their charts. Collaborative documentation practitioners think that engaging service users in clinical documentation is a key way to improve engagement in treatment, reinforce clinical goal setting, and provide service users with health education about their diagnoses and the evidence-based practices being used to treat them. Collectively, these mechanisms serve to increase user satisfaction with services and improve clinical outcomes.

Models of collaborative documentation vary, but the most common model is referred to as the *five and five model*. In this method of collaborative documentation, clinicians use the first 5 minutes of the visit to involve the service user in documenting his or her current symptoms and progress toward established goals. The last 5 minutes of the visit are used to document clinical progress and decisions made during the visit, ending with a plan for the service user to follow in the period before the next visit. The middle part of the visit is carried out as usual (e.g., a clinical examination or counseling session), and during that time the computer may be used to document items considered important to the clinician and service user. Other models of collaborative documentation involve using the computer for documentation throughout the session as important developments occur or at the end of the session to jointly summarize the critical documentation components.

Collaborative documentation is a fairly new model that is still being adopted, but there is evidence supporting its use to improve service user engagement in treatment, including attendance rate, and to improve treatment adherence (Kaufman, 2012; Matthews, 2015; Stanhope et al., 2013). Some evidence suggests that service users prefer collaborative documentation to traditional models of documentation (Schmelter, 2012). Research is looking further into the benefits of collaborative documentation in terms of engagement, user and provider satisfaction, the service user–provider relationship, and treatment outcomes.

Collaborative documentation also serves as a mechanism to help clinicians write and complete progress notes in a timely manner (i.e., by the end of the visit), alleviating work stress for clinicians and promoting organizational efficiency and productivity by reducing the need for additional administrative time. Because collaborative documentation notes are completed jointly in real time, information is more likely to be accurate and to reflect service users' individual values and preferences (Schmelter, 2012). In this way, collaborative documentation can improve the quality of documentation by promoting the inclusion of comprehensive and individualized clinical information rather than impersonal, boiler plate notes that fail to include person-centered information and often lack data necessary for reimbursement, such as symptoms, progress, and clinical criteria necessitating treatment.

Some providers remain hesitant to adopt collaborative documentation models. Common reasons for their ambivalence include a lack of training in this approach, anxiety that service users will not like what they see in their EHR, and unwillingness to use person-centered language in their clinical documentation. More training and on-site support are needed to encourage wider adoption of the various versions of this model. Collaborative documentation is an important approach with a growing evidence base that will be critical in assisting health care providers in this era of health care reform to meet the Triple Aim of better quality of care and better service user experience at a lower cost.

BARRIERS TO ADOPTION OF ELECTRONIC HEALTH RECORDS

Although EHRs are becoming more normative, organizations adopting and implementing these systems still face some common challenges. Despite available incentive payments, purchasing and implementing an EHR requires significant up-front and ongoing costs because organizations often need to build up their information technology infrastructure, including equipment and technical assistance staff, to support system functionality. Financial barriers rank among the most common concerns about adopting a computerized system (DesRoches et al., 2008). This barrier is particularly salient for behavioral health organizations because under current legislation they are ineligible to directly receive any of the incentive payments offered by CMS (National Council for Community Behavioral Healthcare, 2012). Accordingly, funding mechanisms that can alleviate the financial burden of EHR adoption will be critical to the universal implementation of these systems.

After an organization has adopted an EHR, training providers to effectively use EHRs in practice is another challenge of this process. Although EHR adoption has gained speed, effectiveness research and best practices take longer to become established. To facilitate this process, the HITECH Act funded both a workforce development program and the Beacon Community Cooperative Agreement Program, which funds pilot research exploring best practices related to EHR and HIT implementation (DesRoches, Painter, & Jha, 2015).

Other concerns among those preparing to adopt an EHR include the usability of systems and the confidentiality of data (Gold, McLaughlin, Devers, Bersonson, & Bovbjerg, 2012). Because health and behavioral health care systems have traditionally been fragmented, providers' workflows have become quite specialized to their respective discipline or practice. Developing software that is universally applicable to a wide range of health and behavioral health care settings continues to be a work in progress. Inability to overcome this obstacle may have negative implications for provider satisfaction (Buntin, Burke, Hoaglin, & Blumenthal, 2011) and may ultimately reduce the willingness of providers to embrace these systems. Although maintaining the confidentiality of data has been a primary concern for providers, service users have typically reported high levels of satisfaction with the care they receive using EHR systems (Liu, Luo, Zhang, & Huang 2013), suggesting that this concern has not outweighed the perceived benefits associated with computer-supported care delivery.

TELEHEALTH AND MHEALTH

Delivering coordinated health and behavioral health care requires timely access to a comprehensive team of care providers equipped to meet a service user's unique set of needs. Increasingly, the ability to deliver these services does not depend on a provider's physical proximity to the service user or the team of professionals involved in his or her care. Providing care remotely is facilitated by technologies collectively referred to as *telehealth* or *telemedicine*. The Health Resources and Services Administration (HRSA) defines telehealth as the "use of technology to deliver health care, health information, or health education at a distance" (Federal Office of Rural Health Policy, 2015). Alternative terms have been employed to describe the application of this technology in various health-related contexts, including *telemental health* and *telepsychiatry* when the technology is used to deliver behavioral health treatment and *telemedicine* when the focus is limited to the delivery of medical services and diagnoses (Wilson & Maeder, 2015). In the subsequent discussion of these remote technologies, the most inclusive term—*telehealth*—is used.

Telehealth was first developed in the 1960s, and its prevalence and scope have since evolved along with the technology. As research and practice in this area advance, new and innovative ways to deliver services remotely are constantly expanding. However, telehealth services have been most widely used as a mechanism for three primary types of services: real-time consultation or care, remote monitoring, and health and mental health information exchange (American Telemedicine Association, n.d.).

Telehealth technology can take several forms. One of the most common forms of telehealth is the use of telephones or video conferencing software to deliver real-time services at a distance. This type of remote, real-time exchange can be used to provide one-time services (e.g., assessment, consultation) or ongoing services (e.g., care management, counseling). Particularly among those living in rural areas, remote service delivery has been a highly effective mechanism for obtaining a wide range of medical and behavioral health care services. For example, telehealth programs delivering individual and group counseling services have been effective in treating a wide range of populations, including adolescents, older adults, and cultural minorities (Hilty et al., 2013). Remote specialty care consultations have been integrated into various service settings, including emergency departments and outpatient facilities. Particularly in the fields of geriatric and adolescent psychiatry, in which there are shortages of professionally trained workers (Konrad, Ellis, Thomas, Holzer, & Morrissey, 2009), video conferencing has been effective at increasing timely access to psychiatric assessments and medication management that may otherwise have been unavailable. Telehealth conferencing has not been limited to mental health services; it has been used to deliver specialty medical care consultation and to support chronic disease management.

Telephone or video conferencing is being widely adopted as a way to provide ongoing care management. In combination with the other technologies described in the preceding sections, routine telephone or video conferencing check-ins can be an effective way to support disease management, deliver psychoeducation, and provide brief counseling to individuals with chronic conditions (Gellis, Kenaley, & Have, 2014; Gottlieb & Blum, 2006). Although concern has been expressed about the comparative quality and effectiveness of the health care provided, research has found these modalities to be widely accepted by service users and to be equivalent to traditional face-to-face encounters in terms of quality and effectiveness (Bashshur, Shannon, Bashshur, & Yellowlees, 2015).

Remote monitoring is another form of telehealth that allows service users to send health and mental health information directly to a designated health professional. As with video conferencing, the information is typically delivered in real time. Remote monitoring has increased opportunities for service users to remain at home and live independently in scenarios in which doing so may previously have been risky, making these innovations particularly beneficial for the older adult population. From a cost-containment perspective, remote technology can generate savings by reducing the volume and length of stay in skilled nursing or nursing family facilities. Retaining independence can have significant positive implications for service users' quality of life and wellbeing.

Remote monitoring can be conducted using a wide range of devices and applications, and innovation in this area is undergoing rapid growth. A primary form of remote monitoring is through the use of web-based or mobile applications, commonly referred to as mHealth (Tomlinson, Rotheram-Borus, Swartz, & Tsai, 2013). Many mHealth programs have been designed to collect, store, and transmit health information, including vital signs, weight, and test and screening results (e.g., glucose levels, depression screening scores). These programs can be used to facilitate communication between service users and providers, creating new opportunities for users to become informed, active participants in their care. For example, mHealth applications have been used to help service users prepare for upcoming appointments by collecting information about their values, preferences, and important experiences with treatment, such as medication side effects. When this information is transmitted to providers before a meeting, health and behavioral health care professionals can actively address each service user's agenda and encourage them to become active participants in their care (Campbell, 2014).

The mHealth programs can also be used to support medication compliance by delivering reminders to take medication or complete a screening. Specific devices with similar functions have become increasingly available to track and transmit information. *Smart pillboxes* are being used to support medication compliance; they include sensors that alert users when it is time to take their medication and then record and transmit information when the dose is taken. Similar sensors have been incorporated into scales, at-home blood pressure cuffs, and heart rate monitors. As technology continues to advance, so will the number of new software programs and devices to increase the amount of health information that providers have about the individuals they treat.

Web-based programming and mHealth applications have also provided mechanisms for delivering health education and increasing opportunities for social support. Although peer-driven support has been shown to be an effective way to improve illness management and deliver emotional and social support (Fisher et al., 2015), developing peer networks can be challenging for some individuals, such as those living with disabilities or in geographically isolated communities. To address this barrier, mHealth applications use discussion forums, message boards, and online support groups to connect individuals and create virtual communications. In this way, mHealth provides innovative new ways to integrate peer support services into care regardless of geographic proximity.

A current challenge in advancing telehealth and mHealth programming is the development and implementation of best practices to guide the delivery of these services. In telehealth, efforts in this area have been largely spearheaded by the American Telemedicine Association (ATA), an international organization that includes practitioners, researchers, health care organizations, and industry leaders. The ATA created a comprehensive set of resources for telehealth implementation in a wide range of settings, including primary care and behavioral health environments. In addition to refining clinical practices related to telehealth, researchers are developing billing and reimbursement mechanisms. Because many standards for licensing and payment for telehealth services are governed by state agencies, they may vary based on the location of the provider and the recipient of services (Center for Connected Health Policy, 2015). However, as service users and providers use telehealth to collaborate and engage in treatment across state lines, these regulations are becoming increasingly more difficult to implement.

Regulatory bodies overseeing the development of mHealth applications have not yet been formed. As a consequence, although the number of freely available mHealth applications is growing rapidly, most have not been tested for effectiveness and may not adhere to clinical guidelines or best practices (Donker et al., 2013). Although rigorously developed mHealth tools have shown positive effects on health, their impact may be eclipsed by a preponderance of poorly designed or poorly researched applications. Therefore, a critical next step for this field is the development of quality standards and oversight.

IMPLICATIONS FOR SOCIAL WORK

At its core, social work seeks to deliver culturally competent services that recognize the dignity and worth of each individual. This chapter has identified several ways in which HIT serves as a mechanism to make clinical treatment deliberately more inclusive of service users' values, preferences, and choices related to care. HIT and HIT-driven care have provided new and innovative ways to help individuals become informed, activated users of health and behavioral health services. HIT functions are a natural fit with the overarching guiding principles of the social work profession. HIT will play an increasingly large role in the post-ACA era of social work practice. Although social work has long been an interdisciplinary practice, health and behavioral health care reforms are pushing all health and behavioral health care systems to be more collaborative and team based. Technology that facilitates the real-time exchange of information will become a core component of the work of all health care practitioners.

A remaining challenge for the social work discipline is to train existing and emerging professionals to optimally integrate this technology into clinical practice. In the era of rapid HIT expansion, behavioral health professionals have been underrepresented in policy discussions that have shaped HIT implementation and research that is beginning to define best practices. As practitioners with particular expertise in interdisciplinary person-centered practices, the perspective of social workers in both areas is critical.

CASE VIGNETTE

Ellen is a 75-year-old woman living independently in a suburban area about 45 minutes outside a large city. Ellen was diagnosed with type 2 diabetes 10 years ago but continued to manage her illness well by going on daily walks with her husband and cooking healthy meals every night. About 1 year ago, Ellen's husband passed away; shortly thereafter, her own health began to decline. Ellen stopped going for her daily walks and stopped taking her diabetes medication regularly. As a result of her poorly managed diabetes, Ellen's eyesight worsened until she could no longer drive. Without the ability to transport herself to her health care clinic in the city, Ellen began missing her regularly scheduled doctor's appointments. Eventually, Ellen's doctor was able to arrange for a paratransit service to pick her up and drive her to the doctor's office. Ellen shared with the doctor her feelings of social isolation and sadness after her husband's death, which contributed to the changes in her illness management. Ellen's doctor diagnosed her with major depression and prescribed antidepressants. To monitor the diabetes and the depression, Ellen's doctor needed to see Ellen regularly. However, constraints on Ellen's ability to get reliable transportation to the office made this challenging.

As an alternative to traveling into the office regularly, Ellen's doctor recommended enrolling her in the office's telehealth care management program. Ellen now uses a special glucose meter that transmits her blood sugar reading to a nurse care manager and her doctor. Ellen and the nurse care manager have weekly calls on the telephone, during which time they discuss her medication use, blood sugar control, and overall physical and mental health. Ellen also has weekly phone calls with a social worker to focus on goal setting, coping skills, and strategies for managing her depressive symptoms. Once each month, Ellen's nurse care manager comes to her house to check her medical equipment and conduct an in-person visit. Every 3 months, Ellen travels to see her doctor using the paratransit service. During these appointments, Ellen meets with her doctor, care manager, and social worker to talk about her progress, her needs, and her goals. Collaboratively, Ellen and her care team document their discussion in the EHR, and the progress note is uploaded to a secure patient portal. Ellen can log in to her portal from home and review this information, which helps her keep track of her treatment goals and progress.

Since starting in the program, Ellen's depressive symptoms have slowly improved. As a result, she has more energy, has resumed her daily walks, and has met several new people in the neighborhood. The weekly check-ins have helped Ellen to adhere to her medication regimen and lower her blood sugar levels.

CONCLUSIONS

This chapter has reviewed several forms of HIT and how they can be applied in medical, behavioral health, and integrated health care settings. EHRs and telehealth technology offer promising new mechanisms to increase and enhance access to health and behavioral health care services, exchange health information to coordinate care, and guide care decisions that are evidence-based and person-centered. Because these advances have progressed rapidly, particularly since the passage of the HITECH Act and the ACA, regulations about best practices, billing and reimbursement, and licensing have not kept up with the evolving landscapes of health and behavioral health care systems. As technology continues to advance, new and innovative ways of using computerized systems to optimize service delivery will continue to expand, and HIT will continue to become an integral component of routine health and behavioral health care.

RESOURCES

American Telemedicine Association http://www.americantelemed.org/

Office of the National Coordinator for Health Information Technology (ONC), U.S. Department of Health and Human Services (DHHS) www.healthit.gov

REFERENCES

Agarwal, R., Anderson, C., Zarate, J., & Ward, C., (2013). If we offer it, will they accept? Factors affecting patient use intentions of personal health records and secure messaging. *Journal of Medical Internet Research, 15,* e43. doi: 10.2196/jmir.2243

American Telemedicine Association. (n.d.). About telemedicine. Retrieved from http://www.american-telemed.org/about/about-telemedicine

Ammenwerth, E., Schnell-Inderst, P, & Hoerbst, A. (2012). The impact of electronic patient portals on patient care: A systemic review of controlled trials. *Journal of Medical Internet Research, 14,* e163. doi: 10.2196/jmir.2238

Archer, N., Fevrier-Thomas, U., Lokker, C., McKibbon, K. A., & Strauss, S. E. (2011). Personal health records: A scoping review. *Journal of the American Medical Informatics Association, 18,* 515–522. doi: 10.1136/amiajnl-2011-000105

Bashshur, R. L., Shannon, G. W., Bashshur, N., and Yellowlees, P.M. (2015). The empirical evidence for telemedicine interventions in mental disorders. *Telemedicine and e-Health, 22*(2). doi: 10.1089/tmj.2015.0206

Bell, G. C., Crews, K. R., Wilkinson, M. R., Haidar, C. E., Hicks, J. K., Baker, D. K., . . . Hoffman, J. M. (2014). Development and use of active clinical decision support for preemptive pharmacogenomics. *Journal of the American Medical Informatics Association, 21,* e93–e99. doi: 10.1136/amiajnl-2013-001993

Bright, T. J., Wong, A., Dhurjati, R., Bristow, E., Bastian, L., Coeytaux, R. R., . . . Lobach, D. (2012). Effect of clinical decision-support systems: A systematic review. *Annals of Internal Medicine, 157,* 29–43. doi: 10.7326/0003-4819-157-1-201207030-00450

Buntin, M. B., Burke, M. F., Hoaglin, M. C., & Blumenthal, D. (2011). The benefits of health information technology: A review of the recent literature shows predominantly positive results. *Health Affairs, 30,* 464–471. doi: 10.1377/hlthaff.2011.0178

Buntin, M. B., Jain, S. H., & Blumenthal, D. (2010). Health information technology: Laying the infrastructure for national health reform. *Health Affairs, 29,* 1214–1219. doi: 10.1377/hlthaff.2010.0503

Campbell, S. R., Holter, M. C., Manthey, T. J., & Rapp, C. A. (2014). The effect of CommonGround software and decision support center. *American Journal of Psychiatric Rehabilitation, 17.* 166–180. doi: 10.1080/15487768.2014.916126

Carspecken, C. W., Sharek, P. J., Longhurst, C., & Pageler, N. M. (2013). A clinical case of electronic health record drug alert fatigue: Consequences for patient outcome. *Pediatrics, 131,* e1970–e1973. doi: 10.1542/peds.2012-3252

Center for Connected Health Policy. (2015). *State telehealth policies and reimbursement schedules: A comprehensive plan of the 50 states and District of Columbia.* Sacramento, CA: Center for Connected Health Policy. Retrieved from http://cchpca.org/sites/default/files/uploader/50%20STATE%20MEDICAID%20REPORT%20SEPT%202014.pdf

DesRoches, C. M., Campbell, E. G., Rao, S. R., Donelan, K., Ferris, T. G., Jha, A., . . . Blumenthal, D. (2008). Electronic health records in ambulatory care—A national survey of physicians. *New England Journal of Medicine, 359,* 50–60. doi: 10.1056/NEJMsa0802005

DesRoches, C. M., Painter, M. W., & Jha, A. K. (2015). *Health information technology in the United States, 2015: Transition to a post-HITECH world.* Princeton, NJ: Robert Wood Johnson Foundation. Retrieved from http://www.rwjf.org/content/dam/farm/reports/reports/2015/rwjf423440

Donker, T., Petrie, K., Proudfoot, J., Clarke, J., Birch, M.-R., & Christensen, H. (2013). Smartphones for smarter delivery of mental health programs: A systematic review. *Journal of Medical Internet Research, 15,* e247l. doi: 10.2196/jmir.2791

Federal Office of Rural Health Policy, Health Resources and Services Administration, U.S. Department of Health & Human Services. (2015, November). Telehealth programs. Retrieved from http://www.hrsa.gov/ruralhealth/telehealth/

Fisher, E. B., Ballesteros, J., Bhushan, N., Coufal, M. M., Kowitt, S. D., McDonough, A. M., . . . Urlaub, D. (2015). Key features of peer support in chronic disease prevention and management. *Health Affairs, 34,* 1523–1530. doi: 10.1377/hlthaff.2015.0365

Gellis, Z. D., Kenaley, B. L., & Have, T. T. (2014). Integrated telehealth care for chronic illness and depression in geriatric home care patients: The integrated telehealth education and activation of mood (I-TEAM) study. *Journal of the American Geriatrics Society, 62,* 889–895. doi: 10.1111/jgs.12776

Gold, M. R., McLaughlin, C. G., Devers, K. J., Bersonson, R. A. & Bovbjerg, R. R. (2012). Obtaining providers' 'buy-in' and establishing effective means of information exchange will be critical to HITECH's success. *Health Affairs, 31,* 514–526. doi: 10.1377/hlthaff.2011.0753

Gottlieb, S. C., & Blum, K. (2006). Coordinated care, telemonitoring, and the therapeutic relationship: Heart failure management in the United States. *Disease Management & Health Outcomes, 14*(Suppl. 1), 29–31. doi: 10.2165/00115677-200614001-00008

Hilty, D. M., Ferrer, D. C., Parish. M. B., Johnston, B., Callahan, E. J., & Yellowlees, P. M. (2013). The effectiveness of telemental health: A 2013 review. *Telemedicine and e-Health, 19,* 444–454. doi: 10.1089/tmj.2013.0075

Irwin, K. (2013, August 19). Patient portal preferences: IndustryView 2014. Software advice. Retrieved from http://www.softwareadvice.com/medical/industryview/patient-portals-2014/

Jamoom, E., & Hing, E. (2015). *Progress with electronic health record adoption among emergency and outpatient departments: United States, 2006-2011* (NCHS Data Brief No. 187). Hyattsville, MD: National Center for Health Statistics, Centers for Disease Control and Prevention, U.S. Department of Health & Human Services. Retrieved from http://www.cdc.gov/nchs/data/databriefs/db187.pdf

Kaufman, J. M. (2012). *Practitioner perspectives on the impact of collaborative documentation on the therapeutic alliance.* (Master of Social Work Clinical Research Paper No. 44). St. Paul, MN: School of Social Work, St. Catherine University & University of St. Thomas. Retrieved from http://sophia.stkate.edu/cgi/viewcontent.cgi?article=1044&context=msw_papers

Konrad, T. R., Ellis, A. R., Thomas, K. C., Holzer, C. E., & Morrissey, J. P. (2009). County-level estimates of need for mental health professionals in the United States. *Psychiatric Services, 60,* 1307–1314. doi: 10.1176/ps.2009.60.10.1307

Kawamoto, K., Houlihan, C. A., Balas, E. A., & Lobach, D. F. (2005). Improving clinical practice using clinical decision support systems: A systematic review of trials to identify features critical to success. *The BMJ, 330,* 765. doi: 10.1136/bmj.38398.500764.8F

Larsson, S., Lawyer, P., Garellick, G., Lindahl, B., & Lundström, M. (2011). Use of 13 disease registries in 5 countries demonstrates the potential to use outcome data to improve health care's value. *Health Affairs, 31,* 220–227. doi: 10.1377/hlthaff.2011.0762

Liu, J., Luo, L., Zhang, R., & Huang, T. (2013). Patient satisfaction with electronic medical/health record: A systematic review. *Scandinavian Journal of Caring Sciences, 27,* 785–791. doi: 10.1111/scs.12015

Matthews, E. B. (2015). Integrating the electronic health record into behavioral health encounters: Strategies, barriers, and implications for practice. *Administration and Policy in Mental Health and Mental Health Services Research,* 1–12. doi: 10.1007/s10488-015-0676-3

McCoy, A. B., Waitman, L. R., Lewis, J. B., Wright, J. A., Choma, D. P., Miller, R. A., & Peterson, J. F. (2012). A framework for evaluating the appropriateness of clinical decision support alerts and responses. *Journal of the American Medical Informatics Association, 19,* 346–352. doi: 10.1136/amiajnl-2011-000185

National Council for Community Behavioral Healthcare. (2012). *HIT adoption and readiness for meaningful use in community behavioral health: Report on the 2012 National Council survey.* Washington,

DC: National Council for Community Behavioral Healthcare. Retrieved from https://www.thenation-alcouncil.org/wp-content/uploads/2012/10/HIT-Survey-Full-Report.pdf

Office of the Federal Register. (2002). *Standards for privacy of individually identifiable health information* (45 CFR Parts 160 & 164). Washington, DC: U.S. Department of Health & Human Services. Retrieved from https://www.gpo.gov/fdsys/pkg/FR-2002-08-14/pdf/02-20554.pdf

Office of the National Coordinator for Health Information Technology (ONC). (2013, January 15). Basics of health IT. Retrieved from https://www.healthit.gov/patients-families/basics-health-it

Office of the National Coordinator for Health Information Technology (ONC). (2016, September 20). ONC Health IT Certificate Program. Retrieved from https://www.healthit.gov/policy-researchers-implementers/about-onc-health-it-certification-program

President's Council of Advisors on Science and Technology. (2010). *Report to the president realizing the full potential of health information technology to improve healthcare for Americans: The path forward.* Washington, DC: Executive Office of the President. Retrieved from https://www.whitehouse.gov/sites/default/files/microsites/ostp/pcast-health-it-report.pdf

Schmelter, B. (2012). Implementing collaborative documentation: Making it happen! [PowerPoint slides]. Retrieved from http://www.integration.samhsa.gov/pbhci-learning-community/jun_2012_-_collaborative_documentation.pdf

Stanhope, V., Ingoglia, C., Schmelter, B., & Marcus, S. C. (2013). Impact of person-centered planning and collaborative documentation on treatment adherence. *Psychiatric Services, 64,* 76–79. doi: 10.1176/appi.ps.201100489

Tomlinson, M., Rotheram-Borus, M., Swartz, L., & Tsai, A. C. (2013). Scaling up mHealth: Where is the evidence? *PLOS Medicine, 10,* e1001382. doi: 10.1371/journal.pmed.1001382

Wilson, L. S., & Maeder, A. J. (2015). Recent directions in telemedicine: Review of trends in research and practice. *Healthcare Informatics Research, 21,* 213–222. doi: 10.4258/hir.2015.21.4.213

CHAPTER 17

EVALUATING INTEGRATED HEALTH CARE

Benjamin F. Henwood, Elizabeth Siantz, and Todd P. Gilmer

Integrated health care is critical to achieving the Triple Aim of improved health outcomes and service user experience at lower costs (Berwick, Nolan, & Whittington, 2008) (see Chapter 1). Although specific models of integrated health care are supported by empirical research, it remains to be seen whether public health systems that serve vulnerable populations can be successfully redesigned to deliver integrated health care under the Patient Protection and Affordable Care Act (ACA). Although controlled trials can provide an empirical basis for the efficacy of integrated health care models, methods examining the effectiveness of integrated health care in real-world settings are not well established.

This chapter reviews factors to consider when evaluating implementation of integrated health care. They include selecting outcomes to measure the Triple Aim, deciding how to measure the process of integration, determining the importance of and strategies for stakeholder buy-in, and delineating the relationship between evaluations of integrated health care and quality improvement. Throughout the chapter, examples are provided from a large-scale evaluation of integrated health care programs in Los Angeles County (LAC), California, where the Department of Mental Health (DMH) funded three types of integrated models between 2012 and 2015 that were designed for specific subpopulations of people with severe mental illnesses (Gilmer, Henwood, Goode, Sarkin, & Innes-Gomberg, 2016; Siantz, Henwood, & Gilmer, 2016).

The Integrated Mobile Health Team Model provided housing support and team-based services for people who were homeless; the teams followed an assertive community treatment (ACT) model with embedded primary care. The Integrated Clinic Model paired community mental health centers with community health clinics (often Federally Qualified Health Centers) to coordinate mental and physical health care. Finally, the Integrated Service Management Models were designed by and targeted specific racial and ethnic communities that have been traditionally underrepresented or underserved by the public mental health system, such as Latinos, Asians and Pacific Islanders, Africans and African Americans, Native Americans and Alaskan Natives, and Middle Easterners. These programs focused on cultural competency and cultural concordance, community-specific outreach and education, and the use of nontraditional or wellness services. Funding for all of these programs was available through the Mental Health Services Act, which was approved by California voters in 2004 and applies a tax of 1% on incomes higher than $1 million to fund public mental health services (Scheffler & Adams, 2005).

MEASURING INTEGRATED HEALTH CARE

Despite a widespread focus on integrated health care, there is a surprising lack of consensus on how to operationalize and measure integration. Heath, Wise Romero, and Reynolds (2013) observed that "until there is a way to reliably categorize integration implementations, meaningful comparisons of implementations or associated health outcomes cannot occur" (p. 3). Much of the literature that supports the conclusion that integrated health care results in improved outcomes has focused on a specific intervention targeting a single mental health diagnosis (e.g., depression). The Improving Mood—Promoting Access to Collaborative Treatment (IMPACT) model, which is a team-based approach in a primary care setting, has proved effective as a chronic disease management program for older adults with depression (Unützer et al., 2001) (see Chapter 8). Other models that have focused on physical health outcomes among people with severe mental illnesses, such as Primary Care Access Referral and Evaluation (PCARE) (Druss et al., 2010), have also shown favorable outcomes, such as higher rates of screening and improvements in cardiometabolic conditions. But the broader impact of integrated health care on multiple comorbid physical and mental health conditions is not well established.

Health care reform has acknowledged the importance of measuring outcomes that are personcentered when developing novel approaches to integrated health care. The Patient-Centered Outcomes Research Institute (PCORI), which is a private nonprofit corporation, was created by the ACA in 2010. This was done in an effort to produce and promote high-integrity, evidence-based information derived from research guided not only by health care providers and researchers but also by service users and caregivers (Selby, Beal, & Frank, 2012). The main purpose of PCORI is to improve the quality and relevance of evidence available for helping service users, caregivers, clinicians, employers, insurers, and policy makers make informed decisions about health care.

Patient-centeredness is a guiding principle of PCORI's work because findings from traditional medical research are often unavailable to service users and caregivers. The goal is to determine which health care options work best for which service users and under which circumstances. PCORI's approach is engaging service users and other members of the health care community in all aspects of the research process. PCORI has made several funding opportunities available that can be used for projects related to the implementation of integrated primary and behavioral health care services. Findings on integrated health care from projects funded by PCORI have begun to be disseminated (Corrigan, Torres, Lara, Sheehan, & Larson, 2016; Fortney, 2015) and will likely contribute to the evidence base for integrated health care in the coming years. Table 17.1 describes PCORI's current priorities.

Feature	Description
Mission	PCORI helps people make informed health care decisions and improves health care delivery and outcomes by producing and promoting high-integrity, evidence-based information that comes from research guided by service users, caregivers, and the broader health care community.
National priorities	• Assessment of prevention, diagnosis, and treatment options • Improving health care systems • Communication and dissemination research • Addressing disparities • Accelerating patient-centered outcomes research and methodological research
Scientific programs	• Clinical effectiveness research (CER) • Improving health care systems • Communication and dissemination research • Addressing disparities • CER methods and infrastructure • Evaluation and analysis • Engagement

THE NEED FOR PROCESS AND OUTCOMES EVALUATION

The goal of comprehensive system improvement has been described as achieving the Triple Aim of improving health outcomes, reducing costs, and increasing patient satisfaction (see Chapter 1). Some have advocated for a Quadruple Aim, which includes improving the experiences of health care providers and others working in health service systems (Bodenheimer & Sinsky, 2014; Sikka, Morath, & Leape, 2015). Establishing clear goals for integrated health care initiatives is an important step that should drive the selection of outcome measures. Given the limited amount of research on the process of integrating care and the lack of clearly articulated standards of fidelity in an effective or ideal integrated health care model, evaluating the process or implementation of integrated health care initiatives is important and can provide guidance on promising practices. Outcome and implementation evaluations were undertaken for the LAC DMH integrated health care demonstration and are described in the following sections.

OUTCOMES MEASUREMENT

Selecting measures to evaluate community practices can be challenging. Resource availability and response burden are important considerations when selecting outcome measures. Measures must be valid, easy for service users to complete, and easy for staff to administer and evaluate. The use of existing clinical and administrative data for outcome measurement is recommended, although the stage of program development may influence this decision. For example, programs in the beginning stages of developing an integrated health care program may not have established measures or experience in measurement, whereas programs further along in the developmental stages may have established measures. Measures selection must consider the nature of the community and populations being served. Factors that may affect the validity and reliability of such measures include race, gender, culture, community values, language, socioeconomic status, and day-to-day experiences (Barth, Courtney, Needell, & Jonson-Reid, 1994).

To select outcome measures for the LAC DMH integrated health care demonstration project, we followed the recommendations of Cross and McDonald (1995), who described six factors to consider when identifying and selecting appropriate outcome measures for community practices:

1. Identify outcomes related to program goals.
2. Consider the level of program development.
3. Involve stakeholders.
4. Assess resource availability and scarcity.
5. Identify sources of information.
6. Consider the nature of the population.

This resulted in the selection of several key outcome measures, including the Illness Management of Recovery Scale (Sklar, Sarkin, Gilmer, & Groessl, 2012) and measures from the Patient-Reported Outcomes Measurement Information System (PROMIS) (Broderick, DeWitt, Rothrock, Crane, & Forrest, 2013). PROMIS was launched by the National Institutes of Health in 2004 as part of an effort to provide some standardization of service user–reported outcome measures that would enable comparison across studies and illnesses (Broderick et al., 2013). PROMIS is intended to make the selection of measures easier by providing item banks of questions from which researchers can draw. PROMIS items are designed to be *efficient,* so that reliability is maintained even if only a limited number of items is selected; *flexible,* so that one has the option of selecting different items that can be used interchangeably; and *precise,* so that there is minimal estimation error (Cella et al., 2010).

PROMIS can serve as a valuable resource for researchers who are studying integrated health care and examining multiple health outcomes for one or more populations. For the LAC integrated health care project, we selected the global health scale that included subscales for physical, mental, and social health. Items to measure substance misuse outcomes were also derived from the PROMIS system. These measures were sufficient for evaluating whether programs were achieving the project's stated goal of improving physical and behavioral health outcomes (Gilmer et al., 2016).

MEASURING INTEGRATION PROCESS

Another goal of the LAC DMH integrated health care demonstration project was to better understand how programs integrate care. We considered one possible framework that is known as the standard for levels of integrated health care and was proposed by the Center for Integrated Health Solutions (CIHS) of the Substance Abuse and Mental Health Services Administration–Health Resources and Services Administration (SAMHSA-HRSA) (see Chapter 8). This overall framework organizes levels of health care integration into three main categories: coordinated, co-located, and integrated health care. Each category contains beginning and advanced collaboration levels, resulting in six levels of integration. How to assess which level of integration any particular program falls into, however, has not been clearly established.

Because there is limited guidance on how to measure integration, the authors attempted to assess integration in two ways. The first was through the use of the Integrated Treatment Tool (ITT), which was developed through a SAMHSA grant and was intended to provide a framework to guide implementation of a person-centered health home for individuals with severe mental health conditions (Center for Evidence-Based Practices, 2011). The second way in which we attempted to measure integration was through social network analysis (SNA) of teams that were charged with integrating care.

Integrated Treatment Tool. The ITT identifies three main domains of integration: *organizational characteristics*, *treatment characteristics*, and *care coordination characteristics*. Organizational characteristics refer to the structural aspects of implementation, including the operational and fiscal partnerships between primary and behavioral health organizations. Treatment characteristics refer to the clinical components of implementation, including the presence and quality of the services and interventions that are employed. Care coordination characteristics refer to a set of activities designed to increase access, improve health-related outcomes, and decrease fragmentation of care.

To administer the ITT, three trained evaluators spent a full day at each site to rate its integrated program on the 30 items in the ITT (see Table 17.2). Each item is subsumed under one of the three main domains and is rated on a 5-point scale from low to high. Site visits included interviews with staff as the primary source of data, but additional information was obtained through observation of program activities (e.g., service user groups, staff meetings), review of program documents (e.g., policy and procedure manuals, clinical forms, charts), and a tour of the program facility.

Social network analysis of integrated health care teams. Another method we used to measure integration was the SNA of care providers. Interdisciplinary, team-based approaches are essential for delivering integrated health care to people with multiple chronic conditions. SNA techniques illustrate communication between providers and allow researchers to visualize the complex systems of relationships that occur in integrated health care teams. SNA can also examine team cohesion in newly integrated health care coordination networks by illustrating which people in the network communicate with the others (Burt, 2004; Meltzer et al., 2010).

The evaluation team conducted an SNA survey to understand whether and how providers within each integrated program communicated with one another and the extent to which primary care professionals were involved with newly integrated teams. To collect the social network data, survey participants were given a roster of their team members and asked a series of questions related to who they communicated with regarding service user care. They were then asked whether this communication occurred during or outside

Integrated Treatment Organizational Characteristics

IT O1. Organizational philosophy

IT O2. Organizational policies and procedures

IT O3. Integrated health information/technology

IT O4. Multidisciplinary health care approach

IT O5. Interdisciplinary communication

IT O6. Care manager

IT O7. Peer supports

IT O8. Organization-wide training

IT O9. Clinical supervision, guidance, and monitoring

IT O10. Continuous quality improvement

IT O11. Patient-centered approach

IT O12. Patient access and scheduling

IT O13. Executive leadership team involvement

IT O14. Integrated approach

Integrated Treatment Characteristics

IT T1. Comprehensive identification

IT T2. Holistic integrated care plan

IT T3. Integrated stage-appropriate treatment

IT T4. Outreach

IT T5. Stepped care

IT T6. Use of motivational interventions

IT T7. Self-management skill development

IT T8. Pharmacological approaches

IT T9. Involvement of social support network

Integrated Treatment Care Coordination and Management Characteristics

IT C1. Care coordination: activities, elements, and domains

IT C2. Laboratory and test tracking

IT C3. Referral facilitation and tracking

IT C4. Medication reconciliation

IT C5. Reminders

IT C6. Transitions between settings or levels of care

IT C7. Assessing the effectiveness or quality of care received

of team meetings and the extent to which it involved text messages, phone calls, emails, or video conferences.

To understand the degree to which integrated teams are interconnected (i.e., how many people are communicating with one another in a given network), the evaluation team calculated *network density scores* for each integrated health care program. Density scores represent the number of *existing* connections between providers in a network relative to the number of all *possible* connections within that network. Network density can be calculated by counting the number of actual connections or direct lines of communication between providers and dividing that number by the total number of possible connections or direct lines of communication. A density network score of 1 means that everyone is in communication with everyone else, whereas a score of 0 indicates that no one is in communication (Valente, 2010).

Although density speaks to the characteristics of an entire network, positional analyses such as *centrality* focus on the connections of specific network members. Centrality refers to the number of connections an individual network member has; it measures how well connected an individual is within a network (Valente, 2010). We used the concept of centrality to better understand the network positions that medical providers have within and across programs and to achieve a deeper understanding of how medical providers are integrated within team-based care. We did this by calculating the proportion of people who reported working directly with medical staff and comparing that number with the proportion working with other types of staff (e.g., social workers, peer specialists). We found that programs with more central medical staff also scored higher on the ITT. This suggests that SNA may provide a snapshot of the extent to which team members have direct interaction with one another and with medical staff and can serve as a reasonable proxy for the extent of integration within a given health care team. However, measures such as centrality do not necessarily speak to the effectiveness of communications or the quality of care coordination.

Study findings. Although there remains a need for a validated instrument to measure integration, the authors found that programs with higher ITT scores (i.e., higher integration) tended to have better service user outcomes (Gilmer et al., 2016). Using SNA, we also found that integration and high levels of communication are strongly related—one is unlikely to occur without the other. Integrated programs with more dense (i.e., tightly connected) networks were more likely to have higher amounts of communication with medical providers. Most interdisciplinary communication occurred during team meetings, suggesting the value of protected time to improve care coordination. Nevertheless, both formal program infrastructures (e.g., team meetings) and informal modes of communication (e.g., texting, video conferencing) appeared to facilitate integrated health care.

EVALUATION LESSONS LEARNED

In addition to the integrated health care findings obtained over the course of the 3-year LAC DMH project, we learned several lessons related to the evaluation of integrated health care.

USE OF DATA

Providers initially had many practical concerns about the use of data that were being collected to measure service user outcomes and integration. For example, they were concerned that data reported by service users might not be accurate due to translation issues, cultural sensitivity, or social desirability. Because data collection is a time-consuming process, providers were also concerned about how to ensure that data were accurately entered into the system and wanted to understand how to use outcome measures in their clinical practice. LAC DMH and the evaluation team implemented several techniques to encourage the constructive use of data, including discussions at learning sessions, group trainings focused on the clinical use of data, and programs sharing with each other how the data were used.

One important factor that facilitated the use of data was the development by the evaluation team of an electronic data management system that was made available to the programs. This involved close interaction between the designers of the system and its stakeholders. New features were regularly added to the electronic data system based on feedback from providers and LAC DMH, including more efficient ways of tracking service user assessments and more functional reports. This interactive relationship helped ensure that the system's features, such as live reporting and access to raw data, offered value to providers and the LAC DMH. It was important for help desk staff to be consistently accessible because this allowed dialogue between system designers and system users. Along with regular training sessions, the help desk improved providers' comfort and ability to use the system. The dialogue also helped to develop upgrades to the system, such as progress bars and notification alerts, which further enhanced user satisfaction. Today, there are several data management systems and electronic health records on the market for programs to purchase, and they have been tested and are being continually upgraded.

For the LAC DMH integrated health care project, several technical details of the system proved essential for providers—primary among them was a secure connection to the internet. The file share system that was set up was crucial to allow secure transfer of data files. The web-based system allowed access by providers from computers or mobile devices without downloading software or an application. Tablets were distributed to providers at the beginning of the evaluation to determine whether they would streamline the data collection and management process. Although several providers successfully incorporated the tablets into their protocol, they were not widely adopted due to slow page loading and a primarily older population that was more comfortable using paper assessments.

Over time, programs began to use and embrace the data at different levels. Clinicians used the data to improve care and to converse with service users to show change and progress; providers used the data to change and improve aspects of their programs; and LAC DMH used the data to provide additional technical assistance and to decide which programs should continue to receive funding after the demonstration project was over.

The data culture spread as providers began to see the benefits of using data to enhance their services and improve care for service users. For example, several programs reported increased service user engagement and goal setting when they were able to show health status over time. Data provision also brought new transparency in terms of which programs were improving outcomes. It will be important moving forward to continue to use data for learning and not as punishment, which could affect openness to sharing less positive results. Underperformance on outcome measures often prompted providers to implement some of their most successful and engaging service offerings.

While providers learned how to improve their integrated programs, the evaluation team learned how to engage providers in the evaluation and how to meet the needs of a diverse set of stakeholders. There were several barriers to measurement collection that had to be overcome through the course of the evaluation. Despite the differences between programs, the evaluation components were standardized so that the outcomes for each program would be comparable. These components captured most of the goals for the providers but limited our ability to look closer at the unique aspects of each program. It was not until late in the evaluation that some providers expressed a desire to include additional measures. For example, one group of providers wanted to more consistently track the effects of nontraditional services.

Although providers had the opportunity to add measures at the beginning of the evaluation, they were not fully engaged at that point. They might have been more willing to suggest additional measures after receiving the evaluation trainings and learning how the measures would be used by LAC DMH and could be used internally to improve services. Instead of adding new quantitative measures, the evaluation team implemented several qualitative studies that focused on topics such as interagency communication, cultural competency and nontraditional services, and the implementation of peer providers (Siantz et al., 2016). These studies provided great context for the outcome measures, but they could have been supplemented with more targeted outcome measures.

CONCLUSIONS

As health care systems increasingly move to provide integrated behavioral and primary care that is data driven, methods to evaluate the delivery of care are needed. This chapter reviewed a systematic process for selecting outcome measures, new methods for understanding processes of integrated health care and program implementation, and strategies and lessons learned for approaching evaluation efforts.

Although health care reform has offered an opportunity to transform systems of care, innovation and experimentation are still needed to discover evidence-based approaches to integrated health care that can work with diverse populations and settings. Research funded by institutions such as PCORI will increasingly need to include members from these diverse communities, which will ultimately contribute to the development of person-centered, evidence-based integrated health care. The systematic evaluation of integrated health care initiatives and dissemination of the findings will help increase the pace of transformation to more quickly address ongoing health disparities among people with mental and physical health needs.

RESOURCES

About the Center for Integrated Health Solutions (CIHS), Substance Abuse and Mental Health Services Administration-Health Resources and Services Administration (SAMHSA-HRSA) http://www.integration.samhsa.gov/about-us/about-cihs

Academy for Integrating Behavioral Health and Primary Care (The Academy), Agency for Healthcare Research and Quality (AHRQ), U.S. Department of Health & Human Services (DHHS) https://integrationacademy.ahrq.gov

Behavioral Health Integration Capacity Assessment Tool, Institute for Healthcare Improvement (IHI) http://www.ihi.org/resources/Pages/Tools/BehavioralHealthIntegrationCapacityAssessmentTool.aspx

International Journal of Integrated Care (IJIC) http://www.ijic.org

Patient-Centered Outcomes Research Institute (PCORI) http://www.pcori.org/

Resources for Integrated Care Available for Health Plans and Providers, Centers for Medicare & Medicaid Services (CMS) https://www.cms.gov/Medicare-Medicaid-Coordination/Medicare-and-Medicaid-Coordination/Medicare-Medicaid-Coordination-Office/ResourcesforIntegratedCareAvailableforHealthPlansandProviders.html

Social Work and Integrated Behavioral Healthcare Project, Council on Social Work Education (CSWE) http://www.cswe.org/CentersInitiatives/DataStatistics/IntegratedCare.aspx

REFERENCES

Barth, R. P., Courtney, M. E., Needell, B., & Jonson-Reid, M. (1994). *Performance indicators for child welfare services in California: Executive summary*. Berkeley, CA: Child Welfare Research Center, School of Social Welfare, University of California at Berkeley.

Berwick, D. M., Nolan, T. W., & Whittington, J. (2008). The Triple Aim: Care, health, and cost. *Health Affairs, 27*, 759-769. doi: 10.1377/hlthaff.27.3.759

Bodenheimer, T., & Sinsky, C. (2014). From triple to quadruple aim: Care of the patient requires care of the provider. *Annals of Family Medicine, 12*, 573-576. doi: 10.1370/afm.1713

Broderick, J. E., DeWitt, E. M., Rothrock, N., Crane, P. K., & Forrest, C. B. (2013). Advances in patient-reported outcomes: The NIH PROMIS® Measures. *eGEMS, 1*(1), Article No. 12. doi: 10.13063/2327-9214.1015

Burt, R. S. (2004). Structural holes and good ideas. *American Journal of Sociology, 110*, 349-399. doi: 10.1086/421787

Cella, D., Riley, W., Stone, A., Rothrock, N., Reeve, B., Yount, S., . . . Hays, R. (2010). The Patient-Reported Outcomes Measurement Information System (PROMIS) developed and tested its first wave of adult self-reported health outcome item banks: 2005–2008. *Journal of Clinical Epidemiology, 63*, 1179-1194. doi: 10.1016/j.jclinepi.2010.04.011

Center for Evidence-Based Practices. (2011). Integrated Treatment Tool: A tool to evaluate the integration of primary and behavioral health care. Cleveland, OH: Center for Evidence-Based Practices, Case Western Reserve University. Retrieved from http://www.centerforebp.case.edu/client-files/pdf/ipbh-itt.pdf

Corrigan, P. W., Torres, A., Lara, J. L., Sheehan, L., & Larson, J. E. (2016). The healthcare needs of Latinos with serious mental illness and the potential of peer navigators. *Administration and Policy in Mental Health and Mental Health Services Research*, 1-11. doi: 10.1007/s10488-016-0737-2

Cross, T. P., & McDonald, E. (1995). Child and family outcome measures. In *Evaluating the outcome of children's mental health services: A guide for the use of available child and family outcome measures*. Boston, MA: Technical Assistance Center for the Evaluation of Children's Mental Health Systems, Judge Baker Children's Center.

Druss, B. G., von Esenwein, S. A., Compton, M. T., Rask, K. J., Zhao, L., & Parker, R. M. (2010). A randomized trial of medical care management for community mental health settings: The Primary Care

Access, Referral, and Evaluation (PCARE) study. *The American Journal of Psychiatry, 167,* 151–159. doi: 10.1176/appi.ajp.2009.09050691

Fortney, J. C. (2015). Integrated versus referral care for complex psychiatric disorders in rural FQHCs. PCORI. Retrieved from http://www.pcori.org/research-results/2015/integrated-versus-referral-care-complex-psychiatric-disorders-rural-fqhcs

Gilmer, T. P., Henwood, B. F., Goode, M., Sarkin, A. J., & Innes-Gomberg, D. (2016). Implementation of integrated health homes and health outcomes for persons with serious mental illness in Los Angeles County. *Psychiatric Services, 67,* 1062-1067. doi: 10.1176/appi.ps.201500092

Heath, B., Wise Romero, P., & Reynolds, K. (2013). *A standard framework for levels of integrated healthcare.* Washington, DC: Center for Integrated Health Solutions, Substance Abuse and Mental Health Services Administration-Health Resources and Service Administration. Retrieved from http://www.integration.samhsa.gov/integrated-care   models/A_Standard_Framework_for_Levels_of_Integrated_Healthcare.pdf

Meltzer, D., Chung, J., Khalili, P., Marlow, E., Arora, V., Schumock, G., & Burt, R. (2010). Exploring the use of social network methods in designing healthcare quality improvement teams. *Social Science & Medicine, 71,* 1119–1130. doi: 10.1016/j.socscimed.2010.05.012

Selby, J. V., Beal, A. C., & Frank, L. (2012). The Patient-Centered Outcomes Research Institute (PCORI) national priorities for research and initial research agenda. *Journal of the American Medical Association, 307,* 1583-1584. doi: 10.1001/jama.2012.500

Scheffler, R. M., & Adams, N. (2005). Millionaires and mental health: Proposition 63 in California. *Health Affairs, 24,* Web Exclusive 5. doi: 10.1377/hlthaff.w5.212

Siantz, E., Henwood, B., & Gilmer, T. (2016). Implementation of peer providers in integrated mental health and primary care settings. *Journal of the Society for Social Work and Research, 7,* 231-246. Available from http://www.journals.uchicago.edu/toc/jsswr/current

Sikka, R., Morath, J. M., & Leape, L. (2015). The Quadruple Aim: Care, health, cost and meaning in work. *BMJ Quality & Safety, 24,* 608-610. doi: 10.1136/bmjqs-2015-004160

Sklar, M., Sarkin, A., Gilmer, T., & Groessl, E. (2012). The psychometric properties of the Illness Management and Recovery scale in a large American public mental health system. *Psychiatry Research, 199,* 220-227. doi: 10.1016/j.psychres.2012.03.013

Unützer, J., Katon, W., Williams, J. W., Jr., Callahan, C. M., Harpole, L., Hunkeler, E. M., . . . Langston, C. A. (2001). Improving primary care for depression in late life: The design of a multicenter randomized trial. *Medical Care, 39,* 785–799. Available from http://journals.lww.com/lww-medicalcare/pages/default.aspx

Valente, T. W. (2010). *Social networks and health: Models, methods, and applications.* New York, NY: Oxford University Press.

GLOSSARY

ACCOUNTABLE CARE ORGANIZATION (ACO) A financing model composed of a group of doctors, hospitals, primary care settings, and other providers who work together to provide coordinated care. ACOs often utilize patient-centered medical homes to coordinate care across different sectors. The model has been largely targeted towards the Medicare population. Similar to managed care entities, ACOs receive a set amount of "capitated" funding per service user and take on the risk of providing care within this budget. If the ACO reduces costs and provides quality care, they receive financial rewards which are shared among provider entities.

THE AFFORDABLE CARE ACT (ACA) Federal legislation designed to implement comprehensive health care reform. Also referred to as the Patient Protection and Affordable Care Act or "Obamacare," the ACA was passed in 2010. The legislation aimed to reform public and private health care systems through insurance expansion, system redesign, and payment reform using both mandates and incentives.

BEHAVIORAL HEALTH CARE Health care that addresses any behavior-related problems that result in adverse health outcomes (including mental health and substance use conditions, physical ailments that are stress induced, and health behaviors). This care is delivered by providers of various disciplines.

CARE MANAGEMENT A strategy to ensure that service users do not "fall through the cracks" during service delivery. This consists of a set of activities designed to help service users and their support systems in more effectively managing medical conditions and psychosocial problems through measures such as service user activation and education, care coordination, person-centered care plans, and the monitoring of participation in response to treatment.

CENTERS FOR MEDICARE AND MEDICAID SERVICES (CMS) AND THE CMS INNOVATION CENTER CMS is the U.S. federal agency that administers Medicare, Medicaid, and the Children's Health Insurance Program. The CMS Innovation Center is the part of CMS that is responsible for developing ways to integrate primary, acute, behavioral, and long-term care using approaches such as penalizing avoidable hospital readmissions, sharing savings and bonuses with providers when they reduce costs, and improving quality through ACOs.

CHILDREN'S HEALTH INSURANCE PROGRAM (CHIP) Originally known as the State Children's Health Insurance Program, CHIP was established in 1997 as part of the Balanced Budget Act. The program provides health insurance to children from families whose income is modest but not sufficiently low to qualify for Medicaid.

CHRONIC CARE MODEL (CCM) An organizing framework for health homes. This model promotes features of self-management support, delivery system design, decision support, clinical information systems, and community linkages, all of which are aimed at improving health care and health outcomes while simultaneously reducing costs for people with chronic illnesses.

COLLABORATIVE CARE Also known as the IMPACT model, collaborative care is based in primary care settings. Using a team of interdisciplinary providers that includes a depression care manager and a psychiatric consultant, collaborative care screens, tracks and coordinates care for depression in primary care settings. The model was originally designed for older adults but is now employed to treat all adults.

CO-LOCATED CARE A method of care integration in which behavioral health and primary care providers deliver services within the same geographical location. This system also involves professionals working in shared spaces. The aim of co-located care is to achieve shared workflows, culture, and collaboration.

COMORBIDITY When two disorders or illnesses occur in the same person—simultaneously or sequentially—they are referred to as being *comorbid*. Comorbidity also implies interactions between the illnesses that affect the course and prognosis of both.

COORDINATED CARE A method of care in which two or more providers collaborate to appropriately deliver health care services. This involves collaboration among personnel and other resources to carry out all necessary activities as well as an exchange of information among participants who are responsible for the various aspects of care.

DECISION AIDS Tools that facilitate decision-making regarding screening and health care treatment in order to supplement counseling by describing options and outcomes in sufficient detail. Components include exercises for clarification of values, probabilities of outcomes tailored to the service user's health profile, and balanced examples of others' experiences with decision-making.

DECISION SUPPORT A person-centered approach that integrates a service user's individual values, personal resources, and self-determination into health care decision-making. Decision support interventions are currently being developed to supplement counseling by practitioners because of the complexity of many health treatment and screening decisions.

DUAL ELIGIBLES Individuals who are eligible for both Medicare and Medicaid benefits.

ELECTRONIC HEALTH RECORD (EHR) EHRs are computerized systems used to securely store, access, and exchange health information. They facilitate the exchange of information necessary for care coordination, provide mechanisms for guiding evidence-based clinical decisions, and create tools for population management and tracking.

EVIDENCE-BASED PRACTICE (EBP) Clinical practice that integrates the best available research evidence, clinical expertise, and service user values and preferences. EBP is a process of decision-making designed to determine what the best care is for an individual, group, or population. EBP should be distinguished from evidence-based practices or evidence-supported treatments, which refer to clinical interventions that have been rigorously tested using scientific methods such as randomized controlled trials and have been found to be effective.

HEALTH DISPARITIES The differences in health care and health status among populations. Health care disparities are evidenced by irregularities in access to or availability of facilities and services. Health disparities are evidenced by variation in prevalence and severity of illnesses and disabilities among groups based on differences such as race, ethnicity, sexual orientation, gender, socioeconomic status, and geographic location.

HEALTH HOME An integrated care model in which all of an individual's providers and caregivers communicate with one another, ensuring a person's needs are addressed in a comprehensive manner. Promoted by the ACA, Medicaid Health Homes specifically target the needs of Medicaid enrollees who have high volumes of inpatient episodes or complex conditions, including mental health and substance use problems.

HEALTH INSURANCE EXCHANGE One of the ACA's key strategies for expanding access to health care insurance, health insurance exchanges provide a central marketplace where individuals and employers without health insurance can learn about their insurance options, compare plans, and purchase insurance. These can be administered at the federal or state level.

HOME AND COMMUNITY-BASED SERVICES (HCBS) HCBS programs provide opportunities for Medicaid beneficiaries to receive services in their own home or community rather than within institutions or other isolated settings. These programs serve a variety of targeted population groups, including people with intellectual or developmental disabilities, physical disabilities, and/or mental illnesses.

INTEGRATED HEALTH CARE Health care that involves collaboration among providers across settings (e.g., behavioral health and primary care), including frequent communication and the use of one unified treatment plan. This operation is viewed as a single system treating the whole person, and it may result in the physical transformation of a practice or consolidation of multiple practices.

INTERPROFESSIONAL PRACTICE A practice mode in which multiple providers from different disciplines collaborate, often in teams, to deliver services to one person. They all share responsibility for the care provided and adopt a person-centered approach when working with individuals.

MANAGED CARE A system or network of providers that is organized to manage the cost, utilization, and quality of care. Managed care is employed within both the public and private health care sectors; strategies include use of copayments, deductibles, gatekeeping, and capitation payments.

MEDICAID A means-tested government benefit that provides health care insurance for low-income families and individuals. Medicaid is jointly funded by the federal and state governments and is managed at the state level. Because states have some discretion in eligibility requirements and benefits, there is variation in the Medicaid program across states.

MEDICAL MODEL A traditional health care model in which the physician is responsible for diagnosing the illness, deciding on an appropriate treatment, and ensuring that treatment is carried out as prescribed.

MEDICARE A universal government benefit that provides health care insurance for individuals who are 65 years of age or older or who have a disability. Medicare is administered by the federal government and includes plans that cover inpatient care, outpatient care, and prescription drugs.

MENTAL HEALTH PARITY The recognition that behavioral health conditions are equivalent to physical illnesses and should therefore be covered equally by health care insurance. Legislation at the federal and state levels over the past 2 decades has sought to achieve parity in public and private health insurance benefits for mental health and substance use disorders. Parity in health insurance includes conditions covered, co-pays, deductibles, and lifetime caps.

MENTAL HEALTH RECOVERY Although there is no universally agreed-upon definition, the U.S. Substance Abuse and Mental Health Services Administration (SAMHSA) defines mental health recovery as "a process of change through which individuals improve their health and wellness, live a self-directed life, and strive to reach their full potential." Emerging from the consumer movement and psychiatric rehabilitation, the mental health recovery model seeks to move our understanding of recovery beyond symptom reduction and toward the acquisition of a meaningful life within the community.

OPEN ACCESS A system that centers on the use of completely open schedule templates and few restrictions on appointment types, allowing service users to receive prompt appointments, ideally on the same day or the next day.

PATIENT-CENTERED MEDICAL HOME An integrated care model in which the primary care physician leads an interdisciplinary team that is responsible for coordinating the service user's overall health needs. This includes family engagement in care, whole-person care, behavioral health care, and necessary information tools.

PERSON-CENTERED CARE A value-based approach to care that requires people to be actively involved in all aspects of their health care decisions and their care to be determined by their individual values, needs, and preferences. Although it is closely related to patient-centered care within the medical field, the term *person-centered care* is used most commonly in behavioral health.

POPULATION-BASED CARE The practice of enhancing the health of an entire service user population by assessing, tracking, and managing the group's health conditions and treatment responses over time. Health is addressed through informed decision-making, including comprehensive assessments and evidence-based practices based on the clinical data of populations. Population-based care also involves proactive approaches to engage the target group rather than responding only to individuals who actively seek care.

SBIRT (SCREENING, BRIEF INTERVENTION, AND REFERRAL TO TREATMENT) An integrated care approach to the delivery of early intervention and treatment services for people who have (or are at risk for) substance use disorders. People with a positive screening result for problematic use of alcohol or other drugs are provided with brief interventions designed to educate them about their risky behavior and increase their motivation to change, and if warranted, referral to ongoing treatment.

SERVICE USER ACTIVATION The empowerment of individuals to take an active role in managing their own health based on their knowledge, skills, and confidence.

SHARED DECISION-MAKING A decision-making process in which the provider and the recipient of care share information. Service users are viewed as experts in terms of what has worked for them and their values and preferences and providers share their knowledge of treatment options. Both parties work collaboratively to reach a mutually agreed-upon decision about the person's health care.

SOCIAL DETERMINANTS OF HEALTH The factors beyond health care services that shape our health outcomes—including where we live, learn, and work; our level of income; and our social support networks. These social, economic, and environmental factors play an influential role in health outcomes.

TRANSITIONAL CARE Health care services that focus on care coordination for service users moving between different levels and types of care (e.g., inpatient to outpatient) or systems (e.g., pediatric to adult health services).

THE TRIPLE AIM Developed by the Institute for Healthcare Improvement, the Triple Aim has framed the goals for health care reform initiatives. The Triple Aim stipulates that initiatives must simultaneously pursue three objectives: improvement of the service user's experience of care, improvement of population health, and reduction of the per capita cost of health care.

VALUE-BASED PURCHASING A health care model in which payments are based on the value of services, with the aim of improving quality of care and lowering costs. This encompasses purchasing strategies that use alternative payment models to motivate and reward both quality and efficiency and to support delivery system reform. Value-based purchasing represents a shift away from the traditional health care model in which payments were based on the volume of services.

WARM HAND-OFF An approach in which a provider physically and immediately introduces an individual to the behavioral health care provider to whom he or she is being referred. This system aims to establish an initial face-to-face contact between the service user and the behavioral health care provider and to ease the service user's transition. This approach also helps to ensure the service user follows up with the referral.

INDEX

dashboards, 254
data-driven care, 37
data use, 273–274
Daughters, S. B., 120
Davidson, L., 28, 158
decision aids, 160
decision-making
    decision aids, 160
    person-centered care, 158–160
    relational, 159
    shared, 159–160
decision support, 151
Deegan, P., 150, 160, 184
Deficit Reduction Act (DRA), 72
delivery system reform, ACA, 75–79
    accountable care organizations, 76–77
    coordinated care, 75–76
    health homes, 78–79
    patient-centered medical homes, 77–78
    strategy and vision, 75
density scores, network, 272
Department of Health and Human Services
        (DHHS), 98
depression screening, 132–134
Descartes, R., 12
determinants of health
    definition, 36
    population health, 36–40, 37f
dialectical behavior therapy (DBT), children and
        adolescents, 203
differential diagnosis, 22
Dimidjian, S., 175
direct purchase insurance, 51–52
discharge planning, 182. *See also* transdisciplinary care
disease registries, 255
disparities, health care, 3–4, 6–9
    children and adolescents, 196
    gender and sexual orientation, 9
    population health, 35–36
    race and ethnicity, 6–9
Domenici, Pete, 60
Drug Abuse Screening Test (DAST), 137

ecological model, 217
education
    institutions, workforce development, 101–102
    interprofessional, 237, 238, 244
electronic health record (EHR), 219, 251,
        253–259
    adoption, barriers, 258–259
    clinical decision support systems, 253–254
    collaborative documentation, 257–258
    definition, 253

disease registries, 255
    electronic portals, 255–257
electronic portals, 255–257
employer mandate, 70
employer-sponsored insurance (ESI), 51
engagement, transitional care, 183–184
Engel, George, 23, 24
Epstein, R. M., 151, 240
ethnicity, health care disparities, 6–9
evaluating integrated health care, 267–275
    case vignette, 41
    Integrated Clinic Model, 267
    Integrated Mobile Health Team
        Model, 267
    Integrated Service Management Models,
        267–268
    interprofessional practice, 243
    lessons learned
        measurement barriers, 275
        use of data, 273–274
    measuring integrated health care, 268
    measuring integration process, 270–273, 272t
    Patient-Centered Outcomes Research Institute,
        152, 268, 269t
    process and outcomes evaluation, need,
        269–270
Evans, A. C., 28
evidence-based interventions, children and
        adolescents
    cognitive-behavioral therapy, 200–201
    family-focused, 203–205
    mindfulness, 202
    motivational interviewing, 201–202
    trauma-focused, 202
evidence-based practice, 167–176
    behavioral health, 167
    case vignette, 176–177
    cognitive-behavioral therapy, 171–172
    decision-making model, 169
    evidence-based medicine, 168
    history, 167–168
    mindfulness, 175–176
    motivational interviewing, 169–171
    team members, 167–168
    trauma-informed care, 172–174
    wellness self-management, 174–175
evolution, health care policy. *See* policy evolution,
        health care

family-focused interventions, children and
        adolescents, 203–205
family navigator, 104, 221–222
Farley, T., 98, 242